The Birth Partner

The Birth Partner

A Complete Guide to Childbirth for Dads, Doulas, and All Other Labor Companions

THIRD EDITION

PENNY SIMKIN, P.T.

THE HARVARD COMMON PRESS
BOSTON, MASSACHUSETTS

The Harvard Common Press
535 Albany Street
Boston, Massachusetts 02118
www.harvardcommonpress.com

Printed in the United States of America

Printed on acid-free paper

Library of Congress Cataloging-in-Publication Data
Simkin, Penny, 1938-
  The birth partner : a complete guide to childbirth for dads, doulas, and all other labor companions / Penny Simkin. — 3rd ed.
      p. cm.
  Includes bibliographical references and index.
  ISBN-13: 978-1-55832-357-5 (pbk. : alk. paper)
  1. Pregnancy. 2. Natural childbirth—Coaching. 3. Labor (Obstetrics)—Complications. 4. Childbirth. I. Title.
  RG525.S5829 2008
  618.2—dc22
                                                              200702579

Special bulk-order discounts are available on this and other Harvard Common Press books. Companies and organizations may purchase books for premiums or resale, or may arrange a custom edition, by contacting the Marketing Director at the address above.

Photographs by Patty Simanek, Barefoot Photography
Cover illustration by Lola and Bek
Drawings by Shanna Dela Cruz, Penny Simkin, and Childbirth Graphics
Cover design by Night & Day Design
Text design by Cia Boynton

10 9 8 7 6 5 4 3 2 1

Dedication

This book is dedicated . . .

To the thousands of expectant mothers and fathers who have taught me so much while I have taught them;

To the hundreds of women and their loving partners whom I have been privileged to assist during childbirth;

To my eight grandchildren, whose births I have attended in the role of proud grandmother;

To my four grown children, to whom I could not feel closer and of whom I could not be more proud, and to their spouses, who enrich my life;

And lastly but especially to Peter, my husband, father of our children, and my beloved partner for five decades.

Contents

Preface to the Third Edition

I'd like to explain what led me to write the first, second, and now third edition of this book. The first edition was published in 1989, after I learned some truths about what birth means to women and about what it means to be a birth partner who deeply loves the woman giving birth. One of these truths is this: How a woman gives birth matters—to her baby, her family (including her relationship with her partner), and to her self-confidence and self-esteem as a woman and a mother. This is as true today as it was in 1989, and for generations (even millennia) before.

Another very important truth: How a woman is cared for and supported during birth is a major influence, not only in how she gives birth but also in how she feels about it. Yet, medical care before and during childbirth focuses almost exclusively on the physical safety of baby and mother. This medical care places little emphasis on the mother's emotional well-being, her relationship with her partner, and her readiness to parent. Such matters are given much lower priority in our very expensive health-care system, which is beset by nursing shortages, pressure to increase the use of medical and surgical interventions while increasing efficiency, reduction of psychosocial support services, threats of malpractice lawsuits, and other factors that work against personalized, flexible, woman-centered care.

I learned the importance of emotional care during labor when, in the late 1980s, I conducted a study of women's long-term memories of their birth experiences. The women were from childbirth classes that I taught between 1968 and 1974. They had sent me their birth stories shortly after they gave birth. For my study, I contacted the women 15 to 20 years later and asked them (1) to write their birth stories again as they remembered them and (2) to rate their satisfaction as they looked back on their childbirth experiences.

In comparing the two stories from each woman, I was astounded at how clearly they remembered and how consistent their stories were, despite the interval of 15 to 20 years. I then interviewed the women and discovered that they had detailed memories of their doctors and nurses (there were no midwives practicing in my area at that time). All the women vividly remembered specific things that were done and said to them. Many could quote the exact words! Some actually wept as they recalled some of these things—either from joy over the kindness and care they were given, or from sadness or anger over being treated disrespectfully or thoughtlessly.

In a nutshell, those who felt they had been well cared for by the professional staff reported the highest satisfaction, even if their labors had been long or complicated. Those who felt they had been treated disrespectfully or ignored reported the least satisfaction. Also, those who were most satisfied felt a great sense of accomplishment in giving birth. They felt that they had been in control, and that the birth experience had been good for their self-esteem. The less satisfied women did not have these positive feelings.

The presence of the women's husbands was unusual at the time, because it was not customary for men to attend childbirth classes or the births of their babies. Most of these men took as active a role as they were allowed, although they were often required to leave the labor or delivery room for long periods (at the time, only husbands, not other lovers, relatives, or friends, were allowed to be with laboring women at all).

The women's memories of their husbands were also clear and detailed. Here are quotations from some of the women:

> "He was the only reason I got through it."
> "It was one of the finer moments in our life and relationship."
> "He was more patient and took it more seriously than I expected."
> "He's a competitor. He was my coach. It was a very big deal for him."
> "It hurt him to see me in pain."
> "He could feel me tense immediately."
> "He was there 100 percent."
> "He was apprehensive, but wanted to be there."
> "I was very concerned that my husband be there because I didn't trust anybody."

I learned from that study that women need and appreciate loving, familiar people to stay with them, help them, and share the birth—

one of life's most meaningful moments. I also learned that the kind of professional care and emotional support a woman receives during labor determine whether she looks back on the birth experience with satisfaction and fulfillment or with disappointment, sadness, and even anger. I realized that, in the age of high-tech, high-pressure obstetrics, it is unrealistic to expect that busy nurses, doctors, and even hospital-based midwives can provide the kind of professional support—continuous emotional and physical comfort throughout labor and birth—that women need, although many would like to do so.

The lessons from my study have been confirmed over and over again in the hundreds of births I have attended as a doula and in the experiences of thousands of women and partners I have taught in childbirth classes. Their lessons prompted me to write the first edition of this book. I wanted to help partners feel more knowledgeable and confident in their support role, so that women would always appreciate their partners' help. This was also when I decided to train doulas and, with other outstanding doula advocates, founded a local doula organization (Pacific Association for Labor Support) and an international one (Doulas of North America, now DONA International). My goal was to ensure that childbearing women get the kind of care they need, and their partners the kind of practical guidance and tools they need during this challenging and unforgettable time.

This updated third edition bears the same primary message of the previous two editions. This edition is written in a time when, typically, childbearing women are cared for by maternity professionals whom they have never met (or barely met) before. During the span of one labor, because of the timing of shifts and breaks and the staff's need to look after more than one woman at a time, each woman will meet and have to adjust to numerous different professionals. If women are to have any chance at a fulfilling birth in the hospital, they must receive better support and care from their own team of partner, loved ones, and doula.

At this time in North America, a small number of women will choose to give birth outside the hospital—at home or in a birth center. They do so because they want the kind of care that is rarely given in hospitals. They will be surrounded by caregivers whom they know, and will labor in a familiar, low-tech, low-pressure environment. They will also benefit from a capable, confident support team to assist them through the intrinsic challenges that come with birth.

In conclusion, readers, I hope you will find this book empathetic, interesting, and helpful in preparing you for your all-important role, and that you will take pride and pleasure in your own journey through the birth toward parenthood or your career as a doula.

CHANGES IN THE THIRD EDITION

This expanded third edition has a new subtitle, to reflect the large quantity of added information on the doula's role around the time of birth. This added content is a response to the growing demand for and use of doulas in North America and abroad.

There is also much more in the following four major areas: the 3Rs (Relaxation, Rhythm, and Ritual) for coping with the pain and unpredictability of labor; non-drug techniques to relieve pain and enhance the woman's sense of well-being; current medications, tests, technologies, and interventions and how, when, and why they are used; and the rapidly increasing rate of both first and repeat cesarean deliveries.

Throughout the book, the partner's role is emphasized and the doula's role is explained and clarified. Numerous illustrations have been added to enhance the message of the text.

Acknowledgments

I have had my share of support throughout the process of revising this book. I want to thank the following extraordinary people who have made it possible for me to accomplish this in the midst of my busy, distracting life:

Molly Kirkpatrick, Heather Snookal, and Tanya Bake have gone far beyond the call of duty in running my office, helping keep my schedule clear for writing, helping me prepare the extensive revisions, and feeding me licorice as needed.

My friends and coauthors of *Pregnancy, Childbirth, and the Newborn* and *The Simple Guide to Childbirth*, Ann Keppler and Janet Whalley, have spent countless hours with me, sharing their extensive expertise and providing a helpful sounding board for me on many challenging matters relating to childbearing.

Sandy Szalay and Kathy McGrath have stimulated my curiosity and awe regarding the birth process and inspired me with their dedication and commitment to young families and their generosity in providing these families (especially my daughters') with advice and concrete support.

My colleagues and friends at Seattle Midwifery School, Pacific Association for Labor Support, Open Arms Perinatal Services, Great Starts Birth and Family Education, and DONA International have been sources of endless support and patience with me as I follow my passion. Annie Kennedy, Ann Grauer, and Susan Martensen have been especially kind and helpful.

Linda Ziedrich, my editor for all three editions, has been amazing. Her attention to consistency and detail are awesome.

Ruth Ancheta, with whom I coauthored *The Labor Progress Handbook*, holds the copyright to most of the illustrations and donated them for this book.

Shanna Dela Cruz, the artist who drew most of the illustrations, has been fastidious and reliable. I admire her simplicity, accuracy, and individuation of the people in the illustrations.

Childbirth Graphics, producers of teaching materials for expectant and new parents, has allowed me to use some of their classic drawings.

All the women and couples who posed for the photos from which the drawings were made were extraordinarily generous with their time and good cheer.

Patty Simanek of Barefoot Photography donated the perceptive and captivating photographs that open each section of the book.

Phyllis Klaus, my coauthor of *When Survivors Give Birth: Understanding and Healing the Effects of Early Sexual Abuse on Childbearing Women*, Marshall Klaus, and John Kennell are dear friends whose thoughtful and inspiring insights and groundbreaking work on labor support and parent-infant bonding have deepened my understanding.

The birth partners, members of my childbirth classes, who generously shared their personal thoughts for the beginnings of each chapter, have added poignancy and realism to the text.

Finally, and most important, I want to thank my husband, Peter, who has been my loving, patient, and accepting partner throughout the labor and birth of this book and my others.

How to Use This Book

The *Birth Partner* is intended to be useful both as a guide to prepare you in advance for your role as birth partner and as a quick reference during labor. Try to read the entire book before the mother goes into labor. Then, if there is time, you may want to review parts of it during labor.

There may be times during labor when you need immediate help and want to find something quickly in this book. Anticipating which information you may need on the spot, I have indicated certain sections by darkening the page edges. Fan the pages of the book and find those with dark edges. Their titles are listed right on the edge for quick reference. These sections are as follows:

PART ONE

Before the Birth

The birth partner's role begins before the mother is actually in labor. During the last few weeks of her pregnancy, you can learn about labor, encourage her to continue good health habits, help her with last-minute preparations for the baby and for labor itself, and figure out the role you will play as her birth partner.

This is also the time for her to make many important decisions about the birth and to discuss them with her caregiver. If you attend childbirth classes and go to her prenatal checkups, you will not only become informed, but you will also become more comfortable in your role. Together, you will discover many important things, such as what her doctor or midwife is like, the options available in the care of mother and baby, and practical details. You can also get advice and reassurance about anything that is causing anxiety or uncertainty for either or both of you.

During these last weeks, you can prepare for your role through introspection, discussions with the pregnant mother, gathering information, and practicing comfort measures.

CHAPTER 1

The Last Few Weeks of Pregnancy

As the third trimester went on, I had a growing sense of wonder. The big day was coming when I would finally meet my daughter. I had felt her kicks and seen Janna's belly bump around when we spoke or laughed. But, who was she? What would she be like? I just couldn't wait to meet her.

My wife knew she wanted to have a baby naturally. I was worried. I thought, "Why? We have hospitals and medicines to provide comfort. Why turn it away?" My wife told me she just wanted the right to try. This changed my thinking forever. I would not be a roadblock, because my wife should have the right to try to do what her body was designed to do.

—SCOTT, FIRST-TIME FATHER

Early in pregnancy, it seems that nine months is forever and that there is plenty of time to do everything that has to be done. It is all too easy, especially for busy people, to postpone "getting into" the pregnancy. Now, suddenly, the baby is almost due. Time has flown by. As the mother's birth partner, you realize she is counting on you to help her through childbirth. Do you feel ready? Can you help her? What do you know about labor? Do you know what to do when? What should you do now to get ready for the baby?

It is not too late to learn and do what needs to be done. But you had better start right away—a few weeks before the due date is truly the "last minute," especially since many babies arrive early. This first chapter is basically a checklist of things you should do before labor starts to help ensure that you will work well with the mother during the labor and birth. Also included are suggestions about how you can help prepare beforehand for the baby's arrival.

What Kind of Birth Partner Will You Be?

Birth partners come in all shapes and sizes, and they help the laboring woman in any number of ways. Most often the birth partner is the baby's father and the mother's husband or lover. The birth partner may instead be the woman's mother, sister, or friend. Or the birth partner may be the mother's lesbian lover, who will be the baby's co-parent.

A doula is another kind of birth partner, one that is becoming more popular in North America. The number of doulas is increasing rapidly, especially in cities, although doulas are still in short supply in some areas. Sometimes the doula is the woman's only birth partner, but more often the doula helps both the woman and her life partner. The doula is an experienced guide and support person to the woman or couple. (See the description of the doula's role on pages 8 to 9.) In this book you will learn how doulas can help you and the mother in the variety of labor situations that you may encounter.

The role played by the birth partner varies according to many personal factors and the nature of the partner's relationship with the mother. What role will *you* play? What role does the woman want you to play? How much effort do you and she want to put into learning about childbirth and practicing comfort measures? How actively does she want to participate in decision making, in coping with the pain, in helping the labor to progress well, and in delivering her baby? Does she prefer to have a more natural birth or a more medical birth?

If she wants a natural birth, then she is ready to acquire a basic understanding of childbirth, learn many techniques for coping with pain, and plan realistically for the challenges of labor. She expects labor and birth to be challenging, demanding, and also fulfilling, and she feels capable of meeting the challenges with help, guidance, and encouragement from her medical team and her support team. She prefers to rely more on herself and her support team and less on drugs and procedures to get through labor and give birth.

How Will I Feel?

For a realistic idea of the situations and feelings you may encounter as a birth partner, ask yourself these questions. How will I feel if or when:

She asks me to take time off to go to prenatal appointments with her?

She tells me that we are signed up for 12 to 18 hours of childbirth classes?

She asks me to read this book or others?

She wakes up moaning every 10 to 20 minutes during the night, and says she thinks it is labor, and I am very tired?

Her labor begins with a gush of water from her vagina followed immediately by long, painful contractions in her abdomen?

She does not accept my suggestions for relaxation or coping?

I get tired or hungry, but she needs my help with every contraction?

She asks me if we should go to the hospital?

She makes distressing sounds that I have never heard her make?

She expresses discouragement ("This is so hard," "I can't keep on," "How much longer?" "Don't make me do this")?

She clings to me and says, "Help me!"?

She vomits or needs to vomit?

She is in pain and begins to cry, grimace, and tense her muscles?

She criticizes me ("Not like that," "Don't touch me," "Don't breathe in my face," "Don't leave me")?

She needs me to press hard on her back with every contraction, until my arms ache?

She tells me, "I want an epidural"?

Labor goes on for 12, 18, or 24 hours and there is still no baby and I am so tired I can't keep my eyes open, but she needs me?

We are told that a cesarean will be necessary?

Her caregiver says, "Look here! The baby's head is starting to come"?

The baby slides out, wrinkled, soaking wet, streaked with blood, and crying lustily?

I am asked if I want to cut the cord?

The little, squirming, bundled baby is handed to me to hold and cuddle?

The new mother looks at me and says, "I couldn't have done it without you"?

If she prefers or needs (because of health concerns) a more medical birth, she will rely more on her doctor or midwife to make decisions, to use drugs and procedures to control the progress and pain of labor, and to deliver her baby. Although neither preference is right or wrong, your role as birth partner is affected by her approach to labor and birth and your comfort with her choices. Does she have thoughts about what she will want and need from you? Do you feel able and eager to help her as she wishes?

All these questions may be impossible to answer right now. But keep them in mind as you read this book, and start discussing them with the mother. Start imagining her in labor, and the challenges you may face as her birth partner.

Use the exercise "How Will I Feel?" as a reality check. This book will help you prepare for such situations and plan good strategies to handle them. By the time labor begins, you should have a much clearer picture of yourself as birth partner.

Getting Ready for Labor

If you haven't already done the things described in the following pages, try to get them done a few weeks before the due date, or at least before labor starts.

VISIT THE MOTHER'S CAREGIVER (DOCTOR OR MIDWIFE)

If you have not yet met the mother's caregiver, this visit may be more important than you think, for both the caregiver and yourselves. Even a brief meeting helps establish for the caregiver that you are an important person in the mother's life. Although a substitute caregiver (one of the partners in the group practice) may actually attend the birth, this meeting still provides you with an opportunity to ask questions, to get a feel for what doctors and midwives do, and to play a more active role.

VISIT THE HOSPITAL OR OUT-OF-HOSPITAL BIRTH CENTER

Take a tour of the hospital maternity area—triage (the room you and the mother go to first, where a nurse decides whether to admit her to the hospital), birthing rooms, waiting room, nursery, kitchen, and postpartum rooms. You'll get to see much of the equipment that is used during labor. You can find out when tours are available by calling the hospital. Sometimes a tour is included in childbirth classes. This is a good time to ask questions about the hospital's usual way of doing things and any options that the mother may have.

Birth centers are smaller and have fewer rooms than hospitals; labor, birth, and the first hours afterward are spent in the same room. Birth centers also have less equipment, but it is still important to visit and learn the usual practices in the birth center.

On the way to the tour, figure out your route to the hospital or birth center and how long it takes to get there (during both rush hour and slower traffic times). At the hospital, learn which entrances to use during the day and at night; you may have to use the main entrance during the day and the emergency entrance at night. Entrances to birth centers are seldom staffed around the clock and so are usually locked at night. You meet your midwife at the entrance after you call her to announce labor.

If the mother is planning to give birth at home or in a birth center, be sure to visit the backup hospital so that you won't be confused if for medical reasons a transfer becomes necessary.

PREREGISTER AT THE HOSPITAL

Preregistering involves obtaining, reading, and signing preadmission forms and a medical consent form. By registering in advance, you save time and avoid confusion when you arrive with the mother in labor.

CONSIDER ARRANGING FOR A DOULA TO HELP YOU BOTH DURING LABOR

Why consider having a doula? Childbirth is intense, demanding, unpredictable, and painful, and it can last for anywhere from a few hours to 24 or more. Even if you are well prepared, you and the mother may find it difficult to apply your classroom learning in the real situation. If you are not well prepared, all the challenges of labor are baffling and anxiety-producing.

Of course, you will have a nurse and a doctor or midwife who are likely to be kind and caring, but they will probably be very busy with the clinical aspects of the birth, which get the highest priority. Hospital nurses and midwives rarely remain in the room throughout labor, as they have duties outside the room and are often taking care of more than one laboring patient. They work in shifts, so over the course of labor several different professionals are likely to be involved in the mother's care. Doctors rely on the nurses to manage the labor, with phone reports as necessary. They may visit briefly from time to time, and will come if problems arise during labor. And, of course, they are there for the birth.

One of the most positive developments in maternity care is the addition of the birth doula, who guides and supports women and their partners continuously through labor and birth. The doula is on call for you, arrives at your home or the hospital when you need her, and remains with you continuously, with few or no breaks, until after the baby is born. The doula is trained and experienced in providing emotional support, physical comfort, and nonclinical advice. She draws on her knowledge and experience as she reassures, encourages, comforts, and empathizes with the mother. She advises the partner

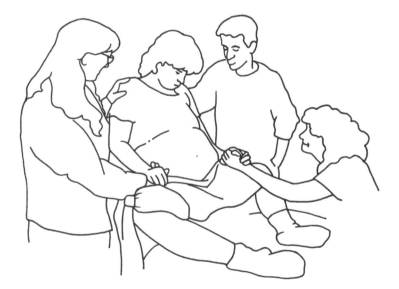

about how to help, suggesting when to use particular positions, the bath or shower, and specific comfort measures.

A doula cannot and does not try to take over your role as the birth partner, because you know the mother better and love her and the baby as no one else does. But there are many times when a woman needs more than one helper in labor, and when her partner needs reassurance, advice, and help.

Besides helping the mother, a doula can help you in numerous ways:

- She can guide you in applying what you learned in childbirth class to the more stressful and unpredictable labor situation.
- She can spell you so that you can get a meal, a short nap, or just a break during a long or an all-night labor.
- She can bring the mother beverages, hot packs, or ice, so that you do not have to leave her side to do so.
- She can reassure you if you are worried about the mother's well-being.
- She can help you understand what the mother might be feeling and interpret the signs of labor progress to you.
- If you do not feel comfortable being the mother's only constant source of support, the doula can help you participate more comfortably by making sure the mother's needs are met.
- By getting to know the two of you before the birth, the doula can discover your priorities, fears, and concerns and help you develop strategies to deal with them.
- She may be able to photograph or videotape the two of you during labor and birth, or all three of you afterward.

The doula does not make decisions for the two of you, or project her personal preferences on you, but she helps you get the information you need to make good decisions. Her goal is to help the mother have a satisfying birth as she defines it.

One father described a doula this way: "She was like my big sister—ready, willing, and able to help me do the best job I could. She showed me how to rub Mary's back, reminded us to try the lunge (see page 136), and got me a bagel when I was really hungry. She kept encouraging us. She seemed so confident. A lot of the time both she and I were helping Mary. I was holding her during the contractions, and our doula was pressing on Mary's back and helping her breathe in rhythm. Our doula even gave me a shoulder rub in the middle of the night. She never left except to go to the bathroom. Without her, the birth wouldn't have been so great for both Mary and me. The doula helped me do a better job."

Numerous scientific trials have compared birth outcomes of women who had doulas and those who did not. In very "high-tech" hospitals with high cesarean and induction rates, women attended by doulas had fewer forceps and vacuum-extractor deliveries and fewer cesareans. They did not request as much pain medication. Also, women attended by doulas were more likely to report that their birth experiences were satisfying than were women who did not have doulas. Although a doula cannot guarantee a normal or an easy labor, statistics show that having a doula results in less need for major labor interventions. Chapter 3 describes what doulas do to help during each phase of labor.

Several organizations train and certify birth doulas. The training, totaling about four intensive days plus reading assignments, emphasizes the needs of laboring women and their partners for emotional and physical comfort, and ways the doula can meet these needs. To become certified, a doula must attend a certain number of births, after which she is evaluated by her clients and their doctors, nurses, or midwives.

Costs of doula services vary greatly. Fees range from $250 to $1500, depending largely on region and the doula's experience. But some hospitals have volunteer doulas available during labor, and some community agencies and charitable organizations employ doulas to care for needy clients. Many trained doulas offer free service while gaining experience to apply for certification. Others offer free service to people in their own ethnic or religious communities. And many private doulas charge a fee to those who can pay but donate their services to those who cannot pay. At present, health insurers rarely cover doula fees.

To learn more about doulas or to locate a doula, contact DONA International (www.DONA.org), search for "doula" or "find doula" on the Internet, or ask new parents, your childbirth educator, or your caregiver for referrals.

Choose and Meet with Your Doula

If you decide to have a doula, it is a good idea to start looking for one a few months before the baby is due, since doulas are often fully booked for weeks or months in advance. Get some referrals, and interview one or more doulas on the phone. Ask whether the doula is available around your due date and whether her fees are in your range, or whether she has a deferred-payment plan or sliding-fee scale. To ensure a good match, interview the doula in person.

There is usually no charge for the first "get-acquainted" meeting with a doula, which usually lasts an hour or so. At this time, you might ask her how she thinks you and the mother would benefit from having a doula. Share some information about yourselves and ask her about the services she offers, her experience, her fees, why she does this work, and how she works with couples.

Once you have chosen a doula, you will probably meet with her at least once more before the birth. In the second meeting, the following topics are usually covered:

- How to reach the doula, day and night.

- Her calendar around the mother's due date (other clients due about the same time, plans to be out of town, unbreakable obligations).

- Arrangements for a backup doula in case she is unavailable when you need her. You should be able to meet the backup doula as well.

- Directions to your home, so that the doula can visit you there in early labor (if you need her and if distance allows).

- Any previous birth experiences the mother has had, and ages of older children.

- How the pregnancy has been, and any problems or concerns you have about it.

- Childbirth preparation classes (see page 13).
- The mother's Birth Plan (see page 26). The doula can help the two of you prepare it, if you wish.
- The mother's preferences regarding pain medication (see page 27).
- Your wishes regarding photographs or video.
- Concerns that you and the mother have regarding the birth.
- The kinds of things the doula can say or do to comfort the mother or help her relax.
- Things the doula should not say or do, because they might bother the mother or make her more tense.
- The doula's visit to your home after the birth to see the baby, review the birth experience with you, and see how all of you are doing.
- Payment arrangements.

Some doulas offer other services, such as private childbirth preparation, massage, birth-related counseling, breastfeeding help, or postpartum doula care (see page 36). There may be additional charges for these services.

CONSIDER AN ALTERNATIVE SUPPORT PERSON

Although doulas are plentiful in many areas in North America, you may not be able to find one locally. Or you may prefer having a friend or family member play a similar role. To choose the right person, think of the mother's needs first. Sometimes family members or friends assume they will attend the birth or ask whether they can come. It may feel awkward to say no, but someone who has never given birth may be a poor choice, especially if she has not taken childbirth-preparation classes. Here are some things to think about:

- Would this person like to help you?
- Is she or he available day and night? Can she or he cancel all obligations on short notice, if necessary?
- Does she or he have transportation to your home, the birth center, or the hospital?

- Is she or he patient, optimistic, calm, unselfish, thoughtful of others, and a good listener?
- What special attributes does she or he bring, such as a comforting touch or tone of voice, comfort with silence, and a positive attitude toward birth?
- Does she or he have stamina for a possibly long labor?
- What experience has she or he had with birth?
- Does she or he have any annoying habits or mannerisms?
- Does she or he recognize and accept the importance of this commitment?

In summary, think of what this person can do for the mother and for you. Ask this person to come not because you think she or he would like to be there, but because you *want* her or him there.

Make Sure the Mother Can Always Reach You by Phone

You can never know when the mother might need you. It's best if both of you carry a cell phone or pager, charged and turned on whenever you are not together. If your job takes you far away or out of cell-phone range, check with the mother often, and have someone else available when you are not. Make sure that person can be reached at all times and will come to the mother's aid, night or day, on very short notice.

Review What You Learned in Childbirth Classes

If you have taken classes, review your handouts and notes. Rehearse comfort techniques. Gather the materials that you might want to refer to during labor—this book, lists, suggestions, questionnaires, information and instructions about the hospital's services, and copies of the mother's Birth Plan.

Gather the Necessary Supplies

What do you pack for the hospital or birth center? What do you need for a home birth? The following lists should help.

Supplies to take to the hospital or birth center. From this list, select only those items that you and the mother feel will be helpful. Try to pack as many of these things in advance as possible.

For the mother during labor:

~~Oil or cornstarch for massage~~

Lip balm

Toothbrush and toothpaste ✓

Hairbrush and comb

Her own short gown and robe, if she prefers them to hospital clothes

Rolling pin, massage device for pressure, or hot or cold pack to relieve back pain

Ponytail holder to keep long hair off her face

Warm socks and slippers

Warm blanket or shawl (hospital beds have only very thin cotton covers)

MP3 player, or compact discs of favorite relaxing music and a CD player (if one is not available in the hospital or birth center) *use mine*

Personal comfort items (pillow, flowers, pictures)

Favorite juice, frozen juice bars, or an electrolyte-balanced beverage (such as Gatorade or Recharge) in a cooler (most hospitals provide juices, but in limited variety)

? Birth ball ("exercise ball," "gymnastics ball"), if the facility does not have one

For the birth partner:

Copy of the Birth Plan (see page 26)

Watch with a second hand

Grooming supplies (toothbrush, breath mints, deodorant, shaver)

Food for snacks, such as sandwiches, fruit, cheese and crackers, beverages (consider what they will do to your breath). Many hospitals have no food available at night except in vending machines.

Sweater

Change of clothes

Slippers

Swimsuit, so you can accompany the mother into the shower
or bath

Paper and pencil

This book

Reading materials or handwork, for slow times when the
mother does not need your help

Phone numbers of people to call during or after labor

Telephone credit card or prepaid telephone card (cell-phone
use might be allowed only in designated areas of the hospital)

Camera (still or video), batteries, charger, etc.

Laptop computer for sending photos and e-mail messages
about the birth (if the hospital allows this)

For the mother during the postpartum period:

Gowns that open in front for breastfeeding, unless she prefers
hospital gowns

Robe and slippers

Cosmetics and toilet articles

Tasty snack foods, such as fruit, nuts, cheese, and crackers

Nursing bras

Money for incidentals

Going-home clothing

For the baby:

Clothing for the trip home—regular or snap-crotch undershirt,
gown or stretch suit, receiving blanket, outer clothing (hat,
warm clothing), crib-sized blanket

Car seat, properly installed (visit www.seatcheck.org or call
1-866-seat-check to locate local car-seat safety-check stations
and to learn about any car-seat recalls)

*For the trip to the hospital or birth center, or in the event of
transfer during a home birth:*

A full tank of gas

A blanket and pillow in the car

Supplies for a home birth.   Look over the preceding lists for ideas about what to have at home. In addition, ask the midwife for a list of special items you'll need, or go over the following lists with her. She may recommend a source for home-birth supply kits.

> *Birthing supplies:*
> Disposable waterproof underpads (Chux pads)
> Sterile 4-by-4-inch gauze pads
> K-Y jelly
> Bulb syringe
> Cord clamps
> Squeeze bottle to cleanse perineum
> Waterproof mattress cover (a shower curtain will do)
> Wet, folded washcloths placed in plastic bags and frozen
> Thermometer
> Basin for the placenta
> Washcloths, hand towels, and bath towels
> At least two sets of clean bed sheets
> Flexible straws
> Trash bags
> Birthing tub, available for rent or purchase, or a kiddie-sized swimming pool at least 24 inches deep (ask your midwife, childbirth educator, or doula whether there is a reliable tub-rental company in your area, or search online for "portable birthing tubs" or "kiddie pools birth")

> *Other supplies:*
> Long, maternity-sized sanitary pads
> Hat for the baby
> Food for the birthing team during labor
> Food and drink for a birth celebration
> A map to your home, for the midwife and doula (give it to them well in advance)

For a home birth, you will want to make some other preparations at the last minute:

◆ Turn up the water heater (to allow a long shower in labor), and make sure everyone knows. Post reminders at every faucet.

- Clean and organize the house.

- Make the bed with fresh linens (that you don't mind getting stained) in the following way: Put a mattress pad, preferably waterproof, over the mattress. Put a cotton sheet over the mattress pad. Put a waterproof mattress cover or plastic sheet over the cotton sheet, and another cotton sheet over the waterproof cover or sheet. During labor and birth, the top sheet may become stained and wet. After the birth, the top sheet and top waterproof sheet can be quickly removed, and the other clean sheet will already be in place.

In case of transfer to a hospital, know the way to the hospital, have plenty of gas in your car's tank, and include in the Birth Plan the mother's preferences in case of transfer (see "Prepare and Review the Mother's Birth Plan," page 26).

ENCOURAGE THE MOTHER TO DRINK PLENTY OF FLUIDS AND CONTINUE TO EAT WELL

During pregnancy, the mother should drink at least two quarts of liquid a day—water, fruit juices, clear soups. This helps support her increased fluid needs. She should maintain a well-balanced diet containing plenty of protein, iron, calcium, and vitamins, and a little fat.

ENCOURAGE HER TO EXERCISE

Regular exercise such as walking, prenatal yoga or aquarobics, or swimming will help maintain or improve the mother's general fitness. Prenatal yoga is especially helpful in enabling relaxation during pain and developing one's inner resources for remaining calm during labor. Encourage the mother to join a class. In addition, you or a friend might take walks or swim with her.

A few special exercises are particularly helpful during late pregnancy and labor: squatting, the pelvic rock on hands and knees (called "cat-cow" in yoga), and the Kegel (pelvic-floor contraction) exercise. These are usually taught in childbirth classes. See page 18 for instructions on squatting and pelvic rocking on all fours, and page 19 for instructions on the Kegel exercise.

Supplies for a home birth

Squatting. This may be very useful in helping the baby come down during the birthing stage. Ten squats per day, lasting for up to one minute each, should increase the mother's comfort with the position. CAUTION: If she has joint problems in her ankles, knees, or hips, or if she develops pain in any of these joints or in her pubic joint (in the middle below her abdomen), she should not practice squatting. Consult the illustrations to see how a partner supports a woman while she squats.

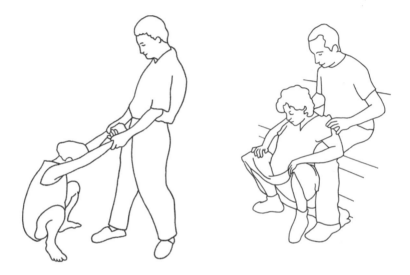

Pelvic rock on hands and knees ("Cat-Cow"). During pregnancy, this exercise helps strengthen abdominal muscles, relieve low back pain, improve circulation in the lower half of the body, and position the baby in the favorable OA (occiput anterior) position (see page 46). During labor, the pelvic rock also helps relieve back pain.

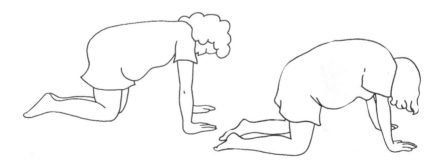

On her hands and knees, the mother should tuck her pelvis under while arching her back for a slow count of five, then return to normal briefly, and repeat for a total of ten times per day. See the illustrations.

The Kegel (pelvic-floor contraction) exercise. Because this is important for both men's and women's lifelong general health, I will describe it in detail here. This exercise strengthens muscles that support the pelvic organs in women and are vital to sexual pleasure and bowel and bladder control in both sexes (for men, this exercise also helps prevent or alleviate an enlarged prostate gland).

During childbirth, good tone in the pelvic-floor muscles helps the baby rotate and descend (see page 54). The mother's ability to relax these muscles in the second stage as she pushes her baby down the birth canal will greatly assist the birth. Well-toned pelvic-floor muscles also recover from childbirth more quickly than do poorly toned muscles.

Men and women perform the exercise in the same way. You contract the muscles of your pelvic floor as you would if you were trying to keep from urinating or to stop the flow of urine once it has begun. You can do some quick contractions, but try to hold others for up to 30 seconds. You may find it difficult at first to do these longer holds, or "super-Kegels," but your stamina will build. If the contraction seems to fade when you have not consciously let go, don't let it go completely, but simply tighten it again. After 20 to 30 seconds, let go and rest. Try not to contract muscles in your legs, buttocks, or abdomen or to hold your breath while doing the exercise.

Do 10 super-Kegels a day. You and the mother can remind each other to do them while riding in the car or bus, waiting in line, or talking on the telephone. Or do one or two while washing your hands after using the toilet.

DO SOME STRENGTHENING EXERCISES, TOO

Labor can be physically demanding for you as well as for the mother. A strong partner is invaluable in helping the mother change and maintain certain positions (see page 135), and in providing steady pressure on her low back or hips to relieve back pain (see page 157).

Furthermore, you will need physical stamina to remain awake and on your feet for hours. If you are not in very good shape, you might want to begin some strength training, particularly for your arms, chest, shoulders, back, and legs. Push-ups, sit-ups ("crunches"), back and leg strengthening exercises, and weight training will all improve your strength. See "Recommended Resources" for suggestions on building strength.

USE PRENATAL PERINEAL MASSAGE

As scientific studies have confirmed, regular massage of the inside of a woman's perineum (the area between the vagina and the anus) in late pregnancy helps prepare the mother to release tension in her perineum during birth (see the illustration on page 44). Prenatal perineal massage can reduce the need for an episiotomy (a surgical incision to enlarge the vagina, done just before the birth) and the likelihood that the mother's tissues will spontaneously tear during birth. Prenatal perineal massage also lets the expectant mother experience sensations similar to those she will feel as the baby emerges, so she can practice relaxing her perineum as she should during delivery.

I advise pregnant women in my classes to use perineal massage four to five times per week for four to six weeks before their due date. Frankly, some women find the massage distasteful and decide not to do it; others find it pleasurable or sexually stimulating, which is a bonus. Most who do it feel it pays off in less soreness and stitching in the perineum after delivery.

CAUTION: If the mother has inflammation, infection, or a herpes sore in her vagina, perineal massage could worsen or spread the condition and should not be done until the problem goes away.

Instructions for perineal massage. Either you or the expectant mother herself can do the massage. It is easier for her to have you do it.

These directions are for you:

1. Make sure your fingernails are short. Wash your hands before beginning. If you have rough skin on your fingers that might scratch her, wear disposable rubber gloves.

2. Have the mother make herself comfortable in a semi-sitting position, with her legs bent and relaxed.

3. Lubricate your index finger with wheat-germ oil, any other vegetable oil that you have in your kitchen, or water-soluble jelly. Do not use baby oil, mineral oil, or petroleum jelly, as they tend to dry the tissue; vegetable oils are better absorbed. To avoid contaminating the oil in the container, squirt a little over your finger instead of dipping your finger into the oil.

4. Start with one index finger. Place your finger well inside the mother's vagina, up to the second knuckle. Bend your finger slightly, and pull down and out (in the same direction the baby will come out) until she tells you she feels a slight stinging. Give her time to relax to the stinging sensation. If she cannot, ease the pressure until she can relax.

5. Maintaining the same pressure, slowly rotate your finger in a U-shaped curve to the left, back to center, and to the right, back and forth for three minutes. If you think of six o'clock as straight down, you'll be moving from about four o'clock to about eight o'clock. The mother should concentrate on relaxing her perineum as she feels the pressure.

6. Once the mother gets used to massage with one finger, try using both index fingers at the same time, in opposite directions—from six to eight o'clock with your left finger, and from six to four o'clock with your right finger.

7. As the mother becomes more comfortable with the massage, increase the pressure just enough to make the perineum begin to sting from the stretching.

8. Ask your caregiver or your childbirth educator to answer any questions you may have after trying the massage.

Perineal massage puts a stretch on the vaginal tissue, the muscles surrounding the vagina, and the skin of the perineum. After doing the massage three or four days in a row, you will probably find that the mother clearly tolerates the stretching better than at first, and that you have to increase the pressure to cause stinging. This is a good sign. During the birth the mother will still feel the stretching as an intense stinging sensation, but by then she will know how to relax despite the stinging.

CONSIDER KEEPING TRACK OF FETAL MOVEMENTS

Although most babies have no problems during pregnancy, some do, and a major purpose of maternity care is to prevent, detect, or treat such problems. On rare occasions, there is a decline in the placental transfer of nutrients and oxygen from the mother's to the baby's circulation. As a result, the baby's growth or activity may slow. Counting fetal movements sometimes detects such a problem.

An active baby is a healthy baby. If a baby is not getting enough oxygen, he will slow his movements to conserve oxygen. There is usually a period of decreasing movement—enough time to act—before the baby is in serious trouble.

The mother's accurate daily account of fetal movements can help the caregiver decide whether other tests of fetal well-being are necessary or whether to deliver the baby early. The mother is most likely to assess fetal movements correctly if she sets aside a period of time each day (an hour or so after a meal) to record how long it takes to feel 10 fetal movements. Such a record is more accurate than the mother's informal impressions, which are influenced by how busy or distracted she is at any particular time.

Some caregivers ask all their pregnant clients, or at least all who are at high risk for fetal problems, to keep a daily or every-other-day record of fetal movements from about the thirty-second week of pregnancy. Others do not ask clients to count fetal movements, but ask mothers to call if they notice that the baby's movements decline. If the mother's caregiver doesn't ask her to keep a record, you and she can decide whether she'll count fetal movements on her own.

Many women find fetal movement counting to be fun, interesting, and reassuring. Not only do they gather helpful information, but they enjoy the time spent focusing on their babies. They learn about different types of movements, their babies' sleep and wake cycles, and other things. Other women find fetal movement counting makes them worry; they feel they are just waiting for something to go wrong.

If the mother decides to count fetal movements, do it with her, at least some of the time. You can learn a lot about the baby too, and you can also support the mother if she finds it stressful.

There are several ways to do fetal movement counting. The "Count-to-10" method, which follows, is simple and can be begun at any time in late pregnancy.

How to count fetal movements. It is most helpful if the mother counts the baby's movements at roughly the same time every day. She can begin any time after the thirty-second week of pregnancy. It makes sense to begin counting when the baby is awake and active. Babies tend to be most active soon after meals.

The mother writes down the time she starts counting. A movement may be a short kick or wiggle, or a long, continuous squirming. She waits for a pause in the activity, and then marks it down as one movement. The pause may last only a few seconds or longer. Hiccups do not count as movements. Some babies may move 10 times in 10 minutes. Others may take much longer to move 10 times. When the mother has counted 10 fetal movements, she writes down the time when the tenth movement occurred, and figures how long it took to count 10 fetal movements. See the chart on page 24.

The important thing is not how quickly the baby gets to 10 movements but whether the baby maintains the same degree of activity from day to day. The mother should call her caregiver if the baby's movements suddenly slow, if over some days the baby takes longer and longer to get to 10, or if the mother has not felt 10 movements in 12 hours. The caregiver will evaluate the baby's well-being with a nonstress test (see page 208), ultrasound (see page 207), and other tests, and prepare to deliver the baby if there are problems. Most of the time there are none, but once in a while a woman has detected real problems with her baby, and her vigilance allows early intervention and a good outcome.

FETAL MOVEMENT COUNTS

Date	Starting time	Movements	Time of tenth movement	Time elapsed
1/1/08	8:45 A.M.	~~HHI~~ ~~HHI~~	9:05 A.M.	20 min.

COMMUNICATE WITH YOUR BABY

Babies can hear, remember what they hear, and even have preferences in what they hear. Sing songs to your baby. I remember one couple who sang "You Are My Sunshine" to their unborn baby for weeks before he was born. The father sang it again when the baby was crying shortly after the birth, and the baby immediately calmed down. He remembered and liked the song! My daughter played her cello (snuggled up to her belly) every day during her pregnancy, and now her son always quiets and pays attention when she plays. In fact, for quite some time he would cry when she stopped practicing!

Besides singing or playing instrumental music to your baby, try reading a simple children's book aloud to the baby during late pregnancy. It is best to read the same story over and over so that the baby can become familiar with its sounds.

Some partners lie with their heads in the mother's lap to talk to the baby, tell stories, and make plans. One father had a lot of fun telling his unborn baby stories about his own childhood and the movies he liked.

PREPARE OTHER CHILDREN FOR THE BIRTH

Things go more smoothly if siblings are prepared in advance for the arrival of a new brother or sister. Children are reassured to know where their mother will be during the birth, where they will be, and who will be with them. Include the children, as appropriate, in preparations for the new baby. Take them on the hospital tour and to some prenatal appointments, and check whether sibling preparation classes are available in your area. These classes teach about birth and prepare older siblings for life with a new baby.

Some parents consider having their older children attend the birth. This can be a very good experience if the child would like to be present, is generally calm and not too needy, and has his or her own adult support person, so the child can come and go.

See "Recommended Resources" for books on the subject of children and birth.

PREPARE A LIST OF KEY PEOPLE

Make a list of the names, phone numbers, and e-mail addresses of the people you may need to reach around the time of the birth. These may include the mother's doctor or midwife, the hospital's maternity unit or the birth center, your employer and the mother's, your doula, your childbirth educator, family members, friends, a babysitter for your older children or a support person for each child who will attend the birth, a dog or cat sitter, the baby's doctor, and a breastfeeding counselor. Enter the list into your cell phone, computer, or both, and post copies in places handy for both you and the mother.

PREPARE AND REVIEW THE MOTHER'S BIRTH PLAN

The mother's Birth Plan tells her caregiver and nurses in writing what options are important to her, what her priorities are, any specific concerns she has, and how she would like to be cared for. The plan should reflect the mother's awareness that medical needs could require a shift from her choices, and it should include her preferences in case labor stalls or there are problems with her or with the baby. Although most useful for birth in a hospital, where the nurses (and often the caregivers) do not know the mother, a Birth Plan can help every couple, even if they are planning a home or birth-center birth, to think through their choices and priorities.

If you are the mother's life partner (lover, husband, father of the baby) as well as her birth partner, the two of you should prepare the Birth Plan together. If you have a doula, she or he can help you to write it so that it reflects your wishes clearly. If you are not intimately involved with the mother, the Birth Plan should be hers, but you should become very familiar with it so you will know how best to help her.

The Birth Plan will be most useful if it is short and concise. I suggest using bulleted sentences or brief paragraphs, with any details that seem appropriate, for each of the relevant items that follow.

Introduction to the birth plan. The plan might begin with the following information:

- *Personal information (two or three sentences).* What would the mother like the staff to know about her? For example, she might describe strongly held beliefs or preferences, relevant previous experiences with hospitals or health care, fears, concerns, or other information that would help the staff get to know her and treat her as a special individual.

- *Message to the staff.* Would the two of you like to express your appreciation for any support, expertise, and assistance the staff can provide to help her have a safe and satisfying birth experience?

- *Names of those on the mother's support team who will attend the birth.*

her

Labor options. The mother can consider the following options for labor. To keep the plan brief, she should try to condense her wishes to general statements.

- *Activity in labor.* Does she want the freedom to walk, change positions, take a bath or shower, or move about in labor to promote comfort or progress? Or will she be content to remain in bed? (See "Positions and Movements for Labor and Birth," pages 135 to 141.)

- *Food and drink.* Does she prefer to eat and drink at will, at least in early labor, or is she comfortable with having intravenous fluids (see page 213) and sucking ice chips?

- *Fetal heart-rate monitoring.* How does she feel about continuous electronic monitoring (internal or external), intermittent monitoring, or, instead, having her nurse or midwife listen with a handheld ultrasound stethoscope or a regular stethoscope? If she must have continuous monitoring, would she prefer wireless telemetry to having her monitor belts connected by wires to the monitor? (See "Electronic Fetal Monitoring," page 216.)

- *Pain medications.* Does she prefer to use them? Does she want them as soon as she goes into labor, or will she try to delay them until mid- to late labor? Does she want to avoid pain medications entirely, if possible? How important is this to her? (See chapter 8, and especially the "Pain Medications Preference Scale" on page 294, for important information and pointers.)

Birth options. The mother can consider the following options for birth:

- *Positions for second (birthing) stage.* Does she want the freedom to move and use a variety of positions? (See "Positions and Movements for Labor and Birth," pages 135 to 141.)

- *Pushing techniques.* Would she prefer spontaneous, nondirected bearing down with her reflexive urge to push, or the prolonged breath holding and straining of directed pushing? (See "Pushing [Bearing-Down] Techniques," page 130.)

- *Perineal care.* Would she like warm compresses on her perineum and other measures to prevent an episiotomy? How strongly does she feel about this? Would she rather risk a tear than have an epi-siotomy? (See "Episiotomy," page 231.) If she has been doing per-ineal massage (see page 20), she might say so.

After-birth options.   The mother can consider the following options in postpartum care:

+ *Immediate care of the baby.* Does the mother want the baby placed skin to skin with her immediately after birth? Do you and the mother have preferences regarding newborn routines (eye care, vi-tamin K, newborn exam, and so forth)? (See "Common Procedures in Newborn Care," page 331, and "The First Few Days for the Baby," page 338.)

+ *Contact with the baby.* Does the mother want to have the baby with her continuously or to have him spend some time in the nursery?

+ *Your presence.* Would the mother like you to stay in the hospital with her? Can you use a cot or fold-out chair and sleep in the room overnight?

+ *Feeding.* Will the baby be breastfed or formula-fed? If the mother will breastfeed, how does she feel about the baby's being given any water, sugar water, or formula? Does she want to feed the baby on cue (that is, whenever the baby indicates an interest)? (See "Getting Started with Breastfeeding," page 361.) If the baby is to be formula-fed, do the two of you want to do all the feeding yourselves or do you want to have the nurses do some of it?

+ *Circumcision.* If the baby is a boy, will he be circumcised or not? (See page 341.)

The unexpected.   You and the mother should think through the possi-bility of such difficulties as the following:

+ *Difficult labor.* Is the Birth Plan flexible enough to apply even if complications or difficulties arise during labor? (Using phrases like "as long as labor proceeds normally" or "unless medically indi-cated" leaves room for changes in the Birth Plan if safety becomes an issue.) If difficulties do arise, does the mother still want to be consulted before procedures are performed, or would she prefer to leave all decisions to the staff? And if labor is very long, who else can help, such as a relative or doula, so that you can eat, sleep, or just take a break?

• *Transfer.* If the mother has planned an out-of-hospital birth but develops complications and has to be transferred to the hospital, does she want you, her midwife, her doula, and any other support people to remain with her? Does she want to keep whatever options from her Birth Plan are still possible? Does she want to be kept informed of the caregiver's concerns, recommendations, and reasons for them, so that she can make informed decisions? Please note that a woman is transferred to a hospital because she needs medications or other interventions that are available only in a hospital. The way she is cared for necessarily changes when she is transferred. (See part 3, "The Medical Side of Childbirth.")

• *Cesarean birth.* If she must have a cesarean, does the mother want you and her doula to be present? Would she prefer to be awake and alert or sedated during and after the surgery? Would she like to see and touch the baby as soon as possible after the baby's birth? After the birth, if the baby needs the higher level of care available in the nursery, would the mother like you to go with the baby or to stay with her? (If she has a doula, the doula can stay with her while you go to the nursery.) What about postoperative sedation? Would she prefer to receive sleep or sedative medications afterward or to accept some trembling and nausea in order to remain awake and to hold and nurse the baby? (See chapter 9.)

• *Premature or sick infant.* Would the mother prefer to be involved, or have you involved, as much as possible in the care and feeding of the baby, even if the baby is in the special-care nursery? Does she want explanations of the baby's problems, the procedures to be done, and the decisions that need to be made? Does she want you to accompany the baby to a different hospital if the baby has to be transferred? If the baby cannot nurse, does the mother want to express her colostrum (the "pre-milk" her breasts make during the first two or three days after birth) and her milk to feed the baby by bottle or tube or to store until the baby can take it?

• *Stillbirth or death of the baby.* Such a tragedy, as rare as it is, leaves the parents so stunned with grief that it is almost impossible for them to make important decisions. Discuss this possibility to-gether, and think about how you and the mother would want the situation handled. Weeks or months after the death of a baby, the things that were done (or not done) at the time will be very important. Consider some or all of the following:

An opportunity to hold and say goodbye to the baby in private

A chance to dress the baby

Mementos—pictures, the baby's clothing or blanket, a lock of hair, hand- and footprints

Help from a counselor or a member of the clergy

An opportunity to discuss the birth and the baby's problems with the doctor, midwife, nurses, and doula

An autopsy to determine the cause of death

A memorial service or funeral—an opportunity for family and friends to acknowledge the baby's life and death and to demonstrate their love, support, and sympathy for the parents

Ongoing support from a group or a counselor

As difficult as it is to face the possibility that the baby could die, it is wise to think through this possibility. I hope you will never need to implement any of the foregoing suggestions. If you do, you will be glad later that you thought about the possibility ahead of time, when you were calm and able to think clearly.

Personal choices. Are there other choices that will help make this birth experience more comfortable or memorable for the mother and for you? Consider doing the following:

Creating a peaceful environment with her favorite music, low lighting, and minimal disturbance

Including others—doula, relatives, friends, interpreter (if needed), or children

Excluding nonessential personnel (for example, students, observers), or requesting that they introduce themselves and politely ask to be present during the birth

Asking the caregiver whether he or she is comfortable having you assist in delivering the baby or cutting the umbilical cord, as long as the birth is going smoothly

Photographing, videotaping, or audiotaping the birth

Using comfort items such as toothbrush, lip balm, cold packs, eyeglasses (if needed), lollipops, ice or fluids, frozen juice bars, massage tool and massage oil, warm socks, blanket, fan, and so forth

Welcoming the baby with private time together, by singing or playing music, or with a religious or personal ceremony

Incorporating traditional or culturally significant birth customs (foods, bathing, contact with baby, and so forth)

The 36-week prenatal appointment is a good time to give the Birth Plan to the mother's caregiver. This gives the caregiver time to review it and to make sure it is realistic and consistent with the options available and the mother's health status. The Birth Plan can then be placed in the mother's hospital chart, where other staff members will have access to it. It is a good idea, however, to take extra copies along to the hospital.

Keep a copy of the Birth Plan with you during labor. Be ready to ask the staff to read and follow the mother's plan, and be ready to remind the mother of some of her prior choices if she forgets them when she is caught up in the intense demands of labor. While using the Birth Plan as a guide, be willing to accept changes if medical circumstances require it.

Preparing for Life with the Baby

Following is a reminder list of some things to do before the baby is born. It is easier to do these things before the birth than afterward, when time and energy will be limited. If you are the mother's partner (husband, lover), you will want to make these preparations together. If not, you might advise her that these need to be done.

TAKE A BABY CARE AND SAFETY CLASS

You'll want to learn about newborns' temperaments, capabilities, and needs; how they communicate their needs; how to soothe newborn babies; diapering and bathing; guidelines for safe sleeping; how to tell whether a baby is sick; making your home safe for your baby; infant cardio-pulmonary resuscitation (CPR); and more. Most hospitals and parent-support organizations offer such classes or can help you find them.

If you can't take a class, get a good book on baby care (see Recommended Resources).

GATHER THE ESSENTIAL SUPPLIES FOR THE BABY

Is everything ready for the baby? Are the necessary supplies on hand? Use the lists that follow as a guide.

Baby equipment
Car seat (install it correctly and have it checked; see page 15)
Crib, bassinet, cradle, or baby bed that attaches to your bed (make sure the bed meets current safety standards)

Bedding (minimum requirements)
Two or more fitted sheets (pillowcases often fit bassinette mattresses)
Two square waterproof pads to fit under the baby's diaper area
Two warm, crib-sized blankets or quilts
Two or three lightweight swaddling blankets (about 42 inches square)

Clothing (Buy baby clothes with room for growing—no smaller than 10- to 12-pound, or three-month, size. Babies usually weigh close to 10 pounds by the time they are one to two months old, if not at birth. Often babies outgrow even six-month-size clothes by the time they are two or three months old.)
Four snap- or tie-front undershirts, or pullover undershirts that snap at the crotch
Three one-piece coveralls (stretch suits, sleepers) or night-gowns
Two or three one-piece footed blanket sleepers, for cold weather
Two sweaters
One hat for use indoors during the first few days

One hat for outdoors
One warm outfit for outdoors
Two pairs of booties or socks
Four Velcro-fastening diaper covers or plastic pants
Two to four dozen cloth diapers and a diaper pail, unless the
  mother plans to use a diaper service, or at least 80 newborn-
  size disposable diapers (even if she plans to use disposables,
  she might want some cloth diapers to use as burp cloths)
Two hooded baby bath towels
Two baby washcloths

Health supplies
Blunt fingernail scissors
Thermometer for taking the baby's temperature
Diaper-rash ointment
Baby wipes

Supplies for feeding the baby
At least three well-fitting, comfortable nursing bras (the
  mother should be fitted for these by a store clerk who knows
  about breastfeeding)
Nursing pads to fit inside her bra (commercially available, or
  she can make her own from six layers of cotton flannel cut
  into 4- to 5-inch rounds and sewn together)
Supplies needed if she will feed her baby formula
Formula if she will not breastfeed (recommended by the baby's
  caregiver)
Eight to twelve bottles with nipples and caps
Nipple brush, for washing nipples

Optional paraphernalia
Mobile (choose one with black and white or other high-
  contrast colors that looks interesting from below)
Infant seat (an infant car seat can double as one of these)
Soft front-carrier or sling (for carrying the baby hands free)
Stroller or carriage
Baby swing
Rocking chair
Baby bathtub

Birth ball ("exercise ball," "gymnastics ball"), for sitting on and
bouncing while holding the baby against your shoulder (see
illustration page 147)

Pacifiers (in case the baby needs to suck a great deal)

Breast pump, for expressing and storing breast milk

Electronic baby monitor (if the baby will sleep beyond easy
hearing range)

Compact discs of soothing heartbeat sounds, nature sounds,
lullabies, other music

Toys (the possibilities are endless)

Books on baby feeding, baby care, and infant development (see
"Recommended Resources")

CHOOSE A CAREGIVER OR CLINIC FOR THE BABY

The baby will need a medical caregiver (pediatrician, family doctor,
nurse practitioner, naturopath, or health clinic) to provide well-baby
care (routine checkups, immunizations) and to treat illnesses if they
occur. Check the mother's health insurance plan for a list of preferred
providers, and get recommendations from friends, your childbirth
educator, or the mother's caregiver. You and the mother can interview
infant caregivers before the birth, often without charge (ask when
making the appointment whether there will be a fee). The following
are important considerations when choosing a caregiver:

+ *Location of the office.* How far away is it? There is a real advantage
  to its being close to home. Traveling a long distance with a sick
  child can be nerve-wracking.

+ *Practical considerations.* Is the caregiver covered by your health insurance? What are the caregiver's educational and professional
  qualifications? What are the fees? Who covers the practice when the
  caregiver is not available? At which hospital(s), if any, does the
  caregiver have privileges?

+ *Philosophy of infant health care.* What are the caregiver's attitudes
  about breastfeeding, introducing solid foods, circumcision, immunizations, feeding and sleeping, daycare, and so on? You won't have
  time to ask about all of these; select one or two topics.

◆ *Personal attributes.* Does this caregiver seem kind, competent, and caring? Is this someone you and the mother like and could trust with your baby's health care?

It can be a great relief to have your child enrolled in a good caregiver's practice. Having a trusted person to consult about your child's development and health issues will bring great peace of mind.

Prepare a Place at Home for the Baby

Whether the baby will have a fully equipped nursery or a corner of a room, you will need to organize space for the baby—for storing clothes, for diaper changing, for sleeping, and for all the equipment that comes along with babies.

Register for Parent-Infant Classes or Peer-Support Groups

Suggest that the mother investigate available classes or drop-in support groups for new parents; her childbirth educator, doula, or caregiver may be able to suggest possibilities. These classes and support groups provide information about child development, emotional needs of parents and infants, and common problems. Parents learn exercises, songs, massage techniques, techniques for soothing crying babies, and games to play with their newborns. If it's convenient and appealing to you, attend with the mother. You may enjoy the opportunity to form new friendships and to share your questions, concerns, and triumphs.

Prepare Meals Ahead of Time

You may be surprised to find that simply going to the store or even figuring out what to eat can seem almost overwhelming in the first weeks after the baby arrives. So stock the kitchen with nutritious foods that are easy to prepare and eat. Cook and freeze food ahead for reheating later. Locate stores and delis where prepared dishes and nutritious convenience foods are available. See page 358 for more suggestions about putting together quick, nutritious meals.

If your friends want to help after the birth, you might ask them to set up a meal train—that is, to take turns bringing you meals every day or two for two or three weeks. (Most people bring enough food for more than one meal, so if you want to avoid accumulating left-overs, ask for meals every other day.) A meal train is usually a very welcome gift for new parents.

Plan to Share Responsibilities

You will probably be astounded by the amount of work and time it takes to feed and care for a new baby and mother, and to keep the household running. Remember that a baby needs almost constant care for the first few weeks. If the new mother tries to do it all, she will get much less sleep than usual. Full-time newborn care is tiring enough, but because the mother will also be recovering from the physical demands of birth, or possibly from major surgery if she gives birth by cesarean, it may take weeks for her to recover.

Plan to share the baby-care responsibilities and to take over much of the housework and cooking, or make arrangements for someone else to help. Many partners use vacation time or family leave to stay at home for the first days or weeks to share the work. The baby's grand-parents or other relatives can also be a great source of help, as long as the mother's relationship with them is good. If the mother and her parents or in-laws do not get along well, their relationship will *not* suddenly improve with the arrival of the baby. Friends can be won-derful about providing meals, running errands, and doing chores. Say yes if they offer to help.

In many communities, postpartum doulas are available to help new families. These doulas come to the home, usually for a few hours each day for a week or two, and do whatever needs to be done in the way of light housekeeping, meal preparation, errand running, and care of older children. More important, they are very knowledgeable about newborn care and feeding, and can teach new parents a great deal. A postpartum doula also can identify problems in the mother or baby and make referrals if necessary. Hiring a postpartum doula can make it possible for you both to spend time enjoying the baby and to relax a bit or get a nap.

You should book a postpartum doula before the birth To find one, visit www.DONA.org, or ask your childbirth educator, birth doula, or caregiver for a referral. Some birth doulas are also postpartum doulas.

The services of a postpartum doula are a popular gift for distant grandparents to give their children. Many grandparents wish they could come and help, but cannot, for various reasons. If a postpartum doula is not available, a house cleaner or a teenage helper may help ease some of the burden on new parents.

On to the Next Step . . .

Once you have prepared as much as possible, enjoy yourselves as you wait for labor to begin. Photograph the expectant mother at the end of her pregnancy; enjoy some evenings out for dinner, movies, concerts, plays, and visits with friends and family. If you and the mother have other children, plan enjoyable activities with them. Make these last days relaxed and enjoyable before your lives change forever.

And now that you know how to really help the expectant mother *before* labor, let's go on to the next step—how you can really help her *during* labor and birth.

PART TWO

Labor and Birth

The climax of pregnancy, the birth of a baby is an everyday miracle—part of a day's work for the doctor, midwife, or nurse, but a deep and permanent memory for the birthing woman and those who love her and support her. Your role as the birth partner is to do as much as possible to *help make this birth experience a good memory for her.* She will never forget this birth. She will not only remember many of the events, but she will also remember and even relive the feelings she had. The kind of care a woman receives and the quality of the support during labor make the difference in whether she looks back on her birth experience with satisfaction and fulfillment or with disappointment and sadness. This is where you come in. Being a birth partner—helping a woman through labor and birth—is clearly a challenge, but it is a challenge that people like you meet all the time.

To be a good birth partner, you need:

▶ A bond of love or friendship with the mother and a feeling of commitment and responsibility toward her.

▶ Familiarity with her personal preferences and quirks, with the little things that soothe and relax her, and the things that may irritate or worry her.

▶ A commitment to help her continuously throughout labor, either by yourself or with the help of a doula or another supportive person.

▶ Knowledge of what to expect—the physical process of labor, the procedures and interventions commonly used during labor, and when these procedures and interventions are necessary and when they are optional.

▶ An understanding of the emotional side of labor—the emotional needs of women during labor and the changing emotions they usually experience as labor progresses.

▶ Practical knowledge of how to help in various specific situations—what to do when. If you have a trained doula, she will help you with this and the two preceding points.

▶ Flexibility to adapt to the mother's changing needs during labor—"leading by following." How you help, and how much you help, is determined by the mother's needs and responses at the time.

If you also love the mother and the baby, you will care for them in the intimate and personal way that only a husband or loved one can. The next few chapters will cover the normal birth process and will explain what happens, how the mother is likely to respond, what the caregiver does, and how you can help. These chapters will also discuss situations that are particularly difficult for the mother and therefore particularly challenging for the birth partner, too. Read these chapters in advance, then use them as an on-the-spot guide during labor.

CHAPTER 2

Getting into Labor

I work in construction. I was at the job site early, eating breakfast with my buddy in my truck. My phone rang. I listened, said, "Hmmm, okay, okay," hung up, and went back to my breakfast. My buddy asked, "Who was that?" I said, "My wife. Her waters broke. . . . HER WATERS BROKE! Get outta my truck, man! I gotta go!"

—CARL, FIRST-TIME FATHER

A few days past her due date my wife started having small contractions. She would have about three every hour. I thought that this was the beginning and anytime now she would be in labor. After a few days the contractions became a bit more intense and very regular, one contraction every ten minutes. I thought that this was the beginning and she would be in labor anytime now. After another week passed, we went for a walk, and the contractions became a bit more intense and frequent, about four to six minutes apart. At this point you know what I thought. I asked my wife if she thought she was going into labor. She said she didn't know but that everyone says you will know when the real contractions hit. That night, at one A.M., she sat up in bed and said, "That was different. I'm in labor."

—SCOTT, FIRST-TIME FATHER

Everyone wonders how to tell whether a woman is in labor. Even those with experience cannot usually identify exactly when labor starts. Often the mother "sneaks" into labor with unclear, on-again-off-again signs—like an orchestra tuning up before a performance. Over the course of many hours or days, the signs intensify, and you and she come to realize that something is different; this is *it*! Step by step, she becomes mentally and physically more ready for the coordinated effort that eventually results in the birth of the baby. Most women experience a period of uncertainty and questioning while they await clear signs that they are truly in labor.

The one situation in which labor is clearly starting is described in the vignette at the beginning of this chapter: The mother's bag of waters breaks with a gush. Then you know. But only about one in ten labors starts this way. (Please note: A gush of fluid is different from leaking of fluid. About two women in ten have leaking of fluid before labor. In such cases, contractions do not usually begin for hours or days. See page 48.)

As long as the two of you eventually put the pieces together, it usually doesn't matter if the mother's labor is vague at the beginning. There is almost always plenty of time, once she is clearly in labor, to get to the hospital or birth center, or settle in for a home birth. Occasionally, however, a woman is caught by surprise, and goes into labor earlier or more suddenly than she anticipated. Because of this possibility, you will want to be able to tell the difference between the tuning up, or prelabor, and the real thing, progressing labor.

This chapter will help you both recognize when the mother is in labor. It explains how she gets into labor both physically and emotionally and describes the role you should play as her birth partner.

The Labor Process

Labor is the process by which a woman gives birth to a baby and a placenta. The labor process involves the following:

1. Contractions of her uterus, the largest and strongest muscle in the woman's body.

2. Softening (ripening), thinning (effacement), and opening (dilation) of her cervix.

3. Breaking of her bag of waters (the membranes or amniotic sac) that surrounds the baby, and the release of her water (amniotic fluid).

4. Rotation of her baby and molding of the baby's head to fit into the mother's pelvis.

5. Descent of the baby out of the uterus and through the birth canal (vagina) to the outside.

6. Birth of the placenta.

Normally, labor does not begin until both mother and baby are ready—between 37 and 42 weeks of pregnancy. The last weeks prepare the mother physically and psychologically to give birth, to breastfeed, and to nurture a baby. During this time the baby acquires the "final touches," preparing him or her to handle the stress of labor and to adapt to life outside the uterus. It is the baby who usually initiates the labor, by producing and secreting the hormones that begin a chain of events that leads to the steps just listed.

About one in eight U.S. babies is born prematurely, before being really ready. Premature birth may be due to conditions in the mother—infection, high stress, heavy smoking, poor nutrition, drug use, or unknown reasons that override the mechanisms initiated by the baby. Multiple pregnancies (twins, triplets, and more) and some fetal abnormalities are other causes.

Sometimes babies are born post-term, after 42 weeks. Of these, most are fine, but the chances of *postmaturity syndrome* increase with longer pregnancies. This cluster of symptoms in the newborn indicate that the placenta was no longer providing adequate nourishment to the fetus. A postmature baby looks, and is, undernourished. He has loose, peeling skin, having lost some fat in the uterus, and long nails. He may have yellow stains on his nails and skin, signs that he passed meconium (fetal stool) in the uterus. Postmaturity is caused by some interference with the hormonal chain of events that normally brings on labor between 37 and 42 weeks. Because of the widespread policy of induction by 42 weeks, very few babies are born postmature today. When they are, they may need special care in the hospital.

How Long Will Labor Last?

It is impossible to predict how long any particular labor will last. A perfectly normal labor can take between two and twenty-four hours.

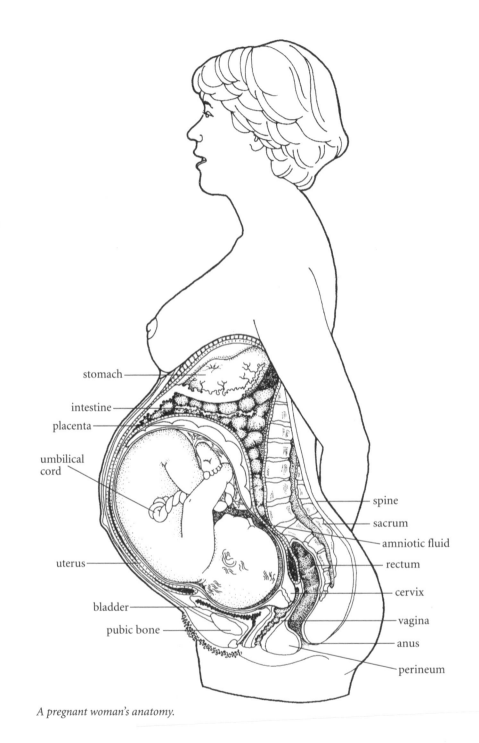

stomach

intestine

placenta

umbilical
cord

uterus

bladder

pubic bone

spine

sacrum

amniotic fluid

rectum

cervix

vagina

anus

perineum

A pregnant woman's anatomy.

In addition, some women experience prelabor contractions for a day or more before labor really begins, that is, before the cervix begins dilating steadily.

Many factors influence the length of labor:

◆ Whether this is a first or later baby.

◆ The condition of the cervix (soft and thin or firm and thick) when contractions begin.

◆ The size of the baby, particularly the head, in relation to the size of the mother's pelvis.

◆ The presentation and position of the baby's head within the mother's body.

◆ The strength and frequency of the contractions.

◆ The mother's emotional state—if she is lonely, frightened, or angry she may have a longer labor than if she is confident, content, and calm.

Presentation refers to the part of the baby—top of the head (the vertex), brow, face, buttocks, feet, shoulders—that will be born first. The top of the head almost always *presents* first; problems occur in delivery if any of the others present first. *Position* refers to the placement of the presenting part within the mother's pelvis. The most common positions are:

◆ OA (occiput anterior): The back of the baby's head (the occiput) points toward the mother's front (anterior).

◆ OT (occiput transverse): The back of the baby's head points toward the mother's side (transverse).

◆ OP (occiput posterior): The back of the baby's head points toward the mother's back (posterior).

Although babies can and do change position during labor and during the pushing (second) stage, at birth the OA position is much more common than OP or OT. When the baby is in the OP position in labor, with the back of his head toward the mother's back, labor is sometimes prolonged, and the mother may experience intense backache. There are many other reasons for back pain in labor, however (see page 185), and you should not assume the baby is OP just because the mother has back pain.

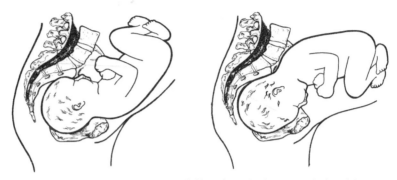

A baby in OA (occiput anterior) position (left) and OP (occiput posterior) position (right).

Signs of Labor

How are you going to know when the mother is in labor? A few clues can help you recognize labor long before the birth is imminent. It is equally important, though, to be able to tell when she is not in labor. There is nothing more frustrating or disappointing for a woman than thinking she is in labor and discovering, after a trip to the caregiver or hospital, that she is not.

If you both know the signs of labor (see the table on pages 47 and 48) and how to interpret them, you will be more likely to react appropriately. Some of these signs are more definite than others. They are categorized as Possible Signs, Prelabor Signs, and Positive Signs.

◆ *Possible Signs (tuning up).* Without other signs, these are not clear enough to get excited about. They can fool and confuse a woman, because they are different from what she was feeling earlier, but, unlike Positive Signs, they do not indicate that her cervix is dilating and that she is therefore in labor. Rather, Possible Signs indicate that her body is *getting ready* for labor. They may go on for days or even weeks before her cervix begins to dilate.

I would not recommend that you or the mother go away on a trip when she has these signs, since at any time she might turn the corner into labor. If the mother has had a rapid labor with a previous birth, she should be particularly alert to the Possible Signs, as they might be all the signs she has before suddenly going into another rapid labor.

◆ *Preliminary or Prelabor Signs.* These are more important than the Possible Signs, but real labor could still be hours or even days away.

◆ *Positive Signs.* These are the only certain signs that the mother is truly in labor—that is, her cervix is dilating.

If you know the significance of these signs, chances are very good that you will be able to correctly interpret what is going on. Sometimes, though, couples need the help of the caregiver to figure out whether the mother is really in labor or not. You or the mother should certainly call the caregiver if she is having any of these signs before 37 weeks, since they could indicate the onset of premature labor.

SIGNS OF LABOR

SIGNS AND SYMPTOMS	COMMENTS
Possible Signs (Late Pregnancy Changes)	
Vague nagging backache causing restlessness—a need to keep changing positions.	• Different from the fatigue-related backache that is common during pregnancy.
Several soft bowel movements—sometimes accompanied by flu-like, "sick" feelings.	• When this sign accompanies others, it is probably associated with an increase in hormone-like substances in the bloodstream (prostaglandins). These substances soften and thin the cervix and stimulate bowel activity. By itself, however, this symptom may be due to a digestive upset.
Cramps, similar to menstrual cramps, that come and go; the discomfort may extend to the thighs.	• May be associated with prostaglandin action and early contractions. • May go away and return several times over weeks or progress steadily to Positive Signs.
Unusual burst of energy resulting in great activity (cleaning, organizing); this is termed the "nesting urge."	• Ensures that the mother will have strength and energy to handle labor (but she should try to curb exhausting activity).
Preliminary or Prelabor Signs	
Blood-tinged mucus discharge ("show" or mucus plug) released from the vagina; mother continues passing this discharge off and on throughout labor.	• Associated with thinning of the cervix. • May occur days before other signs or not until after progressing contractions have begun.

SIGNS OF LABOR *(continued)*

SIGNS AND SYMPTOMS	COMMENTS
Preliminary or Prelabor Signs (cont.)	• A discharge, often mistaken for show, may also appear within a day after a prenatal pelvic examination or sexual intercourse and is not a sign of labor. Show is pink or red; the discharge after a pelvic exam or sex tends to be brownish.
Bag of waters leaks, resulting in a trickle (not a gush) of fluid from the vagina. (See "If Her Bag of Waters Breaks Before Labor Begins," page 49.)	• Leaking fluid occurs before labor in about 2 of every 10 women. • A signal to call and report to the caregiver.
Continuing, nonprogressing contractions—that is, they do not become longer, stronger, and closer together over a period of time. These are prelabor, or Braxton-Hicks, contractions. (See "'False' Labor, or Prelabor," page 51, and "Timing Contractions," page 55.)	• Accomplishes softening and thinning of the cervix, preparing the cervix to begin dilating. • Should not be perceived as unproductive. • These are usually not painful, but they may be tiring or discouraging if they continue for many hours.

Positive Signs

Progressing contractions—that is, contractions that become longer, stronger, and closer together over time. These usually continue until it is time to push. Some women having second or subsequent babies, however, have periods of progressing contractions that come and go over a few days before they settle into a continuous pattern.	• A clear sign that the cervix is opening are 10 to 12 contractions that (1) consistently average 1 minute in length, (2) occur 5 or fewer minutes apart, and (3) feel painful or "very strong." • It is an even clearer sign if these contractions are combined with a "show" (blood-tinged discharge). • The mother cannot be distracted from these contractions. • She may feel these contractions in her abdomen or back, or both.
Spontaneous breaking of the bag of waters (rupture of the membranes) with a pop or gush of fluid followed by progressing contractions within hours. (See "If Her Bag of Waters Breaks Before Labor Begins," page 49.)	• Often associated with rapid labor. • The bag of waters usually breaks in late labor. Rupture of the membranes with a gush occurs before other signs of labor in only about 1 in 10 women.

CAUTION: If a mother who is less than 37 weeks pregnant experiences noticeable contractions every 15 minutes or less for more than two hours, combined with *any* of the other Possible, Preliminary, or Positive signs of labor, she should consult her caregiver. She might be in *premature labor*, which can sometimes be stopped if it is caught early. If she is beyond 37 weeks of pregnancy, she should wait for the Positive Signs before calling her caregiver.

If Her Bag of Waters Breaks Before Labor Begins

If the mother's membranes rupture—if water leaks or gushes from her vagina—before labor begins, make the following observations to report to her caregiver:

1. The *amount* of fluid. Is it a trickle, a leak, or a gush? A "leak" is a squirt that occurs when a woman changes position; about two in ten labors begin this way. A "gush" is an uncontrollable heavy flow that may start with a popping noise or feeling. About one in ten labors begins this way.

2. The *color* of the fluid. Normally, the fluid is clear. If it is brownish or greenish, the baby may have emptied his bowels (passed meconium), which happens when a baby is stressed in the uterus. Such stress is caused by a temporary lack of oxygen.

3. The *odor* of the fluid. Normally, the fluid is practically odorless. If it has a foul smell, there may be an infection within the uterus, which could spread to the baby.

This information helps the caregiver plan what to do next—have the mother stay home, with some precautions; go to the hospital; or come into the caregiver's office so some of the fluid can be collected and tested to determine whether it is amniotic fluid or something else (liquid mucus or urine). To collect fluid from the vagina, the caregiver uses a sterile speculum and a sterile swab. This test is important if the status of the membranes is not clear.

A concern with ruptured membranes is whether the mother is a carrier of Group B streptococcus. If so, her caregiver will want to start treatment with antibiotics and, if labor does not begin spontaneously, induce labor in a matter of hours. For more information on Group B strep, see page 206.

Also, once the bag of waters has broken, the mother should take precautions to prevent bacteria from entering her uterus, since this would increase the chance of infection. She should put nothing in her vagina: She should not use tampons; she should not have sexual intercourse; she should not check her cervix with her fingers. She *can* take a tub bath, which will not increase the chance of infection, provided that the tub is clean.

Until the mother is clearly in active labor, the caregiver and nurses should be very cautious about doing vaginal exams to assess the mother's cervix for dilation. Such exams tend to push bacteria up through her cervix into her uterus and increase the chances of infection. Without recognizing the risks and curious about dilation, mothers in this situation, and their partners, sometimes request vaginal exams. Don't do this, and question the nurse or caregiver who wants to do one. Collecting fluid for testing is an exception to this rule; because the speculum is sterile and nothing is placed in the vagina, this procedure poses little risk of infection.

If precautions are followed and the mother does not carry Group B streptococcus, she can probably safely wait for labor to begin spontaneously, and the caregiver probably won't think that it is necessary to induce labor, at least for a day or more. Most caregivers have a policy regarding their management of ruptured membranes (broken bag of waters); some want to induce labor within hours after the bag breaks, whereas others wait. It is wise to find out this policy ahead of time. If the mother is at low risk for infection (for example, she has tested negative for Group B strep and she has had no vaginal exams), she can reasonably ask to delay induction for a day or more.

CAUTION: On very rare occasions when the bag of waters breaks, the baby's umbilical cord slips out of the uterus as the water escapes. This is called *prolapsed cord* and is a *true emergency*. See "Prolapsed Cord," page 256.

If her bag of waters breaks before labor begins

"False" Labor, or Prelabor

Frequently, women have contractions that are quite strong and frequent, but they are *non-progressing*—that is, the pattern of contractions remains the same. When examined, these women may be told they are in "false" labor, which means the cervix is not yet opening (dilating). The term *prelabor* is much more appropriate, because there is nothing "false" about these contractions, and they are accomplishing changes that allow "true" labor (that is, dilation) to occur. Prelabor contractions are also called Braxton-Hicks contractions. Many women who are examined in prelabor and told it is not labor feel discouraged and embarrassed at their error and may lose faith in their ability to recognize labor. The kind of support the mother receives from you or the doula under these circumstances is critical to her ability to cope with "true," progressing labor later on. Here is how you can help:

◆ It is most important to point out that "false" labor does not mean that what the mother is experiencing is not real. All it means is that her cervix has not yet begun to open. Refer to the contractions as "prelabor."

◆ Remind her that opening (dilation) of the cervix beyond about 2 centimeters is one of the *last* things to happen, after the cervix has moved into position, ripened, and effaced (see page 53). The fact that her cervix is not yet opening does *not* mean that she is not making any progress.

◆ If the mother becomes discouraged with a prolonged period of non-progressing contractions, remind her of the six ways that labor progresses (see "Labor Progresses in Six Ways" on page 52).

◆ Ask the caregiver who examines the mother whether the cervix has moved forward, softened further, or thinned more. Sometimes the caregiver is so focused on the opening of the cervix (dilation), he or she fails to mention these other important signs of progress.

◆ See "Prelabor," page 63, and "The Slow-to-Start Labor," page 180, for some strategies to help the mother cope with these early contractions.

You can be sure that, if the mother has either of the Positive Signs of labor listed in the table on page 48, her cervix is opening. She cannot be in "false" labor if, over a period of time, her contractions have become (1) longer, (2) stronger, *and* (3) closer together, or at least two of those three. See "Timing Contractions," page 55.

Labor Progresses in Six Ways

A woman makes progress toward birth in the following ways. Note that significant dilation does not take place until step 4. The first three steps usually occur simultaneously and gradually over the last weeks of pregnancy.

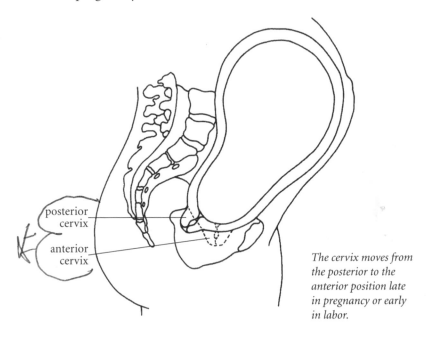

posterior
cervix

anterior
cervix

The cervix moves from the posterior to the anterior position late in pregnancy or early in labor.

1. *The cervix softens (ripens).* While still thick, the cervix, through the action of hormones and prostaglandins, softens and becomes more pliable.

2. *The position of the cervix changes.* The cervix points toward the mother's back during most of pregnancy, then gradually moves

forward. The position of the cervix is assessed by a vaginal exam and is described as posterior (pointing toward the back), midline, or anterior (pointing toward the front).

3. *The cervix thins and shortens (effaces).* Usually about 1¹/₂ inches (or 3 to 4 centimeters) long, the cervix gradually shortens and becomes paper-thin. The amount of thinning (effacement) is measured in two ways:

    - *Percentages.* Zero percent means no thinning or shortening has occurred; 50 percent means the cervix is about half its former thickness; 100 percent means it is paper-thin.

    - *Centimeters of length.* Three to 4 centimeters long is the same as 0 percent effaced; 2 centimeters long is the same as 50 percent effaced; and less than 1 centimeter long means 80 to 90 percent effaced. Be sure not to confuse centimeters of cervical length with centimeters of cervical dilation!

4. *The cervix opens (dilates).* The opening (dilation) of the cervix is also measured in centimeters. Dilation usually occurs with progressing contractions—after the cervix has undergone the changes just described—but it is common for the cervix to dilate 1 to 3 centimeters before the woman has Positive Signs of labor. The cervix must open to approximately 10 centimeters (almost 4 inches) in diameter to allow the baby through.

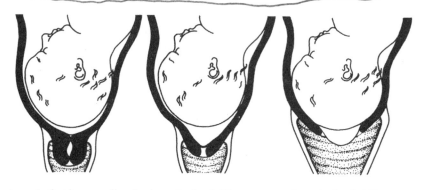

A cervix that has not effaced or dilated, and is 3 to 4 cm long.

A cervix that is 75 percent effaced (about 1 cm long), and 1 cm dilated.

A cervix that is 100 percent effaced (or paper-thin) and 4 cm dilated. The bag of waters is bulging.

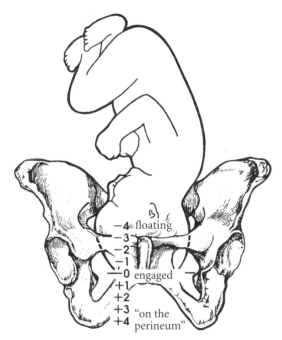

Station—a measure of the baby's descent.

5. ***The baby's chin tucks onto his chest (this is called** flexion) **and his head rotates.*** The rotation makes it easier for the baby to pass through the birth canal. (Sometimes, especially if the head is large, it must "mold" before it can rotate. This means that the head changes shape, becoming longer and thinner. Molding is normal, although some babies' heads look somewhat misshapen for a day or two following birth, after which time the head returns to a round shape.) The most favorable position for birth is usually the OA (occiput anterior) position. See page 45 for information on other positions.

6. ***The baby descends.*** The head continues to mold as necessary to fit and descends through the cervix, the pelvis, and the vagina to the outside. The descent is described in terms of "station," which (a) tells how far above or below the mother's mid-pelvis the baby's head is (or buttocks or feet, in the case of a breech presentation; see page 190); (b) is measured in centimeters; and (c) ranges from minus 4 to plus 4. A "zero station" means the baby's

head is right at the mother's mid-pelvis. Minus 1, 2, 3, or 4 means the head is that number of centimeters above the mid-pelvis. The greater the "plus" number, the closer the baby's head is to the outside and to being born.

Some descent usually takes place before labor begins, especially with first-time mothers. When the baby "drops," it settles into the pelvis to about minus 2 or minus 1. Most of the descent occurs late in labor.

Steps 4 through 6 (dilation beyond 2 to 3 centimeters, rotation, and descent) cannot take place until the first three steps are well underway. In other words, a cervix that is firm, thick, or posterior won't open. It simply is not ready. And a baby won't rotate and descend significantly until the cervix is open. For many women the first three steps take place imperceptibly and gradually in late pregnancy. For others they take place in a relatively short time, with strong or even painful non-progressing contractions, which are referred to as "prelabor" or Braxton-Hicks contractions.

Timing Contractions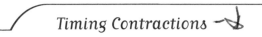

In early labor, one of the important jobs of the birth partner is to time contractions. Since changes in the length, strength, and frequency of contractions are the all-important hallmarks of true, progressing labor, it is a good idea for you to (1) know how to time correctly and (2) keep a written record. Then, when you call the mother's caregiver, you will have accurate and concrete information to provide.

Time contractions in this way:

1. Use a watch or clock with a second hand.

2. Use a written form similar to the sample "Early Labor Record," page 56.

3. You do not need to time every contraction. Instead, time and record five or six contractions in a row and then stop for a while (a few minutes to several hours depending on how quickly the contractions seem to be changing). Draw a line across the page to

separate the timing periods. Later, when the mother thinks the contractions have changed or when she has experienced some of the other signs of labor, time and record another five or six contractions.

EARLY LABOR RECORD

DATE _____

TIME CONTRACTION STARTS	DURATION (SECONDS)	INTERVAL (MINUTES FROM START OF ONE TO START OF NEXT)	COMMENTS (CONTRACTION STRENGTH, FOODS EATEN, COPING METHOD, VAGINAL DISCHARGE, ETC.)

Early labor record

4. Always note the time each contraction begins (specify when the times change from A.M. or P.M.). Record this time in the column headed "Time Contraction Starts."

5. Time the length of each contraction in seconds, and record this time in the column headed "Duration." Contractions usually range from 20 to 50 seconds long in pre- or early labor and 1¹/₂ to 2 minutes in late labor. Knowing when a contraction begins and ends is tricky. The best way is for the mother to signal when she feels the contraction begin and end. The mother can usually feel a contraction longer, from the "inside," than can a nurse, who by palpating her abdomen probably feels only the peak.

6. Figure out how frequently the contractions are coming by subtracting the time at the start of one contraction from the time at the start of the next. Record the number of minutes between contractions in the "Interval" column. (For example, if one contraction begins at 7:32 and the next one begins at 7:38, they are 6 minutes apart.) Do the same for each subsequent contraction.

7. In the "Comments" column, record anything else that may be significant: how strong the contractions seem now compared with earlier, the mother's appetite and what she has eaten, what she is doing to cope (see chapter 4), whether she has back pain or blood-tinged discharge ("show"), whether fluid is leaking or gushing.

When you call the mother's caregiver or the hospital's labor floor, be prepared to report what you have recorded on the "Early Labor Record." Have it near the phone. (Make sure you know whom to call. Some caregivers prefer that you call them directly; others want you to call the hospital's labor-and-delivery area and talk to a nurse.)

See page 71 for the discussion "When Do You Go to the Hospital or Settle In for a Home Birth?"

Now that you know how to tell when the mother is in labor, you're ready to read the next chapter about what happens during labor.

Timing contractions

CHAPTER 3

Moving through the Stages of Labor

At home with my wife in labor, I couldn't wait to get the doula to the house. Shortly after she arrived, I wanted to get to the hospital. In the end, it was 16 hours from the first contraction that woke my wife until we went to the hospital. You probably have way more time than you think.

—SCOTT, FIRST-TIME FATHER

The class described a step-by-step process and walked me through what I needed to know. Afterward, I was nervous because I did not remember the stages and how I could help. Then labor began, and it all came flooding back in one rush of a major contraction. We are told that a woman has the instincts to birth and care for her child, but I think the partners during these experiences are also enabled with such gifts. We just need the knowledge and facts to go along with these instincts.

—HOWARD, FIRST-TIME FATHER

Labor and birth rate among the most intense of all normal human experiences, because they are so demanding—physically, emotionally, and mentally. This is true not only for the woman, but also for those who love and care for her. Labor is unpredictable, empowering, and fulfilling, and it comes with a great prize at the end!

Compare Labor to Running a Marathon

Childbirth has many similarities to a marathon or other physical endurance event. Both include pain and psychological demands for the participant. Both require stamina and patience. Both become much more manageable when the participant is well prepared and flexible and has the following:

- Knowledge of what to expect.
- Prior planning with a knowledgeable guide.
- Physical health and fitness.
- Encouragement and support before and throughout the event.
- Confidence that muscle pain and fatigue are normal side effects of such effort.
- Fluids and adequate nourishment.
- The ability to pace herself.
- The availability of expert medical assistance, in case it is needed.

The meaning of the event (the race or the labor) varies among endurance athletes and childbearing women alike. For some athletes, running a marathon means not only finishing, but also trying to come in at the front of the pack. For others, finishing is the goal and the reward. For some childbearing women, labor and birth mean not only having a baby, but also doing it without medical or surgical intervention. For others, having the baby is the goal and the reward.

It is true for both athletes and birthing women that if they develop complications, or begin to worry about the tough challenges ahead, or become preoccupied with their pain, or lose confidence, or become overwhelmed, they will have to adjust. The athlete may have to slow down or drop out; the laboring woman may have to change her plans and rely more on her caregiver to help her give birth in a safe and satisfying way.

The analogy between an endurance sporting event and childbirth breaks down, however, when we look further. One of the greatest differences is the matter of choice. Marathon runners do not have to run the race. They choose to do so. Healthy pregnant women, however, must go through labor and delivery (or another demanding and painful process—cesarean delivery) if they are to have a child. The other enormous difference between the two events is their degree of predictability. The marathon runner knows when the event will take place and how long the course is, and can study and jog the course ahead of time. The course doesn't change and is the same for all participants.

(The most predictable thing about childbirth is its total unpredictability.) A pregnant woman does not know when it will begin, how long it will take, or how painful it will be, and she certainly does not know whether or how it might be similar or different from her mother's labors or the labors of other women. She cannot even be sure she can get a good night's sleep beforehand! And she certainly cannot predict what her postpartum course will be like.

This unpredictability of childbirth may be a source of frustration as you try to learn what to expect and how to help. Partners in my childbirth classes often ask me questions like these:

- Once the cervix has begun to ripen, how long does it usually take before labor starts?
- After contractions begin, how many hours before we should go to the hospital?
- How long is the pushing stage?
- When should I take time off from work?
- How bad will the pain get?
- When do babies sleep through the night?
- How long do women breastfeed?

When I get questions like these in my childbirth classes, I feel like an evasive politician with my answers: "It may be hours or days. You can be sure it is a sign that she is moving in the right direction." "It varies." "We can't be sure." "People experience things differently." "It's hard to say."

Birth partners would like to know exactly what to prepare for, but it is simply not possible to answer these questions precisely. Variations are inherent in childbirth because each human being and each labor are unique. The key is to accept the unpredictability and pace yourselves while the labor process unfolds. There is good news, however. Despite all the uncertainties, there are some things you can count on. This chapter will give you a broad idea of what you can expect from this mysterious process. You will learn the wide range of normal possibilities, and how you can be truly helpful. The emotions experienced by laboring women constitute a large part of the discussion, along with the emotional responses that you as the birth partner may have. I will give you practical and useful suggestions to help you with the challenging task of providing the mother with emotional support as well as physical comfort. Finally, I will describe how a doula may help both of you throughout the labor.

The following terms describe what is happening during labor and how the mother is progressing:

- *Prelabor* refers to the time before labor actually begins, when the mother is having non-progressing contractions (see page 63) and her cervix is not dilating. The contractions may come and go for a period of hours to days.

- The *first stage* of labor (often simply called *labor*) is the *dilation stage*, during which the cervix dilates completely—to about 10 centimeters in diameter. The contractions progress; that is, they become longer, stronger, and/or closer together.

- The *second stage* is the *birthing stage*, during which the baby is born.

- The *third stage* is the *placental stage*, during which the placenta, or afterbirth, is born.

See the illustrations of each stage and phase of labor on page 90.

The dilation (first) and birthing (second) stages are further subdivided into three phases each. With every new phase, labor changes its rhythm, and the mother must make an emotional adjustment. This chapter describes each stage and phase, and includes suggestions for how you and a doula can help the mother cope. See the table "Normal Labor—in a Nutshell," pages 107 to 110, for a brief summary of this information.

Prelabor

I devote much attention to the phase that precedes actual labor because, unless you have a doula, you and the mother are likely to be coping on your own during this time. If you understand what is going on and how to help the mother handle it, you have a better chance of getting to the hospital or birth center or gathering the birth team for a home birth at the appropriate time—not too early nor too late. Getting to the hospital too early means either that the mother will be sent home or that medical interventions to start labor may be performed essentially out of impatience ("she's here; let's get labor going"). Medical interventions don't always succeed, and then they tend to pile up; one intervention leads to another. If you can avoid this cascade of interventions by going to the hospital at the proper time, the mother will have a better chance of a normal delivery.

What is prelabor like for the first-time mother? During prelabor, the first-time mother may have very regular uterine contractions as the uterus begins "tuning up." These may continue in an unwavering pattern for many hours. Contractions may be regular and strong, and sometimes even fairly close together (every 5 to 8 minutes), for hours. However, they do not progress (by becoming longer, stronger, or closer together over a period of time), and they may stop. The cervix softens, moves forward, and thins, but does not dilate beyond 1 to 2 centimeters. Until the contractions are clearly progressing (which you can best discover by timing them for a while, as described on page 55), the mother is in prelabor, and her cervix is not ready to begin dilating significantly.

Before going on, I should mention that a minority of mothers, first-time and not, never experience much of what I just described. They skip over the preliminaries and begin having progressing contractions as soon as they are aware that they are having contractions. Sometimes when they look back, they realize that the restless night's sleep, or the crampy, soft bowel movements that they had must have been their prelabor. Others have no warm-up. They plunge immediately into labor.

What is prelabor like for the mother having a second or subsequent child?
Prelabor is often different for the experienced mother. Strong contractions may continue for a while, especially at night, even progressing enough to convince her that she is in labor, but then subside by morning, and resume the next night for more hours. I call this an "on-again-off-again" contraction pattern. It is not unusual for an experienced mother to be 3 or 4 centimeters dilated but not yet be in labor! While such a pattern can be frustrating, help her think of it this way: "You're already dilating, and you aren't even in labor!" Once labor actually gets going, it is usually faster than her first, though there are exceptions.

As you can see, prelabor can be a confusing time for the mother, her birth partner, and even for her caregiver. You may find it difficult to distinguish between this tuning up and the "real thing." Then, without warning, and perhaps without either of you recognizing it, prelabor contractions will become the "real thing": They will begin to get longer, stronger, and/or closer together. The cervix will begin to dilate.

How long does prelabor last? Prelabor may last from a few hours to many hours, or it may come and go over several days.

What will the mother feel? During prelabor, the mother may feel one or more of these emotions:

◆ Confusion about whether she is in labor or not.

◆ Excitement and anticipation, as she realizes she will have the baby soon.

◆ Overreaction, as she assumes that she must be dilating more than her signs would indicate.

◆ Fear or dread, especially if she is not mentally prepared, if labor is earlier than she expected, or if her contractions are more painful than she expected.

If prelabor goes on for days, the mother may feel one or more of these emotions:

◆ Frustration over not knowing what is happening and feeling tricked by the confusing signs.

- Discouragement over the long wait.
- Fatigue, if she has missed sleep.
- Doubt or anxiety about her body's ability to function properly, especially if the contractions are painful but not progressing.
- Worry about being too tired to handle the progressing contractions when they begin.

What does the caregiver do? Depending on your report, the caregiver may suggest that the mother wait at home, come into the office for a progress check, or go straight to the hospital or birth center. In addition, the caregiver may do any of the following:

- Come to your home to check the mother, if she is having a home birth.
- Offer advice and encouragement to help her handle this frustrating phase.
- Suggest a warm bath or drugs for rest or to slow contractions if prelabor has been going on for a long time. See page 296 for information about drugs used for these purposes.
- Try to speed labor with drugs or by breaking the bag of waters (see "Induction or Augmentation of Labor," page 224).

What might you feel? As the birth partner, you may experience:

- Confusion, since you have no frame of reference against which to compare the mother's present behavior or verbal expression of pain ("This seems easy" or "How much harder can this get?" or "I can't believe the nurse told us not to come in yet").
- Anxiety about packing the car and getting to the hospital or birth center in time.
- Frustration that prelabor seems to be taking a long time or that the signs of labor are not clearer.
- Concern over whether you are helping the mother enough or that she is not handling it very well.
- Excitement that the big day is here (or near)!

- Eagerness to help the mother and see the baby.
- Worry, if the mother is tired and discouraged because she missed a night's sleep.
- Exhausted, if you stayed up with her.
- Guilty, if you slept.

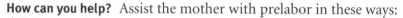

How can you help? Assist the mother with prelabor in these ways:

- Realize that a long prelabor is not a medical problem in itself. Therefore, it is mostly up to the two of you to handle it, perhaps with the help of a doula, friends, or family members.

- Recognize prelabor for what it is. Help the mother determine whether her contractions are progressing by timing them occasionally. If they are not progressing, point out that labor will feel clearly different from what she is currently experiencing. (See "Timing Contractions," page 55; "Signs of Labor," page 47; and "'False' Labor, or Prelabor" page 51.)

- Check with the caregiver for advice and reassurance, and possibly to arrange for an examination.

- Encourage the mother to eat when she is hungry and drink when she is thirsty.

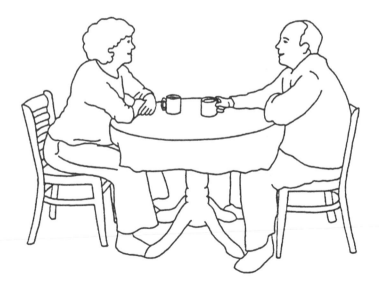

◆ Do projects or activities together to help get your minds off the contractions. You might give her a massage, or the two of you might prepare food, go for walks, visit with friends, or read a book aloud to each other.

◆ Consult "The Slow-to-Start Labor," page 180, for specific coping techniques if prelabor continues for a long time.

How does a doula help? If you have a doula, give her a heads-up call during prelabor even if you don't need her yet, especially if prelabor goes on for a long time. Depending on the situation and the mother's needs, the doula may simply talk with you by phone, or she may join you at this time. She will listen to both of you describe what is going on and give concrete suggestions for raising your spirits if you are discouraged, pacing yourselves if progress is slow, and getting some rest, even if neither of you can sleep. She may review how you will know when labor is progressing, and remind you of comfort measures that help during prelabor. If she lives close enough to come to your house, she can go for a walk with the mother, suggest and help with activities such as packing the car and baking cookies or bread, or just stay a while so that you can run errands, take a nap, or shower. She may go home if contractions slow down and you no longer feel the need for her company. If she leaves, she will make sure you know how to reach her immediately when you need her. She can also help you decide when you should call the caregiver or go to the hospital.

The Dilation Stage

What is dilation? Dilation, or the opening of the cervix, occurs in the first stage of labor. Dilation begins when the prelabor contractions change from their non-progressing pattern to becoming longer, stronger, and closer together (or at least two of those three). The first stage ends when the cervix has dilated completely (to approximately

10 centimeters). The dilation stage can proceed very quickly, unevenly, or slowly. It has distinct phases: the latent phase (also called
early labor); the active phase (or active labor); and the transition
phase (or just "transition"). See the illustrations on page 90.

The change from prelabor to the dilation stage may be gradual,
so don't expect that you or the mother will know the moment her
cervix begins to open.

In a "textbook" labor, the contractions gradually and steadily
increase in intensity and duration and come closer together. Early
contractions may last from 30 to 40 seconds and come anywhere from
5 to 20 minutes apart. Although there are exceptions, these early contractions are usually painless. But by the time the cervix has opened to
8 or 9 centimeters, the contractions may last 90 seconds or more, feel
very intense (almost surely very painful), and come every 2 to 4 minutes. The pain of labor usually reaches its maximum by 7 or 8 centimeters. Second-stage contractions are different and may not be
painful or may be painful in another way. See pages 94 to 96.

How long does dilation last? The dilation stage lasts from two to 24
hours, although for first-time mothers it rarely lasts less than four
hours.

You cannot know in advance how long dilation will take, but the
way labor starts may give you some clues. If the mother starts right
off with contractions that seem very long or very painful and close
together, you may wonder whether these are the relatively easy ones
you've been expecting: "If this is early labor, what will active labor be
like?" You must trust her perceptions and yours. Her labor might be
one of those uncommon very fast ones. Call her caregiver or the hospital, give an accurate idea of what is happening, and get the caregiver's or nurse's advice. Try not to worry; a very fast labor usually
means everything is normal (almost too normal!). Turn immediately
to chapter 5, page 171, for a discussion of the very rapid labor.

In a slow labor, contractions continue as quite manageable and
progress very gradually over a long period of time. This can lead to
discouragement, fatigue, and worry. You'll both need to pace yourselves through an extra-long labor. (See "Arrest of Active Labor
[Dystocia]," page 253.)

When should you call her caregiver or the hospital? Make sure you have the correct numbers to call on hand (see chapter 1, page 25)! Call under any of the following circumstances:

♦ If the mother may be in premature labor, that is, if she has signs of labor before 37 weeks (see "Signs of Labor," page 47).

♦ If she has leaking or a gush of fluid from her vagina (see "If Her Bag of Waters Breaks Before Labor Begins," page 49).

♦ When the mother's contractions are clearly becoming longer, stronger, and closer together (see "Signs of Labor," page 47; "The 5-1-1 or 4-1-1 Rule," page 72; and "Timing Contractions," page 55).

♦ Whenever you or the mother has questions or concerns.

♦ If the mother has had a child before, she should call the caregiver or hospital whenever she thinks or knows she is in labor. A second (or later) labor is usually faster than a first one.

EARLY LABOR - Here

What is early labor? This first phase of the dilation stage lasts until the cervix is dilated to 4 or 5 centimeters. Medical professionals call this the *latent phase* of the first stage.

The big difference between prelabor and early labor is that during early labor the cervix begins to gradually open. For the mother and the birth partner, this shift to early labor is signaled by progressing contractions. The caregiver uses vaginal exams as necessary to determine changes in the cervix during this phase.

How long does early labor last? Typically, early labor takes from two-thirds to three-quarters of the total time of the dilation stage. In other words, it could take from a few hours to 20 hours or so for a woman to reach 4 centimeters of dilation. The length of early labor depends largely on the state of the cervix, the position and station of the baby within the pelvis at the time labor begins, and the strength of the mother's contractions. Chances for more rapid progress are increased if the following conditions exist:

♦ The cervix has moved forward and is very soft and thin. See page 52.

- The contractions are intense and close together.
- The baby is in the occiput anterior (OA) position, with her head down, her chin on her chest, and the back of her head toward the mother's front (see page 46).
- The baby's head has begun to move down into the mother's pelvis (see page 54).

These favorable conditions increase the likelihood of an average or shorter-than-average early labor. Under any other conditions, early labor is likely to take longer than the rest of labor. Labor is not a race against time, however. A normal early labor can last from a few hours to many hours.

How will the mother feel? The mother's response to early labor will probably not be all that different from her response to prelabor. She is still likely to feel somewhat uncertain as she begins to recognize the positive signs of labor.

Getting into labor emotionally takes time. How the mother adjusts will depend on the circumstances—whether labor is early, on time, or late, and whether early contractions are hard and fast or vague and slow.

Reactions to labor range from relief, elation, or excitement to denial, disbelief, or panic. As labor settles into a rhythmic pattern, the mother settles down emotionally, pacing herself and finding routines for handling each contraction.

Sometimes, in the excitement of early labor, the mother rushes the labor along in her mind. She may overreact to these relatively mild contractions. If she concentrates hard on each one, she can feel it for a longer time, and so it seems longer and more intense than it would if she were distracted by some other activity. This results partly from her desire for labor to go quickly and partly from not knowing what level of intensity to expect. Without this frame of reference she may easily become convinced that her labor is progressing more rapidly than it really is.

When a woman rushes her labor mentally, she may want to go to the hospital too early, start using rhythmic breathing and other labor-coping measures before they are really needed, and speculate that her cervix is dilated much more than it really is. Then, when she has a vagi-nal exam and finds that she's not as advanced in labor as she had hoped, she becomes discouraged and may lose confidence that she can cope.

How can you tell whether the mother is (1) overreacting to early labor, (2) reacting appropriately, or (3) having a particularly diffi-cult or rapid labor? Without vaginal exams, you cannot really know whether labor is progressing quickly or not. The best you can do is make an educated guess. Refer to "Signs of Labor" (see page 47), time the contractions, and see whether the mother can be distracted. Try a walk outside, or phone or visit with friends or relatives. If labor seems to "slow down" or become easier when the mother is dis-tracted, she may have overreacted. Keep up the distractions (see "How Can You Help?," page 66, for other ideas for handling over-reaction to early labor). Above all, try not to overreact yourself. It is just as easy for you to make this mistake as it is for her.

If you are unable to distract her, or if labor does not slow down when you do, then the mother is not overreacting. Stop trying to dis-tract her, and help her cope instead. Encourage her to focus on her contractions and begin using her prescribed (or planned) ritual—slow breaths combined with relaxation and positive mental focus (see page 121). If strong contractions are coming one on top of another, and nothing that you and she try to do helps her to cope, she is likely having a fast, intense labor (see page 171).

What does the caregiver or labor-and-delivery staff do? During early labor, the caregiver or hospital staff can help in the following ways:

- ◆ By giving advice over the telephone. When you call, be prepared to provide the information recorded on the Early Labor Record (see page 56).
- ◆ By helping the mother decide when to go to the hospital or, if she is having a home birth, when to settle in at home for the labor.
- ◆ By doing a vaginal exam to give you both an idea of how dilation is progressing.

When do you go to the hospital or settle in for a home birth? Under most circumstances, the first-time mother should go to the hospital or birth center or settle in for a home birth when she has had 12 to 15 consecutive contractions that:

- ◆ Last at least 1 minute.
- ◆ Are 4 to 5 minutes apart (or closer).
- ◆ Are strong enough that she *must* use a breathing, relaxation, or attention-focusing ritual (see page 115) to get through them.
- ◆ Are strong enough that she cannot be distracted from them.

Usually it takes about an hour to time the contractions and determine whether they fit this pattern. If they are less than four minutes apart and advancing quickly, however, you needn't wait an hour before going to the hospital or birth center.

THE "4-1-1" OR "5-1-1" RULE: Before going to the hospital or birth center, wait until the contractions have been four or five minutes apart and one minute long for one hour. Whether you use 4-1-1 or 5-1-1 depends on the caregiver's preferences, the mother's preferences, whether this is her first or a subsequent labor, how far she lives from the hospital or birth center, and whether she is considered at high risk of complications.

Sometimes there are special reasons for the mother to go to the hospital earlier. For example:

- ◆ The mother lives a long distance from the hospital.
- ◆ She has medical problems that require early admission. Her caregiver will advise her whether these problems exist.
- ◆ The mother has given birth before (especially if she had a rapid labor), and recognizes that she is in labor. A woman's second (or later) labor usually goes faster than her first one did.
- ◆ She is anxious and really wants to be at the hospital or birth center.

NOTE: If she is planning to give birth in an out-of-hospital birth center, do not go there without calling her midwife to set a time to meet at the birth center. The place may be locked and unstaffed, especially if it is nighttime.

When do you go to the hospital or settle in for a home birth?

Because early labor can take a long time, it is often a good idea to spend the time relaxing together by yourselves or with friends until the mother's contractions fit the pattern described here. It is usually best not to arrive at the hospital (or call the caregiver to the home) too early because:

- The mother may feel "performance anxiety"—pressure to start producing some good contractions. Feeling watched by her caregiver or nurse, who seems to be waiting for something to happen, she may feel embarrassed that labor is so slow.

- The mother may become unnecessarily preoccupied with the contractions and the apparent lack of progress, and this may make labor seem longer or more difficult than it is.

- The mother may become bored, anxious, or discouraged.

- The staff may offer or suggest medical interventions to speed up this normally slow part of labor. You and the mother should ask the Key Questions on page 202 before considering these interventions. They all carry some risks, including the possibility that they will not succeed and other interventions will be required. Without a medical need, these interventions may carry more risk than benefit.

Sometimes the caregiver will suggest that the mother leave the hospital and come back later. For a home birth, everyone except you may have to leave for a while. Although discouraging, this measure allows the labor to settle into its own pattern and takes pressure off the mother.

How might you feel? You may have many of the feelings described for prelabor, plus:

- Hope and elation, now that you notice the contractions progressing.

- Concern, especially if the mother is tired, discouraged, or having trouble dealing with the pain.

- Eagerness to get word from "the experts" that this is labor, that it is time to go to the hospital or for the midwife and others to arrive for a home birth.

- Tired, if you have missed sleep.

How can you help? Your role now is very similar to the role you played during prelabor. You should remain close by; supply the mother with food and drink; time five or six contractions, as described on page 55, when the pattern seems to change; and help the mother pass the time with pleasant and distracting activities (see "The Slow-to-Start Labor," page 180).

Talk with the mother if you feel you must leave for work, errands, or other activities. Whether you go depends on her feelings and the following considerations:

◆ How important is it that you go now?

◆ Can you be reached by phone or pager at all times?

◆ How far would you have to travel to reach the mother? How long would it take you?

◆ Is there someone else available (a friend, a relative, your doula, a neighbor) to help out if the mother needs someone right away?

◆ What are the pressures on you—from work, school, or other responsibilities?

◆ Will a few more hours really let you clear up pressing obligations?

If you still feel you should leave, and the mother agrees, make sure someone else stays with her until you are free. This should be a last resort, as labor can change quite suddenly.

Sooner or later, the labor pattern will intensify and the mother will become preoccupied with the contractions. She will no longer be able to walk or talk through them without pausing; the contractions "stop her in her tracks." From this point on it is inappropriate to leave her or to distract her. Instead, you now need to do the following:

◆ Give the mother your undivided attention throughout every contraction. Stop what you are doing, and stop talking so you can focus on her. Do not ask her questions during contractions.

◆ Watch her during the contractions and, if she tenses, help her to relax her entire body during each one (see "Relaxation," page 121).

◆ Suggest that she begin using her planned ritual—slow, rhythmic breathing and focusing on something pleasant or positive, such as letting go of tension with each out-breath (see page 115).

◆ Encourage her slow, rhythmic breathing through comforting touch and verbal encouragement during each contraction ("That's good. . . . Just like that"), and helpful comments when the contraction is over ("You relaxed very well that time," or "I noticed you tensed your shoulders with that contraction; with the next one, try to keep your shoulders relaxed").

◆ Help her decide when to call her caregiver.

◆ If you have hired a doula but have not called her yet, call her now, either to alert her that you expect to need her soon or to ask her to join you.

What does a doula do? Beginning with your phone call to her, the doula will probably:

◆ Ask what's going on. Tell her about the signs of labor, the contraction pattern, and how you both are feeling and coping.

◆ Ask to speak to the mother, and assess her distractibility.

◆ Listen to her through a contraction to get an idea of how she is coping (does her breathing or moaning sound relaxed or tense?) and to encourage her in her planned ritual, perhaps by breathing audibly with her through the contraction. This will help the mother relax and breathe rhythmically.

◆ Ask the mother the all-important question: "What was going through your mind during that contraction?" As she listens to the mother's response, the doula assesses whether the mother is positive and coping well or feeling distressed.

If the mother is coping well and you do not tell her otherwise, the doula will probably conclude that you do not need her to come yet. She will remind you of things to do and make a plan for staying in touch.

If the mother is distressed or asks the doula to come, the doula may suggest some coping strategies to try until she gets there, and then hurry to join you. She should tell you just when and where she'll arrive—at your home, the hospital, or the birth center.

When the doula joins you, she will:

◆ Wash her hands, and, if you are at the hospital or birth center, introduce herself to the staff.

- Assess the mother's needs and how you are feeling.

- Assist as appropriate, keeping in mind your planned support role, which you, the mother, and the doula will have discussed in a previous meeting.

- Sit quietly through a contraction or two to observe the two of you working together, so that her role will fit with what you are doing. She may fix a cup of tea for each of you, give the mother a shoulder or foot rub, or in other ways create a calming atmosphere.

- Help you figure out when to go to the hospital or birth center, if you are still at home.

Early labor eventually evolves into a more intense pattern of progressing contractions. As the cervix dilates from 3 to 5 centimeters, the rhythm and pace of labor change. Contractions often accelerate and intensify for an hour or more before the mother's cervical dilation begins to speed up. When her cervix responds to the increasing pace of her contractions by beginning to dilate more rapidly, the mother has turned the corner into active labor.

ACTIVE LABOR

What is active labor? The active phase of labor begins when the cervix has dilated to about 5 centimeters. At this point the cervix is thin and soft, and contractions are closer and stronger. The cervix usually begins to dilate faster. Active labor lasts until cervical dilation reaches 8 to 9 centimeters.

During active labor, contractions consistently last more than one minute and come every three to four minutes. The contractions are usually very intense, and most women describe them as painful.

It is important to recognize the positive meanings of active labor. As demanding as the contractions are, they mean that labor is progressing well and that the mother's body is doing exactly what it needs to do. The pain is not a danger sign; rather, it is a side effect of the strong contractions, the pressure in her uterus, and the stretching of her cervix that will bring the baby into the world.

[handwritten note: last 1 min't - Every 3 to 4 minutes]

Active labor last 3 to 7 hours

How long does active labor last? Normally, active labor is much shorter than early labor. For first-time mothers, active labor usually ranges from three to seven hours. It is usually much faster for mothers who have had babies before—from 20 minutes to 3 hours.

What does the mother feel? The mother must make an emotional adjustment to the changing rhythm and sensations of labor. She is focused on coping with the more frequent and intense contractions, and she may not realize that the pace of dilation is also picking up, or will soon. She may respond to the changing rhythm of labor in the following ways:

- She may feel tired and discouraged as she realizes that the tough part is just beginning. She may lose confidence in her ability to cope with these more frequent, intense contractions.

- Her sense of humor fades. Your funniest jokes don't amuse her.

- Extraneous conversation becomes annoying. She may feel very alone if you and others do not recognize this change and continue trying to distract her, or, worse yet, ignore her and talk to one another.

- For many women, the active labor phase is a moment of truth. Suddenly it sinks in that this labor is real; there is no way out except

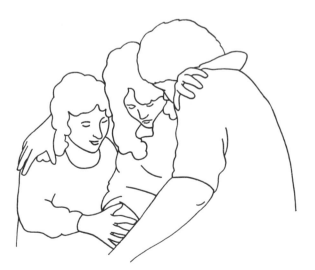

to keep going and have the baby. Realizing this may at first frighten or depress the mother.

- As she realizes that she is not in control of this relentless process, she may struggle a bit, feel panicky, or break down temporarily, weeping and saying that the labor is too hard, that she cannot go on, or that she wants pain medications.

- She, and the room, may become quiet.

- With your understanding and good support, she will be able to get past this crisis, let go of her need to be in control, and work with, not against, her contractions, by letting her body take over. Her mood will turn to acceptance, and she will discover her own ways to handle the contractions. I call these unplanned coping techniques "spontaneous rituals."

A *ritual*, in labor, is a series of comforting rhythmic actions repeated during every contraction. Some rituals, such as breathing, relaxation, and attention-focusing techniques, are learned in advance, and are especially helpful in early labor. In active labor, if the mother feels safe and uninhibited, she releases the need to control the process. Then she adapts her ritual or comes up with a completely new one. This is a very good sign that she is no longer "thinking" her way through labor but has reached deep within herself to find her own instinctual way of coping. For examples, see "Spontaneous Rituals," page 119.

When the mother lets her body take over, she becomes serious and focused on herself and her contractions. She devotes all her attention to maintaining her ritual—releasing tension, breathing, moving, and, perhaps, moaning rhythmically during her contractions. When a contraction ends, her conversation, if any, is likely to consist of reviewing it with you and talking about what to do for the next one.

At this time, the mother benefits from a quiet room, freedom to move around in and out of bed, and as little disturbance or interruption as possible. She may want to be held or stroked, or, conversely, not touched at all. This is when laboring women become more instinctual, more focused, less verbal. You might think that when labor is steadily advancing, women would find it more and more difficult to cope. But this is not the case when women feel well supported. They find it easier to cope once they release the need to be in control and can let their bodies take over.

What does the caregiver do? In a hospital birth, generally, the doctor isn't in the birth room during active labor but is available nearby or by telephone. A nurse provides most of the direct clinical care, following the doctor's orders. If the caregiver is a midwife, she is likely to provide more care herself than a doctor would, but sometimes, a nurse carries out the midwife's orders.

As labor advances, the midwife or nurse becomes more actively involved. Now that progress is faster and the contractions are more intense, closer surveillance is needed. The nurse or the midwife checks:

◆ The mother's blood pressure, pulse, and temperature.

◆ Her fluid intake and urine output.

◆ The baby's heart rate.

◆ The length, intensity, and frequency of the contractions.

◆ The dilation of the cervix.

◆ The baby's position and station (see page 54).

Routines vary depending on the management style of the caregiver. Some obstetricians rely heavily on routine interventions and medical technology. For example, they might break the bag of waters, keep the mother in bed, give intravenous (IV) fluids, use electronic fetal monitors to continuously check the fetus and the contractions, give the mother medications to speed the labor and to relieve pain, perform an episiotomy (a surgical incision to enlarge the vaginal opening just before birth), and use forceps, a vacuum extractor, or cesarean surgery to deliver the baby.

Other obstetricians and most midwives and family doctors rely on simpler methods. They might encourage a healthy mother at low risk for complications to drink liquids and move around. They might listen to the fetal heartbeat with a hand-held doppler ultrasound device or use the electronic fetal monitor off and on through the labor rather than continuously. They might suggest comfort measures (see page 111) to relieve pain before offering an epidural or other drugs.

Midwives and family doctors tend to intervene less than do most obstetricians partly because of training, but also because midwives and family doctors care for women with healthy pregnancies and few risks of medical problems in labor. Obstetricians care for women at both low and high risk for problems, and they tend to use procedures for all their patients that are really needed for only the high-risk women. See both the introduction to part 3 and chapter 6 for information about commonly used tests and procedures, and also for key questions to ask and alternatives to consider.

The nurse or caregiver may offer helpful advice and reassurance. Having someone there with expertise and experience—someone you both trust—can be immensely reassuring. Don't hesitate to ask for help or advice if you feel uncertain about the labor or about how you can help the mother.

How might you feel? Although you may be excited to recognize that labor is progressing faster, active labor may be hard for you in several ways:

◆ Seeing the mother in pain, weeping, or asking you for more help may make you feel ineffective, helpless, worried, or even a little guilty that she has to go through so much.

◆ If you do not recognize that her progress is probably speeding up, you may worry about how long the labor is taking, especially because it is so intense.

◆ You may feel cruel if you encourage her to endure the pain, even if that is what she wants to do. You may feel so anxious to relieve her pain that you are tempted to request an anesthesiologist to give her an epidural.

◆ If you recognize that the mother is making good progress, you may feel encouraged and confident that she can get through labor as she prefers to and that you can help her.

How can you help? Your role during active labor is very important. How you respond to the mother's needs will determine to a large extent how well she copes and how satisfied with her labor experience she will feel later. Here are some guidelines for helping the mother during this phase:

- *Take care of yourself.* How long has it been since you ate? If labor has gone on for a long time already, do you need to freshen up with a shower, brush your teeth, or change your clothes? Do you need a rest? If you're exhausted, hungry, or feeling grungy, you may need a break. Try not to be gone for long, and make sure the mother is not left alone.

- *Make sure the staff is aware of the mother's Birth Plan,* especially with regard to her preferences for pain medications and other interventions.

- *Follow the mother's lead.* Take your cues from her; match her mood. When she becomes serious or quiet, you should become serious or quiet. Don't try to jolly her out of this mood or distract her in any way. The labor takes almost all her attention, and she needs you with her both physically and emotionally.

- *Acknowledge her feelings.* If she says, "I can't do this," you might reply, "This is rough. Let me help you more. Keep your rhythm."

- *Give the mother your undivided attention* throughout every contraction, even if her eyes are closed and she seems not to need it. Do not ask her questions during contractions; they could interrupt or disturb her ritual. Do not chat with others in the room, and discourage others from engaging in nonessential conversation. Such talk could make the mother feel very alone and ignored, even if she is coping well.

- *Help her with comfort measures.* Hold her and slow-dance; rub her shoulders or press on her back; walk with her; stay beside the shower or bathtub or get in with her (bring a swimsuit for the purpose). For more suggestions, see chapter 4.

- *Offer her liquid to drink after each contraction or two.* Don't disturb her by asking her what she would like to drink; just hold the beverage where she can see it. She will take it if she wants it, ignore it if she doesn't, or tell you whether she wants a different beverage.

- *Support her "ritual".* Help her maintain a rhythm through each contraction. See "Relaxation," page 121, and "Rhythmic Breathing and Moaning Patterns," page 127.

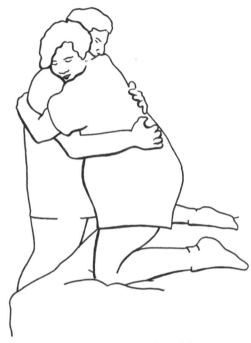

Rhythm is the key to coping in the dilation stage. If there is rhythm in whatever the mother does during contractions (moaning, swaying, tapping, rocking, chanting, even silent self-talk) or whatever she wants you to do (holding her, stroking her, swaying with her, talking, nodding your head, moaning with her), she is coping.

In other words, *rhythm is everything.* If the mother loses her rhythm and tenses, grimaces, writhes, clutches, or cries out, she needs your help (or the doula's or nurse's) to regain the rhythm she had or to find a new one. At times you might help her by making eye contact or by rhythmically talking, stroking, or swaying along with her (see "The Take-Charge Routine," page 166).

Do give rhythm top priority as a way to keep the mother from feeling overwhelmed and to help her maintain a sense of mastery during this challenging part of labor. Let her stick with the same ritual for as long as it helps. Don't be afraid to suggest something new, though, if the mother loses her rhythm and has real trouble getting back to it. Labor may become so stressful that she will need to follow someone else's lead. She will let you know whether she wants to go back to the previous ritual.

What does the doula do? It is a good idea for the doula to join you before the mother rounds the corner into the active phase. Once the mother is in active labor, the doula does the following:

- She recalls the mother's Birth Plan and uses it to guide her own actions and suggestions.

- She remains calm, and models patience and confidence.

- She reminds the mother that labor is progressing and makes other positive comments and suggestions.

- If the mother has wanted to use little or no pain medication but worries that she cannot hold out, the doula will remind her to stay in the present and not look hours into the future. ("Let's take the contractions one at a time. Your job is to keep a rhythm during the contractions, and you're doing it. We'll help you.")

- If the mother has planned to use pain medications and now acts distressed or frightened, the doula supports her if she asks for medication.

- The doula might suggest appropriate comfort measures (see chapter 4). She may ask you to offer the mother a drink or ice chips and help you to become a part of the mother's ritual—by holding or stroking her, for example, or by moaning, walking, or swaying with her.

- If the doctor or midwife suggests an intervention, the doula assists you both in asking the right questions so you can make good, informed decisions.

- Knowing that the mother will never forget this birth experience, the doula asks herself frequently, "How will she remember this?" She uses this thought to guide her in what she says and does.

- She may photograph some tender moments in labor, if you have requested this beforehand.

With your love and understanding of the mother, the knowledge you've gained from your childbirth classes and this book, and your dedication to the baby, combined with the doula's continuous presence, perspective, knowledge, and commitment to a satisfying birth as the mother defines it, you and the doula can be a terrific support team.

TRANSITION

What is transition? The transition phase is a turning point in labor, from the dilation to the birthing stage. In this phase, the mother's body seems to be partly in the dilation (first) stage and partly in the birthing (second) stage.

During transition, the cervix dilates the last 1 to 2 centimeters (from about 8 or 9 centimeters to about 10) and the baby begins to descend. The head moves from the uterus through the cervix and down into the vagina (see the illustrations on page 90). Contractions have reached their maximum intensity, last one and a half to two minutes, and occur very close together.

Sometimes a "lip" of cervix delays the last bit of dilation. A "lip" occurs when a part of the cervix remains thick after most of the cervix has completely dilated. This may be caused by the position of the baby's head, which may press unevenly against the cervix. Several contractions or more may be needed to draw the cervix out of the way so the baby's head can come through.

The uterus may begin its expulsive action even before the cervix is completely dilated. We call this action the "urge to push." It makes the mother catch her breath, grunt, or hold her breath and strain; this is what is meant by the terms "pushing" and "bearing down."

The urge to push is an involuntary reflex; the mother does not make it happen and cannot prevent it from happening. Yet if the cervix is not completely dilated, she may be best off bearing down very slightly—just enough to satisfy her urge. I call this "grunt-pushing." She may do this instinctively or be asked to do this by the nurse or caregiver. Pushing very hard before the cervix is dilated could cause the cervix to swell and the labor to slow (see "Avoiding Forceful Pushing," page 130).

How long does transition last? The transition usually takes from 5 to 30 contractions, or from 15 minutes to a couple of hours. If the cervix has a lip or the baby's head is not well positioned (or both), the transition phase is likely to take longer.

What does the mother feel? For most women, the peak of pain in the dilation stage seems to be reached by 7 or 8 centimeters. Electronic recordings made from within the uterus (with an intrauterine pressure catheter, see page 217) show that after 7 or 8 centimeters contractions do not continue to increase in intensity, though they sometimes come closer together. Contrary to most people's assumptions, the contractions do not keep getting worse until dilation is complete or the baby comes out.

Transition poses other challenges, however. Even though the contractions are not more intense, their frequency, combined with the sensations of the baby's head moving down, may cause the mother's legs, or even her whole body, to tremble. She may feel nauseated and may vomit; vomiting usually brings relief from nausea. She may feel cramps in her thighs or pressure in her pelvis. Even her skin may be sore. She may feel she needs to pass a bowel movement. She may feel very hot, then cold. She may weep or cry out, feeling that she cannot handle any more, that labor will never end. She may feel overwhelmed and frustrated, and react by saying, "Don't touch me! My skin hurts!" or "I can't go on!" or "Stop doing that!" or "I want an epidural right this minute!" Or she may withdraw into herself, dozing between contractions and moaning, groaning, or whimpering during them, all the while relaxing her body quite well. Transition affects women differently, but all are relieved when this phase is over.

Many of these symptoms are caused by a normal outpouring of adrenaline (also called epinephrine) and other stress hormones that occurs late in labor. Stress hormones cause the "fight or flight" response, which gives people great strength and stamina when they must exert themselves—for example, when they are afraid, in danger, or about to take part in competition or a demanding feat like pushing a baby out. Thus, the unpleasant symptoms of transition are followed by a second wind and the strength needed for the hard work of pushing a baby into the world. It helps to know that the symptoms of transition mean the woman is getting close to the birthing stage.

Even though stress hormones help the mother in late labor, if they are produced as a result of great fear, anxiety, or unmanageable pain in early or active labor they can slow progress and put stress on the baby. This is why calmness, rhythm, and relaxation are so important in early and active labor—not only to give the mother a sense of mastery during her contractions but also to prevent excessive production of stress hormones.

What does the caregiver do? During the transition phase, a nurse or a midwife is in constant attendance. The doctor is not necessarily with the mother, although when informed that the mother is approaching delivery, the doctor soon comes.

The nurse or the midwife may do any or all of the following:

♦ Check the cervix to confirm the mother's progress in labor.

♦ Ask the mother not to push, or to push only gently, with little grunts, if the cervix is not fully opened.

♦ Reassure the mother that she is all right and that labor is moving rapidly.

♦ Help you in your role as birth partner and reassure you that the mother is all right and behaving normally.

♦ Begin arranging the room, bringing in the equipment for the birth, and setting up the warmer for the baby (see page 336).

This is an exciting moment, when everyone begins preparing for the infant. Finally, even the staff is acting as if a baby is really coming!

How might you feel? You may feel as if you are caught up in a flurry of activity and intense feelings:

♦ You may be tired, especially if the labor has gone through the night.

♦ You may feel surprised that the mother is finally reaching complete dilation.

♦ You may feel helpless in the face of her pain, and wish you could do something to erase it.

◆ You may feel frustrated or hurt, if she seems to find fault with everything you try to do to help.

◆ You may want to take a break (but she may plead, "Don't leave! I need you!").

◆ You may worry, wondering whether such a demanding labor is normal.

How can you help? Your role during transition is all-important. You can truly relieve some of the mother's burden if you know what to do:

◆ Help her maintain a rhythmic ritual (see page 117).

◆ Stop worrying about relaxation. It is unrealistic to expect the mother to relax when labor is this intense.

◆ Stay calm. Your touch should be firm and confident. Your voice should remain calm and encouraging.

◆ Stay close to the mother, with your face near hers.

◆ If she is panicky and scared, use your "Take-Charge Routine" (see page 166).

◆ Remind her that this difficult phase is short, that she is almost in the birthing stage, and that the contractions are as painful as they will get. Help her get through one contraction at a time.

◆ Remind yourself that it is normal for the transition phase to be difficult, that the mother's mood will improve when her cervix is fully dilated, and that if you are to reassure her you must not worry about her. Her behavior is not abnormal; her pain is not more than one should expect at this time. The rest of labor will not be this intense.

◆ If the mother has wanted to avoid pain medications (see the "Pain Medications Preference Scale," page 294), do not mention them. Instead, help her get through this phase without them, as tough as it may be. If, however, she cannot maintain any rhythm and seems panicky, even though you and others are helping her all you can, and the nurse or midwife says it will be some time before she will have the baby, this might be a good time to suggest pain medication or ask if she wants to use her code word (see page 295).

◆ If the nurse or caregiver isn't in the room when the mother has an urge to push, summon help right away (see page 84). The caregiver will observe the mother's behavior or check her cervix to determine whether pushing is appropriate.

◆ If the caregiver says the mother isn't ready to push yet (because she is not quite completely dilated), help her to avoid pushing, or to push with little grunts (see page 130).

◆ Try not to take it personally if the mother criticizes you or tells you to stop doing something that you expected to be helpful. Just say, "Sorry," and stop doing it. Don't try to explain why you did it or express frustration with her. She is really saying that labor is so difficult right now that nothing helps. You are the safest person for her to lash out at. Later, she will probably apologize.

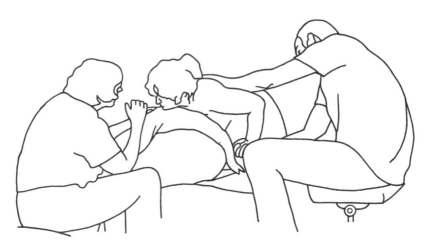

What does a doula do? A doula, with her training and experience, does not worry over the normal distress that often comes with transition. She can be very helpful to both of you in understanding what is happening and what to do.

◆ If you are tired or anxious, or if you lack confidence in calming the mother, the doula can either spell you in your role or show you what to do.

◆ She can reassure you and the mother that the intense reactions are not signs of danger but of good progress, and that this phase will not go on forever.

◆ The doula can assist if the mother needs two people to help her through the contractions—one holding her or pressing on her sore back, and the other in front of her, making eye contact and helping her maintain a rhythm.

◆ The doula can bring her calmness and confidence into play during the "Take-Charge Routine" (see page 166) and between contractions.

The mother may at times respond better to the experienced doula than to you, especially when you feel tired, uncertain, anxious, or frustrated and need a break.

The Birthing Stage

What is the birthing stage? This stage begins when the cervix is fully dilated and ends with the birth of the baby. During this stage the baby rotates, descends through the vagina (or birth canal), and is born. Medical professionals call this the *second stage*.

During the birthing stage the mother works very hard: She bears down—actively pushes—by holding her breath and straining or breathing out forcefully and vocally with the urge to push that comes several times in every contraction. In this way she works with her uterus to press the baby down and out.

The birthing stage has three distinct phases: the resting, the descent, and the crowning and birth phases. Each phase is characterized by different physical developments, and each requires that the mother make an emotional adjustment.

Care of the mother and baby during the birthing (second) stage varies among caregivers. Some are guided by patience and assessment of the mother's and baby's well-being. These caregivers feel it is best to let the birth unfold spontaneously, without interference, if the

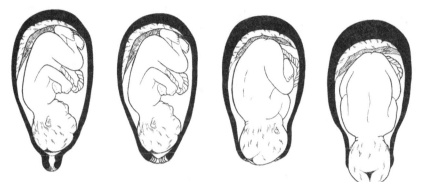

Prelabor and dilation (first) stage.
The cervix effaces (thins) and dilates; the baby rotates.

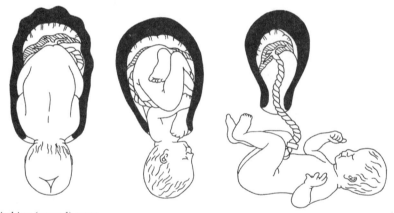

Birthing (second) stage.
The baby's head enters the vaginal canal; there may be a "rest" while the uterus tightens around the baby's body, and the baby descends and rotates, then is born.

mother and baby are doing well. Instead of rushing the mother to push, these caregivers await the mother's spontaneous urge. They encourage her to bear down when the urge compels her to do so. If the resting phase lasts a long time, they may encourage the mother to change positions.

Other caregivers want to speed the baby's descent as much as possible. They coach the mother to push (hold her breath and strain) during contractions while they count to 10. Then they tell her to quickly take another breath and push for 10 more counts, and to repeat this pattern until the contraction ends. These caregivers tend to place a time limit on the second stage (usually two hours for a first-time mother and one hour for an experienced mother) and use drugs, instruments, and episiotomy to meet this limit.

How long does the birthing stage last? A normal birthing stage may last from 15 minutes (three to five contractions) to three hours or more. For most first-time mothers, the birthing stage is completed in less than two hours; for most women who have given birth before, in less than one hour. A longer birthing stage may be due to the position of the baby's head in the pelvis; some babies need time for the gradual molding of their heads, or for tucking their chins and wiggling or rotating into the best-fitting position. Other reasons for a prolonged birthing stage are described on page 253.

THE RESTING PHASE

What is the resting phase? The resting phase is an apparent pause in the labor. Although not all women experience this phase, you and the mother should both be ready for it.

The resting phase is a "catch-up break" for the uterus; it comes after the cervix is completely dilated and the baby's head has passed through the cervix into the birth canal. The uterus had been tightly stretched around the baby before the head slipped out. Now, suddenly, only the baby's body remains inside the uterus, and the uterus fits more loosely around the baby. The uterus needs time to tighten around the rest of the baby. See the illustration on page 90.

During this phase, the muscle fibers in the uterus shorten, making the uterus smaller, without noticeable contractions and without the mother having an urge to push. After the tumult of transition, the resting phase provides a welcome break. Sheila Kitzinger, the well-known British teacher and author, has termed this the "rest-and-be-thankful phase."

One woman I worked with looked up at her husband during this phase and asked, "Did you feed the cats?" Only 10 minutes before she had been moaning and tensing during contractions. (Incidentally, he had fed the cats.)

How long does the resting phase last? The resting phase usually lasts from 10 to 30 minutes. If it lasts longer than that, the caregiver will probably ask the mother to change position or to push (bear down), in the hope that this will bring on stronger contractions or an urge to push, and so speed the labor along. The caregiver won't want labor to slow down for very long at this point.

What does the mother feel? The start of the birthing stage is always a milestone. The mother will probably welcome this rest, especially after the tumult of transition. She gets a second wind. If she was confused, her head is now clear. If she was discouraged, she is now optimistic. If she was withdrawn, she is now outgoing and aware of her surroundings. Sometimes a woman feels anxious if the resting phase seems to go on for too long or if the staff is imploring her to push before she feels an urge to do so. She may also feel inadequate or apologetic if everyone is commanding her to push, making her feel as if she is not doing well enough. In fact, no one should be expecting her to push if she feels no urge. She should be allowed to rest.

Even women who do not experience the pause in contractions that comes with the resting phase feel an improved mood and greater alertness at the beginning of the birthing stage.

What does the caregiver do? During the resting phase:

- The midwife or nurse remains close by, offering encouragement, praise, and positive suggestions.

- The nurse will probably call the doctor to come soon. If the mother has had a child before, the doctor will try to arrive soon after she begins pushing. If this is her first child, the doctor will probably not rush.

- The midwife or nurse may become more directive at this time, telling the mother what positions to try, or coaching her in how or when to push.

- The midwife or nurse listens frequently to the baby's heartbeat and continues assessing the mother's welfare.

- The midwife or nurse may do a vaginal exam to assess the progress of the baby's descent.

◆ The midwife or nurse may apply warm compresses on the mother's perineum to help her relax her pelvic floor muscles and improve her sense of how and where to push, and she may pour some oil over the perineum to lubricate the vaginal outlet.

How might you feel?

◆ You may be excited by the lifting of the mother's mood as she passes into the birthing stage, and you will probably be relieved that she seems more like her usual self.

◆ You may be baffled that her labor has apparently stopped. Do not worry. The pause is temporary and will give the mother a second wind.

◆ You may feel overwhelmed at the realization that you are about to witness a miracle—the birth of this beloved baby.

How can you help? The birthing stage is an exciting time. Even though you have your own powerful emotional reaction to the birth, if you are the mother's major source of support you must remain calm and continue to encourage and assist her. Here are some guidelines:

◆ Be patient during the resting phase. Don't try to rush the mother through it or make her push too soon.

◆ If the nurse or caregiver wants the mother to push without a contraction or an urge to push, ask whether she can wait until she feels the urge.

◆ Match the mother's mood. As she leaves the emotions of transition behind, you should do the same.

◆ If you are confused, ask the midwife, nurse, or doula what is going on.

What does a doula do? During this resting phase, the doula encourages the mother to take advantage of the break. She can help in these ways:

◆ She reminds you both about the resting phase if you are puzzled over this pause.

◆ She points out that this break will be short and prepares both of you for the next step—pushing the baby down and out.

- While patiently awaiting the next step, she may suggest that you re-mind your nurse of items in the mother's Birth Plan that pertain to the birthing stage, such as the kind of bearing-down efforts and po-sitions the mother wants to use and her feelings about episiotomy.

- If the resting phase goes on for a long time, the doula may suggest changes of position to see whether this helps bring on an urge to push.

THE DESCENT PHASE

What is the descent phase? This is the longest of the three phases of the birthing stage. During the descent phase, the uterus resumes con-tracting strongly, and the mother usually feels an increasingly strong urge to push. The baby descends through the birth canal to the point where the top of the head is clearly visible at the vaginal outlet. The mother alternately pushes and breathes lightly during contractions, and rests between contractions.

By *pushing*, I mean that she takes in a breath and bears down for five to six seconds at a time. While bearing down, she either holds her breath or lets air out with a moan or bellow. The pushing may be directed, which means that she does it when she is told, regard-less of whether she has an urge; this technique is used for women who have had epidurals, since they usually feel no urge to push. Or the pushing can be spontaneous, which means that the mother bears down with the reflexive urge to push. By this time, a rhythmic ritual is no longer possible or desirable, as the woman's behavior is being guided by her pushing urges, which come three or four times over the peak of each contraction. The urges last about five or six seconds, with three to five seconds in between.

Many women tell me that the term *urge to push* does not come close to describing what they feel. One woman cried out during this stage, "It's like a vomit in reverse!" That, crude as it is, is a much bet-ter description. The urge to push can be as involuntary and as uncon-trollable as vomiting, except that all the force moves downward instead of upward (and the result is a lot more rewarding!).

Sometimes, especially early in the descent phase, the urge to push is a much milder sensation, like a catch in the breath and a grunting sensation. Occasionally, a woman who hasn't had an epidural lacks the urge to push. She may be simply having a long resting phase, and a change of position and some patience usually result in an urge to push. Or perhaps her uterus is not contracting with enough intensity to bring on an urge to push; Pitocin might be used in such a case. If a woman is having good contractions and no urge to push, the caregiver tells her when to push.

It can take an hour or two of pushing before the baby's head is visible at the vaginal opening. Before it becomes visible, there is progress in rotation and molding of the baby's head, and some descent, but these changes are undetectable from the outside. Then, the mother's perineum bulges as she bears down. Soon thereafter her labia part, and the tiny vaginal outlet gradually enlarges as the baby moves down. Next, the head becomes visible, though at first it looks more like a wrinkled walnut. The walnut seems to grow bigger with the mother's bearing-down efforts. But rather than moving steadily downward the baby moves down when the mother bears down and slips back during the pauses between her bearing-down efforts. If you watch this incredible process, you will likely find yourself totally engrossed. You almost hate to see the baby slip back each time because you're so anxious to see him born. You must remember that progress is being made, and this gradual stretching is easier on both baby and mother than constant pressure on the baby's head and continuous stretching of the vagina.

The mother may change positions during the descent phase. The most common positions are semisitting, lying flat on one's back, side-lying, hands-and-knees, and squatting. Supported squatting, lap squatting, "the dangle," and sitting on the toilet are also useful at times. See "Positions and Movements for Labor and Birth," pages 135 to 141, for illustrations of each of these positions and descriptions of their benefits.

How long does the descent phase last? The descent phase usually takes up most of the total time of the birthing stage—from a few minutes to as much as four hours.

What does the mother feel? The mother will find strength and determination during the descent phase, even after a long labor. The imminence of the birth will hearten her, and she will be receptive to suggestions and to praise. Mothers often say they enjoy the descent phase because they are doing something active—working hard—to help their baby be born.

The mother may have other feelings as well:

◆ Early in the descent phase, especially, she may feel uncertain about what to do and how to do it. She will be thrown off her rhythm by the involuntary urges to push (in fact, at this time rhythm is no longer important). She may ask how to push, and she may need reassurance that her sensations are normal and that she and the baby are all right. She will feel better after a few contractions, as she gets the idea of how to push.

◆ She may feel afraid to let go. This is the most difficult thing to do at this time—to let the baby come out. The sensations of descent and of the large, solid head stretching the birth canal are gratifying and yet alarming and painful. It is scary to let the baby come *because it hurts.* Alarmed by the pressure in her vagina, she may instinctively hold back, that is, tense her pelvic floor against the baby's downward movement. It may take several contractions before she wills herself to let go of the tension in her vagina. If the mother has done perineal massage (see page 20) during pregnancy, she will find it easier to relax to the stretching sensation of birth.

◆ If the baby's descent is extremely rapid, the mother may feel shocked and frightened by the intensity of the pain, her total lack of control over her body, and the suddenness with which it is all over and her baby is born.

◆ If the descent is very slow, she will become discouraged. This may be the most demanding work of her entire life, and she needs to feel she is making progress.

What does the caregiver do?   During the descent phase:

◆ The midwife or nurse continues as before, encouraging the mother's efforts and reassuring her.

◆ The doctor usually arrives during this phase, sometimes to your great relief.

- The doctor or midwife performs occasional vaginal exams to confirm the baby's progress through the birth canal. The nurse, midwife, or doctor checks the baby's heart rate and the mother's vital signs periodically.

- When the birth is imminent, the doctor or midwife scrubs and dons surgical gloves, special hospital clothing, and a mask.

- The nurse, doctor, or midwife may place drapes beneath the mother, may cleanse the mother's vaginal area, and may massage her perineum or place warm compresses on it.

- If it will be a medicalized birth, the nurse, doctor, or midwife prepares the bed for delivery by removing the foot section and placing the woman's legs in rests on each side of the bed. The doctor or midwife then sits close to the mother's perineum. This setup is helpful if the woman needs medical assistance with the birth (through the use of forceps, a vacuum extractor, or an episiotomy), but many doctors prefer it for all births. It is uncomfortable and restrictive for most women. If the mother prefers not to be in this position unless necessary, she should say so in her Birth Plan, and you can request a more comfortable position.

- The doctor or midwife uses his or her hands to control the emergence of the baby's head.

How might you feel? You may react in various ways:

- Your fatigue may disappear, and you may feel ready to do whatever you are asked to do.

- You may feel divided between wanting to remain at the mother's head to support her and wanting to watch the birth (or even catch the baby, with the help of the midwife or doctor).

- You may find yourself holding your breath right along with the mother!

- You may find yourself in an awkward position as you support her upper body or her leg. Your arms or back may tire. (This is one reason to try to improve your physical fitness before the birth; see page 19.)

- Your initial excitement may fade to discouragement if progress seems too slow.

How can you help? If there are more people around during the descent phase, you may feel less vital to the mother than you felt earlier. It is true that she now receives much of her direction and praise from the professionals. This may be a relief to you because it allows you to become absorbed in your own experience of the birth. You are, however, still the mother's birth partner—the one who has seen her through all this—and she still may rely on you despite all of the attention from others. Here are some suggestions:

- Don't leave at this time if you want to see the baby's birth. Things can change quickly.

- Stay close to the mother, where she can see, feel, and hear you. You may support her from behind or by her side.

- Don't try to keep her in a rhythm now, because her urge to push takes over and she must respond to that.

- Compliment her—tell her how well she is doing—after every contraction.

- Mop her brow and neck with a cold washcloth. Pushing is hard, sweaty work!

- Stay calm. Try to maintain a steady and reassuring tone of voice and a confident, firm touch. (Don't rub her or squeeze her too hard in your excitement.)

- Do not keep telling her to push harder; you would only make her feel inadequate. Instead, encourage her: "That's the way! Come on, Baby."

- Help her get in and out of positions for pushing, such as squatting or hands-and-knees, or the less common dangle or lap-squatting (see pages 140 and 141). If she is on her side or semisitting, hold one of her legs up (someone else will need to hold her other leg if she is semisitting; see page 137).

- If progress is slow, suggest that she try a different position. Help her change positions every half hour or more often, if she or her caregiver wants this. Be ready to support her in these positions.

- Using whatever suggestions work, remind her to relax her perineum: "Let go," "Relax your bottom," "Open up," "Let the baby out."

You might remind her to relax as she did during perineal massage (see page 20).

- Request warm compresses to place on her perineum.

- Remind the mother that the baby is almost here! Sometimes, believe it or not, the mother almost forgets she is doing all this for her baby.

- Remember that during the first few contractions after the baby's head becomes visible at the vaginal opening, the head may appear wrinkled and spongy. One birth partner thought he was seeing a brain without a skull or scalp! Pressure on the head by the vaginal wall squeezes the skin of the scalp toward the top of the head until the head moves down more. Then it looks more as you would expect—hard and smooth.

- If the descent phase seems slow, remember that sometimes more time is needed for the baby's head to mold or to take the best position in the mother's pelvis. If you are discouraged, don't let the mother know.

What does a doula do? If the mother agrees, the doula can stay at her head to encourage her while you watch or even help with the birth, take photos, or take a break if you are tired or feel squeamish. I have served as doula for a number of couples in which the partner has worried about feeling faint or sick with the intense emotion, sights, sounds, and smells of birth. The couples have wanted to be sure the mother's needs for support would be met while the partner would be able to participate as was comfortable for him or her. In most of these cases, the partners have become swept up in the excitement of the moment and have felt fine, but some have had to sit down and put their heads between their knees or take a break now and then. Attending a birth can be demanding and stressful. This is a very good reason to have a doula.

- The doula encourages the mother through every contraction and makes her comfortable between contractions.

- She assists you in your role as needed—for example, by getting cold cloths and taking pictures of both of you.

◆ She helps the nurse or midwife by getting blankets for the mother, fetching hot water and cloths for compresses to apply to the mother's perineum, and doing whatever else needs to be done to get ready for delivery.

Few people are prepared for the power of the moment: the mother's superhuman effort, the sounds she makes, the bulging of the vagina and the peek at a wet and wrinkled scalp before the baby retreats yet again, the charged atmosphere of the room as everyone anticipates the birth. It is impossible to describe the awe, excitement, and tension you will feel as you await the moment of birth.

THE CROWNING AND BIRTH PHASE

What is the crowning and birth phase? The crowning and birth phase is when the baby is actually born. This phase begins when the baby's head *crowns*—that is, when it remains visible at the vaginal opening even between contractions, no longer sneaking back between the mother's bearing-down efforts—and ends when the baby is born.

During the crowning and birth phase, the baby's head stretches the mother's vagina and perineum, and she feels burning and stinging. Her tissues might tear at this time. Protecting her perineum now becomes a major focus of the caregiver's role.

Until now, the baby's head has appeared wrinkled and spongy. Once the head crowns, the skin evens out over the scalp. The head seems to lurch forward a few times, and then it emerges—first the top of the head, then the brow and ears, and then the face. The head rotates to one side; one shoulder appears; and the rest of the baby slides out with a gush of water.

The baby may immediately cry and appear vigorous, or she may appear bluish and lifeless at first. But within seconds she begins breathing, usually with a gurgle and then a lusty cry. Immediately, the baby begins to turn more pink, and very soon she will be a healthy pink or ruddy color.

How long does the crowning and birth phase last? The crowning and birth phase takes only a few contractions.

What does the mother feel?   The mother's body gives mixed messages during the crowning and birth phase: On the one hand, she knows the baby is almost here, and she is anxious to push hard to get him out quickly. On the other hand, she feels the stretching and burning (the "rim of fire") that signal her to stop pushing. To prevent her vagina or perineum from tearing, she should pay attention to this feeling and listen to her caregiver, who will tell her to stop pushing in order to ease the baby out. The mother should *not* push hard.

Although the crowning and birth are exciting for everyone else, this phase may be acutely painful for the mother, who has to devote all of her attention to getting the baby out. By the time the head is about to slip out, the pain may have disappeared, because gradual stretching of the vagina, in some women, causes numbing. If this happens, the mother may become alert, calm, and totally engrossed in greeting her baby. If not, she will be relieved and surprised to have the pain go away the moment the baby is born.

Some mothers watch in a mirror, or touch the baby's head or body as it emerges. The mother may glow with joy or withdraw her hand in surprise if the baby doesn't feel the way she expected.

After the birth, it may take her a few moments to realize that labor is over (or nearly so), and to shift her attention to the baby. This may take longer for some women than others. One woman yelled, as soon as her baby was out, "Yay! It's over! I did it!" Then, "Hi, little baby! Oh baby, oh baby," and she kissed her baby and her husband.

What does the caregiver do?   During the crowning and birth phase, the caregiver:

- Supports the mother's perineum and controls the passage of the baby's head as it crowns.

- Asks the mother to stop pushing as the head emerges. In fact, the mother should stop pushing whenever she begins to feel the burning and stretching. The uterus will still contract and give the mother an urge to push, but to help avoid a tear, the mother can try to keep herself from holding her breath and straining. To do this, the mother raises her chin and blows lightly throughout the contraction. (See "Avoiding Forceful Pushing," page 130.)

◆ May consider doing an episiotomy (see page 231 for a discussion of this controversial procedure).

◆ Holds the baby's head as it emerges. The caregiver may encourage both you and the mother to touch the baby or even hold her as she comes out.

◆ Dries the baby and places her either on her mother's abdomen, so her mother can hold her, or in a heated crib nearby, depending on the caregiver's routine and your preference.

A nurse or doctor checks the baby quickly and gives her an Apgar score (see page 210) when she is 1 minute old and again when she is 5 minutes old. Five signs are evaluated in order to decide whether the baby needs extra immediate care, close observation, or no extra attention at all. A total score of 7 points or above is very good. If the score is below 7, at both 1 and 5 minutes, the baby needs extra ob-servation and care until the problems are corrected.

How might you feel? The suspense mounts as the baby's head becomes more and more visible:

◆ You may be barely able to contain your excitement.

◆ You may feel more love and awe for the mother than you ever thought possible.

◆ You may feel stunned, overwhelmed with emotion, or even queasy with so much going on at once.

How can you help? During the crowning and birth phase, you can help the mother in the following ways:

◆ Stay close by.

◆ Help her with her position, by holding a leg, lifting her shoulders for pushing, or letting her lean on you in a squatting position. See pages 137 to 141 for illustrations of positions for pushing and ways to support a woman while pushing.

◆ If the midwife or doctor tells the mother to stop pushing so that she will not injure herself or the baby with too rapid a delivery, the mother may find it difficult to comply. Help her avoid pushing by getting her to follow your directions: "Lift your chin, look at me, blow . . . , blow . . . , that's the way . . . , blow . . . ," and so forth.

◆ Help her understand the caregiver's instructions if she is unsure about what to do.

◆ Remind her to look in the mirror (to see the baby's head crown and to see the baby being born) and to touch the baby's head, especially if she has said earlier that she wants to do these things. But do not be surprised or upset if she refuses. She may be unable to take in more than she is already experiencing.

◆ Participate in this miracle in the way that is most comfortable for the two of you. Stay at the mother's head and focus on her face if she needs you, or if you feel squeamish about watching the baby come out. Or take it all in by watching in the mirror or by moving so that you can watch closely. Please, though, don't get so caught up in the birth that you ignore the mother!

◆ Remember that although the baby's initial appearance may be dusky (bluish) and almost lifeless, it will begin to change within seconds as the baby breathes and cries.

What does a doula do? The doula is right there, supplementing your efforts to help the mother physically and emotionally as needed.

◆ If there is a crowd around the mother at this time, the doula steps aside, knowing it is important that you be where you want to be and that the nurse and doctor or midwife have room to do what they need to do.

◆ She may take photos or a video, if you have asked her to do this and if the staff allows.

◆ If the mother has planned to have particular music playing as the baby is born, the doula starts the music.

◆ She will share in your excitement when the baby is born!

THE PLACENTAL STAGE

What is the placental stage? The placental stage begins when the baby is born and ends after the placenta, or *afterbirth*, is born.

This stage is usually anticlimactic when compared with the baby's birth, and many women barely notice their few contractions and the emergence of the placenta. Others feel sharp cramps. The two phases of the placental stage, the separation of the placenta and the expulsion of the placenta, are usually indistinguishable to the mother. Medical professionals call this the *third stage* of labor.

How long does the placental stage last? The placental stage is the shortest stage of labor. It usually lasts only 15 to 30 minutes.

What does the mother feel? A flood of deep emotions sweeps over the mother during the placental stage. The apparent end of labor, the new baby, the rest of the job to be done—all vie for her attention.

- She may be caught off guard when her caregiver tells her, "Now push for the placenta." She thought she was all done. Pushing out the placenta, however, is nothing compared to pushing out a baby!

- She may be so caught up in the baby and you that she hardly notices when the placenta comes out.

- Some women are unable to pay much attention to the baby for a few minutes, because all they can feel is relief that the ordeal is over: The pushing, the pain, and the contractions have all stopped. Once this sinks in, the mother can focus on the baby.

- She may marvel at her new shape and her very soft abdomen.

- She may become preoccupied with the baby or with establishing suckling at the breast.

- She may begin to tremble all over and feel weak.

What does the caregiver do? During the placental stage, the caregiver:

- Attends to the umbilical cord, clamping it and either cutting it or inviting the partner to cut it. Sometimes the caregiver withdraws some blood from the cord, to analyze for the baby's blood type or, if the parents wish, to donate it or to store it privately in a blood bank. (Umbilical cord blood is a rich source of stem cells that can be used for children or adults with certain cancers or blood disorders, as an alternative to a bone marrow transplant. Consult your caregiver to learn more about this procedure and the options in your area.)

◆ Dries and checks the baby.

◆ Checks the mother's birth canal to see whether stitches are needed.

◆ Attends to the placenta. When the placenta has separated from the uterine wall (the caregiver can tell by feeling the uterus and pulling gently on the cord), he or she may ask the mother to push gently to deliver the placenta.

◆ Carefully inspects the placenta to make sure that all of it has been delivered.

◆ Palpates the mother's abdomen to feel whether the uterus is firm. If it is "boggy," the nurse or midwife vigorously massages the uterus through the abdominal wall. This is painful for the mother but very effective in contracting the uterus and protecting against excessive blood loss. The nurse can teach the mother to do this herself; see page 330.

How might you feel? At this time you will probably be engrossed with the baby and mother, and letting out your emotions—pride, joy, relief, love. You may find yourself weeping with joy and relief and showering kisses on the mother and baby.

How can you help? During the placental stage you can do the following:

◆ Cut the cord, if you want to; the caregiver will probably invite you to do this. The symbolism of separating mother and baby appeals to many women and their partners. You may be surprised at how firm and slippery the cord is. When you cut it, don't snip gently; make a decisive effort.

◆ Enjoy the baby and help the mother to do the same—this is your main role now. Make sure the mother is comfortable, that she can see the baby, and that she is warm enough.

◆ Make sure the baby stays warm. The warmest place for the baby (and the place where he will be happiest) is against his mother, skin to skin, with the two of them covered by a warm blanket. Unfortunately, many hospitals customarily keep a baby in a warming unit while the nurse does all the newborn procedures (see page 210). Then the baby is usually wrapped and given a hat. If the baby is presented to the mother all wrapped up, she should ask whether she can place the baby naked against her skin with a warm blanket over both of them. You should not uncover the baby or remove the hat. If a newborn gets chilled, it may take a long time (often in the nursery, away from the mother) for him to regain his temperature.

◆ Go along if the baby has to be removed to the nursery (either because of a health problem or because it is hospital policy), unless the mother needs you to remain with her.

◆ Jump at the chance, when the mother is ready to let you, to hold the baby close. Talk or sing to her, and begin getting acquainted. The baby already knows and loves your voice.

◆ Congratulate yourselves on a job well done, and start making those phone calls, as the after-birth care (see page 104) of mother and baby begins.

What does a doula do? After the baby is born, the doula may:

◆ Support the mother during the birth of the placenta and the caregiver's massage of her uterus and inspection of her vaginal canal, since these can be painful. The doula's help allows you to focus on the baby.

◆ Remind you to ask the nurse to bring your baby to the mother, if the nurse is keeping the baby in the warmer.

◆ Remind you both to talk or sing to the baby, keep her warm against the mother's skin, and keep her hat on and a blanket over her.

◆ Stay with the mother, so that you can hold the baby if the mother can't. If the baby must go to the nursery you can go along, knowing that the doula will remain with the mother.

◆ Assist the mother with initial breastfeeding, especially if the nurse or midwife is too busy with other tasks to help (see chapter 11).

◆ Photograph the first precious moments of the baby's life.

◆ Point out some of the baby's capabilities—feeding cues, attention to parents' familiar voices, alert state, and more.

Normal Labor—in a Nutshell

The following table summarizes the events in normal labor and the ways you can help. You may find this table useful as a quick reference during labor.

NORMAL LABOR—IN A NUTSHELL

WHAT HAPPENS	HOW YOU CAN HELP
PRELABOR Off-and-on or constant non-progressing contractions for hours or days.	
• The cervix softens, thins, and moves forward. • The mother has some possible or preliminary signs of labor (see page 46), or both. • The mother may become anxious, discouraged, or tired if it lasts a long time. • You're both in danger of overreacting to contractions.	• Encourage normal activities in the daytime, as long as they are not strenuous; rest at night. • Distracting activities are appropriate. • The mother should eat whenever she feels like it. • Time the contractions off and on. Use the "Early Labor Record" (see page 56). • Be patient; do not get overexcited or preoccupied with the contractions. • The mother can use music, massage, or a shower to relax. • Call the doula if you need coping ideas.
DILATION (FIRST) STAGE (2 TO 24 HOURS) *Early labor (a few hours to 20 hours)* • The cervix continues thinning, and opens to about 4 or 5 cm. • The mother has one or both positive signs of labor (see page 48). Progress usually begins slowly. • Between 3 and 5 centimeters comes the challenge of getting into active labor; this is the mother's "moment of truth," as she realizes she cannot control the labor. • Contractions are close and intense by the end of this phase. • She may seem discouraged, weep, or feel labor will never end.	• Continue as in prelabor. • Suggest a ritual of slow breathing, relaxation, focusing on a visualization, counting breaths, etc., when the mother cannot walk or talk through contractions without pausing. • The doula should join you. • If the bag of waters breaks, take precautions (see page 49); call the caregiver. • Remain with the mother and encourage her. Match her mood.

Normal labor—in a nutshell

NORMAL LABOR—IN A NUTSHELL *(continued)*

WHAT HAPPENS	HOW YOU CAN HELP
Early labor (a few hours to 20 hours) (continued)	• Do not ask questions during contractions.
	• Using the 4-1-1 or 5-1-1 rule (see page 72), go to the hospital, or call the midwife to your home.
Active labor (¹/₂ hour to 6 hours)	
• The cervix dilates from about 5 to 8 cm.	• Present the mother's Birth Plan to the nurse or midwife (see page 26).
• Contractions become intense or painful, last 60 seconds or more, and come closer—every 4 minutes or less.	• Give the mother your total, undivided attention for every contraction.
• Progress speeds up.	• Match her quiet, serious, focused mood.
• The mother becomes quiet, serious, and focused on her labor.	• Encourage her. Point out the more rapid progress.
• She may find a spontaneous ritual involving the 3 Rs (see page 115).	• Use comfort measures (see page 142). For backache, use cold or heat, counterpressure, and positions (see page 135). Use "The Take-Charge Routine" (see page 166), if necessary, to help her maintain her rhythm. Suggest a long bath in warm water.
• The pain of the contractions peaks by 7 or 8 cm of dilation.	• If you are worried or uncertain, ask the doula, staff, or caregiver for help, explanations, or reassurance.
	• Remind the mother to urinate every hour or two.
	• Offer a beverage after each contraction.
Transition phase (10 to 60 minutes)	
• The cervix dilates from about 8 cm to complete (10 cm). This usually takes 5 to 20 contractions, but the presence of a cervical lip (see page 84) may prolong this phase.	• Continue the same rituals as in the active phase.
	• Stay very close.
	• Focus on one contraction at a time.
• The mother has long, painful contractions, with short breaks.	• Let the mother doze or relax *between* contractions. It is okay if she does not relax *during* these contractions.

NORMAL LABOR—IN A NUTSHELL *(continued)*

WHAT HAPPENS	HOW YOU CAN HELP

Transition phase (10 to 60 minutes) (continued)

- The baby may begin descending, causing pressure in the mother's rectum and, possibly, the urge to push.

- The mother becomes restless, tense, overwhelmed, irritable, despairing. She may weep, cry out, want to give up, or fight contractions. She may doze during the few seconds between contractions.

- The mother may tremble and vomit; her skin may hurt when rubbed; she feels hot, then cold.

- Remind the mother that transition is short, that she is almost ready to begin pushing her baby out.

- Use "The Take-Charge Routine" (see page 166), if necessary; talk her through contractions.

- A firm touch usually helps; rubbing or touching may be annoying.

- Call the nurse or caregiver if the mother begins pushing.

- Help her push or keep from pushing (see pages 86 and 88) according to the advice of the caregiver or nurse.

BIRTHING (SECOND) STAGE (15 MINUTES TO MORE THAN 3 HOURS)

Resting phase (10 to 30 minutes)

- The baby's head may be in the birth canal.
- The cervix is fully dilated.
- The contractions may subside or seem to stop for up to 30 minutes.
- The uterus is "catching up" with the baby.
- The resting phase may not occur if the baby is very low.
- The mother becomes clear-headed, optimistic, and determined. She may wonder why labor has "stopped."
- The staff may want the mother to begin pushing even without contractions.

- Be patient; remind the mother of the lull of the resting phase.

- If a staff member tells the mother to push without the urge, ask whether she can wait for the urge to push.

- Encourage the mother to relax and take advantage of the rest.

- If 20 minutes pass without pushing contractions, suggest that mother change position.

- Try hands-and-knees, squatting, a supported squat, or standing (see pages 139 to 140).

Descent phase (30 minutes to 3 hours)

- Strong contractions resume.
- The baby moves down the birth canal.
- The urge to push becomes stronger and more frequent with each contraction.

- Remind the mother to relax her pelvic floor. Say, for example, "Open up," or "Let the baby come."

- Encourage the mother to bear down and push when she feels the urge.

Normal labor—in a nutshell

NORMAL LABOR—IN A NUTSHELL *(continued)*

WHAT HAPPENS	HOW YOU CAN HELP
Descent phase (30 minutes to 3 hours) (continued)	
• The mother cannot avoid pushing. The urge is strong and involuntary; it comes from inside. She cannot make the urge happen, although she can push without the urge. • The mother may be alarmed at feeling the baby's head in her vagina. She may "hold back" by tensing her pelvic floor. • The baby moves down during each pushing effort, and slips back between pushes.	• Suggest that the mother sit on the toilet for a few contractions if she seems to be holding back. • Warm compresses may help relax her perineum. • Reinforce her efforts. Tell her how well she is doing. • Suggest that she touch the baby's head (she may or may not want to do so). • The baby's head appears wrinkled; do not be alarmed. • Help the mother change positions (see page 134) if she needs to.
Crowning and birth phase (2 to 20 minutes)	
• The baby's head no longer slips back between pushes. • The birth of the head is imminent (it will emerge within a few contractions). • The mother feels an intense burning or stinging in her vagina ("the rim of fire"). She may be confused, wanting to push very hard to get the baby out right away but feeling she may split if she pushes. • The baby's head emerges, and rotates; then the shoulders and the rest of the body are born.	• Don't rush the mother; remind her to stop pushing and "breathe her baby out," or pant (with her chin up) to keep from pushing (see page 131). • Help her tune in to the caregiver's instructions. • Help the mother hold the baby, preferably skin to skin. • Keep the baby warm; cover him with blankets.
PLACENTAL (THIRD) STAGE (5 TO 30 MINUTES)	
• The mother may be very shaky. • Her uterus cramps. • The placenta separates from the wall of the uterus. • The cord is clamped and cut. • The mother may hardly notice the expulsion of the placenta.	• Enjoy the baby. • Cut the cord, if you like. • Make sure the mother and baby are warm and comfortable. • Hold the baby if the mother is not ready or has pain during contractions or stitching.

Normal labor—in a nutshell

CHAPTER 4

Comfort Measures for Labor

I'll tell you, while practicing that "take-charge routine" in class I thought, "Is the teacher trying to make us look stupid?" It seemed so phony, "conducting" Lynn's breathing . . . Well, in labor, I used it a lot. It helped Lynn stay on track with her rhythm. I don't think she could have done it by herself.

—JEFF, FIRST-TIME FATHER

That rhythm rocks!

—GREG, FIRST-TIME FATHER

The pain of labor has many physical causes. In the first stage, pain is caused by:

- Contractions of the uterus—the strongest muscle in the human body—which reach maximum intensity during this stage. (Try doing several chin-ups for a minute at a time. The muscle pain in your arms is similar to the kind of pain caused by uterine contractions.)
- Stretching of the cervix as it opens. (Try sitting on the floor with your legs out straight, and bending forward as far as possible with your hands grasping your lower legs. This will give you a sense of the nature of the pain caused by the cervix stretching.)

◆ Stretching of pelvic ligaments, from the pressure of the baby's head within the pelvis. This causes mild to severe back pain. One-fourth to one-third of laboring women have back pain during labor.

In the birthing stage, pain is caused by uterine contractions, pressure in the pelvis, and also by stretching of the muscles of the pelvic floor, the vaginal canal, and the skin of the vaginal outlet.

Labor pain also can have many emotional causes. These can affect the woman as much as physical causes and can turn pain into suffering.

Pain vs. Suffering

Although the terms *pain* and *suffering* are often used interchangeably, there is a big difference between the two. Labor, even when long and painful, does not inevitably cause suffering. Pain is an unpleasant physical sensation that may or may not be associated with suffering. For example, the pain people feel when working out at the gym or jogging uphill is not suffering. Consider the motto "No pain, no gain." Suffering is a distressing psychological state that may include feelings of helplessness, anguish, remorse, fear, panic, or loss of control and that may or may not be associated with pain. For example, being jilted by a lover or emotionally abused (ignored, insulted, or humiliated) or witnessing another person being hurt or injured may cause one to suffer, even though one may feel no physical sensation of pain.

Many women tell me that what worries them most about labor pain is that they will be overwhelmed, helpless, and out of control. They worry that the pain will take them beyond their limits and make them behave in a shameful way. This is a fear of suffering. If they carry this fear into labor, the fear will augment their pain, and they will likely suffer in the ways they fear. These women do not have confidence that labor pain can be manageable and that it does not inevitably lead to suffering.

When women recognize that labor pain is really a side effect of a normal process, not a sign of damage or injury, fear cannot increase their pain. Most of us have had pain that we did not understand, and it frightened us. For example, when I turned my ankle with an awful crunching sound, I was terrified that I had broken it. In great pain, I was rushed to the emergency room, where I was told there was no break, only a bad strain that should clear up if I wore a stabilizing boot for a couple of weeks. I immediately felt better and was able to walk (or limp) out of the hospital that I had entered in a wheelchair. Knowledge replaced my fear, and my pain diminished.

Some laboring women will cross from pain to suffering if they become exhausted or if something interferes with their confidence or their way of coping, such as frequent disturbances, rigid hospital routines, thoughtless or demoralizing remarks, lack of emotional support, or clinical complications. If a woman understands why contractions hurt; if she is continuously nurtured and encouraged by humane, caring, confident people in a peaceful and safe environment; if she is free to move about to find greater comfort; and if she knows healthy ways to respond to her contractions; fear gives way to mastery, confidence, and a sense of well-being as she responds to her pain. She copes; she does not suffer.

We discuss the difference between pain and suffering in my childbirth classes. After giving birth, one of my students told me that when she was considering an epidural she asked herself, "Am I suffering?" and answered herself, "I'm in a lot of pain, but I am not suffering." She decided she could manage without the epidural, and she did so without suffering.

How to Decrease Pain and Prevent Suffering in Labor

There are many ways that you and the mother can reduce her labor pain. Through childbirth education (classes, this book, video media, and Internet resources), you can learn about the birth process, self-help comfort measures, the wide range of other measures to relieve labor pain, and other options regarding the mother's care in labor. She can use relaxation techniques, rhythmic breathing or moaning, attention focusing, movements, and positions. You can help by never leaving her alone in labor; by attending to her emotional needs; by comforting her with massage, hand holding, and hot or cold packs; by suggesting a shower or bath; and by assisting her in the use of self-help comfort measures.

This chapter will tell you more specifically what you can do to help ease the mother's pain in labor. These numerous techniques do not take away all pain, but when combined with caring and skilled labor support they enable many women to cope successfully with their pain. Some women use these techniques in combination with pain-relieving medications; others rely totally on the techniques.

Make sure, before labor begins, that you know and respect the mother's preferences regarding her use of pain medications. Use the "Pain Medications Preference Scale," page 294, to help find out how she feels and whether your feelings are different from hers. Then you will know how to react if and when she approaches the limits of her tolerance of pain. You will either (1) ask for pain medication (see "Medications for Pain During Labor," page 269) or (2) redouble your efforts in encouraging, guiding, and helping the mother to continue handling her pain. For the latter, you will find many of the comfort measures described here to be highly effective.

The techniques described in this chapter work in different ways:

◆ By actually eliminating or reducing factors causing the pain.

◆ By increasing other pleasant or neutral sensations to dampen the mother's awareness of the pain.

◆ By involving her in activities that focus her attention on something besides the pain.

◆ By showing her that she is cared for, respected, and heard.

Using a variety of techniques seems more helpful than doing the same thing for the entire labor.

Learning about the following techniques before labor will enable you to suggest them when appropriate and help the mother use them. Along with the lists in chapter 1, the information in this chapter will also help you in packing a bag of comfort items to take to the hospital (or to have ready in your home) to use during labor.

As you learn these many techniques and positions, please keep in mind that there are other ways to help a woman through labor besides doing things to or for her. Sometimes the best thing to do is to simply be there, quietly standing by while labor unfolds and the mother searches within herself for her best way to respond. If she seems withdrawn and incommunicative, do not be concerned. You don't need to engage her in discussion. Let her discover what she needs from you. Take your lead from her rather than trying to figure it all out in advance.

The Three Rs: Relaxation, Rhythm, and Ritual

Coping well with the pain and indeterminate length of labor involves the use of the Three Rs—relaxation, rhythm, and ritual. The concept of the Three Rs arose from my observations as doula for hundreds of laboring women. I have learned that some women cope well with pain and stress in labor; others are overwhelmed. I have noticed that these three characteristics are shared by most women who cope well:

- They are able to *relax* during or between contractions or both. In early labor, relaxation *during* contractions is a realistic and desirable goal; later in labor, however, many women cope much better if they move or vocalize during the contractions, or even tense parts of their bodies. They do, however, relax or stay calm *between* contractions.

- They use *rhythm* to cope.

- They find and use *rituals*—that is, personally meaningful rhythmic activities repeated with every contraction.

How and when does a woman use the Three Rs? In prelabor and very early labor, a woman who is coping well uses distracting activities until the contractions become intense enough that she can no longer continue walking or talking through them. When she finds she has to stop everything for 30 seconds or so at each contraction's peak, she stops trying to distract herself and begins using a ritual.

While she is still in early labor, her ritual is usually one she has learned in advance, perhaps in childbirth class. If she hasn't learned a ritual in advance, her nurse or doula may teach it to her at the time. This "planned" or "prescribed" ritual usually involves sighing (breathing slowly, audibly, and rhythmically), releasing muscle tension with each out-breath, and focusing her attention in some positive way.

As labor intensifies, the woman may adopt another planned ritual. She may change to a light rhythmic breathing pattern, move rhythmically (sway, rock, slow-dance with her partner [see page 136] or tap or stroke herself, her partner, or her pillow or another object), and focus her attention by staring into her partner's face, counting her breaths, using imagery, or chanting, singing, moaning, or talking to herself, audibly or not.

By this time in labor, however, many women stop thinking and behave more instinctually as they give up trying to control the labor. The planned ritual gives way as they discover their own personal, spontaneous rituals. These become very powerful aids in getting through each contraction. Once women discover these rituals, they repeat them for many contractions. Then, as labor changes, they may change rituals spontaneously once again.

It is a good sign when a woman goes into a more instinctual state, almost a reverie. It means that the thinking part of her brain, her neocortex, is calm, and this allows the more primitive parts of her brain—her midbrain and brain stem, which guide all basic bodily functions—to prevail. Michel Odent, a French physician, has explained the need to avoid stimulating the neocortex in laboring women. When they are in a state of reverie, being asked questions or touched unexpectedly, having bright lights come on, or having people coming and going is a disturbance that tends to activate the neocortex and inhibit the primitive brain. When a woman finds her own spontaneous ritual, she has found a way to deal with the pain of contractions. If anyone disturbs her ritual, she becomes more aware of the pain, and finding her way back to her ritual might take her a while.

Of course, in modern hospitals disturbances are common. I often marvel at how well some laboring women block them out and labor for long stretches without appearing to notice the busyness around them.

What do labor rituals have in common? As I have described, they always seem to involve rhythm in some way. I have come to realize, in fact, that rhythm is the the most essential element in the Three Rs. Sometimes the rhythm is supplied by someone or something else, in the form of murmuring, rhythmic stroking or pressure, pouring water over the mother's belly, or moaning or swaying with her.

INTERNAL AND EXTERNAL RITUALS

Some women close their eyes and either become very still or rock, tap, or sway and moan during contractions. Their rituals are internal; they involve relaxation, rhythmic breathing or moaning, and some kind of mental activity. These women seem hardly aware of those around them. Other laboring women keep their eyes open and focused, move their bodies, vocalize rhythmically, and depend on someone else to be a part of the ritual. These are external rituals, in which a woman receives help from outside herself. It is quite common for a woman to use an internal ritual early in labor and shift to an external one later, or vice versa.

HOW TO HELP WITH LABOR RITUALS

As birth partner, you can help a laboring woman develop or continue her ritual. First, observe her behavior during contractions. Is she remaining still, with relaxed muscles? Or is she moving or vocalizing with rhythm? If she is doing any of these, she is coping well, even if her ritual involves moaning loudly or swaying vigorously. If she has lost her rhythm, your job (or the doula's) is to help her find or regain a ritual (see "The Take-Charge Routine," page 166, and "How Can You Help?," page 87). Do not interrupt her ritual during a contraction by asking a question or telling her to try something else.

Your assistance will probably be more active when she uses an external ritual than when she uses an internal ritual. For example, with an external ritual you might:

◆ Maintain eye-to-eye contact with her.

◆ Help her keep her rhythm by moving your head or hands, stroking her, or murmuring soothing words to her in the rhythm of her breathing or moaning.

◆ Press firmly on her upper arms, hands, thighs, or feet to anchor her.

◆ Press her hips or low back (see "Counterpressure for Back Pain," page 157).

◆ Hold her close, walk, sway, or slow-dance with her.

If she uses an internal ritual, you might:

◆ Remain close by, holding her hand quietly and calmly.

◆ Refrain from, and ask others to refrain from, disturbing her during contractions.

If you have prepared yourself for a very active support role, you may feel useless if the mother uses an internal ritual. You may want to do more, to have her look at you or allow you to stroke her or talk to her. You must realize, however, that she still needs you, but more as a calm, caring presence than as an active helper. If she is coping (relaxing during contractions and remaining still, with eyes

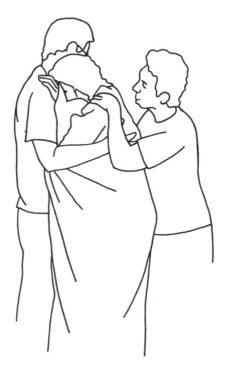

Her ritual: burying her face in her partner's chest with the doula rubbing her shoulders and all three swaying together.

closed), trying to get her to look at you or follow your rhythm would disturb her.

Even if she doesn't seem to need much help from you at the moment, you should continue to observe her during contractions. If she begins to wince or tense or vocalize or loses her rhythm, then you should get her attention and help her regain a ritual.

If there are continual interruptions—a nurse or caregiver examining her, checking her pulse, taking her temperature or blood pressure, drawing blood, monitoring her—the mother may become too unsettled to be able to keep a rhythm or regain her ritual. In this case you might tell the nurse, "If we could get through a few contractions without interruption, I think she could get back on top of them. Is this possible?" If the procedures cannot be postponed, you may need to play a more active "coaching" role. Use the "Take-Charge Routine" (see page 166), and tell the mother, "All that matters during this contraction is that you keep your rhythm. Let me help you through this." Help her with her rhythm until the mother has some quiet, undisturbed time to develop her ritual.

Once the mother's cervix has dilated completely and she is in the birthing stage, she will become more alert and focused. She is less likely to use the same ritual now, and her rhythm will give way to her powerful urge to push. Her contractions will now dictate whether, when, and how she pushes, and she will approach birth in a crescendo of emotion, excitement, and sensation. Instead of trying to help her maintain a ritual during the birthing stage, help her maintain a good position for birth and encourage her to relax her perineum as she pushes. See "The Birthing Stage" in chapter 3.

EXAMPLES OF SPONTANEOUS RITUALS

The following examples illustrate some spontaneous rituals developed by women and their birth partners. You can see how people add their personal touches to get the most out of the comfort measures.

One couple found themselves handling the contractions with the birth partner scratching the mother's back during each contraction while she knelt on the floor and leaned forward onto his lap. The mother had always loved having her back scratched, and she found that during contractions it really helped to have him scratch lightly, moving gradually upward from the left buttock to the left shoulder, over to the right shoulder, and down to the right buttock. Following the changes in her breathing, he timed his scratching so that when he reached her right shoulder the contraction had peaked, and when he reached her right buttock it had ended. This back scratching was a helpful focus for the mother; she could tell where she was in the contraction by where her birth partner was scratching! Later she said, "He cut my contractions in half! I knew I just had to cope until he got to my right shoulder. Then I knew I was on my way out of the contraction."

Other birth partners have helped mothers know when a contraction has passed the halfway point by counting breaths. Once you know about how many breaths it takes the mother to get through a contraction, you can tell her when she is "on the downside." In active labor, if you listen carefully to her rhythmic breathing or moaning, you'll notice that it sounds more strained at the peak and seems to relax and sound easier once she is over the peak. You can then tell her, " It's peaking now," and, when you are sure she is well past the peak, "You're on the downside," or "You're on the way out. Good job."

In another case, the ritual involved hair brushing. The woman had long, straight, silky hair, and she found that she could cope well as long as her mother brushed it rhythmically during the contractions. If her mother stopped, the woman felt more pain. It happened that her mother had often brushed the woman's hair when she was a child and teenager, and during those times they had felt very close to each other. The daughter had felt safe and content then, and these same feelings surfaced during her labor.

An example of the importance of detail is the woman who found herself staring at a hole in her husband's T-shirt during every contraction, and repeating to herself, "Blow out the hole and you're in control. Blow out the hole and you're in control." When her husband turned away to get a drink of water during a contraction, she fell apart. She said, "You can't do that!" He thought she meant he couldn't drink water. "I need your hole!" He had no idea how important the hole in his T-shirt was!

Here is a heartwarming ritual. A laboring woman and her partner would pace slowly between contractions, and when a contraction began they would face each other and slow-dance (see page 136), swaying together silently. When the contraction ended, they would resume the pacing. Later, at the childbirth class reunion, he described this ritual with tears in his eyes: "I've never felt so manly in all my life. Holding her close, I could feel every contraction while she pressed against me."

One last ritual shows how relaxation can give way to rhythm: The woman was having a very rapid, painful labor. While reclining in the tub, she discovered that it really helped to slam her open hand against the wall in the rhythm of her moaning. Slam, slam, slam. I was worried that she would injure her hand, but I knew I should not try to stop her. Soon the slams began to turn the bathroom light off, then on. This went on for an hour. Somehow she had created a short circuit. Later the nurse told me, "I thought you were doing that—some fancy new ritual!" (Incidentally, the woman did not injure her hand. I don't know whether the hospital fixed the light.)

The development of rituals is a truly creative aspect of labor, although it is largely unrecognized by caregivers and by childbirth educators and authors. It is not comfort measures by themselves that reduce pain; rather, it is the mother's unique adaptation of these measures to suit her personality and her needs at the time.

Self-Help Comfort Measures

Self-help comfort measures are skills that the mother masters before labor to help relieve her pain and enhance labor progress. Many are taught in childbirth classes, on audio or video electronic media, or in books. You should learn how to help her use these. They can make the difference between feeling overwhelmed by the pain and coping in a positive way. This section covers many self-help comfort measures. Practice them together and adapt them to work best for her.

RELAXATION

Relaxation, rhythmic breathing, and attention focusing have long been the cornerstones of childbirth preparation. Relaxation is the goal of most comfort measures. If a woman lets her body go limp during her contractions, she will feel less pain or will be less overwhelmed.

The mother's attempt to relax, even if not completely successful, is helpful in itself because it serves as a positive focus away from her pain.

In active labor, relaxation during contractions may be more difficult than it was in early labor; the mother may need to keep moving in rhythm. At this phase her goal should be to relax between contractions and to carry on a ritual (see page 115) during them.

During the last weeks of pregnancy, help the mother learn to recognize and release tension in all parts of her body. By practicing with her, you can learn what tone of voice, which words, and what sort of touch help her relax. Try the following:

◆ While she lies still, tell the mother which parts to focus on and relax. Start at her toes, and gradually go through the parts of her body to her head.

◆ Help her to identify any "tension spot" and to release the tension at will. A tension spot is a part of her body where tension seems to settle whenever she is stressed. This same spot (or spots, since she may have more than one) is likely to be the seat of tension during labor. Her tension spot might be her shoulders, neck, brow, jaw, low back, or buttocks. Help her to let go of tension when you touch the spot with your whole hand or when you say, for example, "Relax your right shoulder," or "Let go right here." If the mother has difficulty relaxing, she can learn to let a particular part of her body go limp by first tensing it (for example, tightening her arm or leg as much as possible) and then relaxing it. Repeating this exercise trains both of you to recognize when her body is tense and trains the mother to relax it.

◆ Try "floating" an arm or a leg. While the mother sits or lies comfortably, gently lift her arm, with one of your hands just above her wrist joint and the other just above her elbow. Gently move her arm up and down and around in circles. Encourage her to "let go," to avoid helping or resisting your movements. She can try to imagine being a rag doll, loose and floppy. This exercise teaches trust as well as the difference between tension and relaxation.

Good childbirth preparation classes emphasize relaxation techniques. CDs and DVDs are also available to help people master the skill of relaxation for childbirth. See "Recommended Resources" for a description of some helpful aids for relaxation.

During labor you can help the mother to relax in the following ways:

- When she feels a contraction start, remind her to begin her ritual immediately (if she doesn't do so spontaneously), using her rhythmic out-breaths to release tension.

- If she tenses in any parts of her body as the contraction intensifies, remind her with soothing words or touch (or both) to let go of the tension in those places. Don't just say, "Relax." She needs you to be more specific than that. Instead say, "Let go right here," as you touch her hands, brow, shoulders, and so forth. Your touch should be comforting, not tense or tentative. When she responds by releasing tension, tell her. Say, "Good," or, "Just like that."

- Try "floating" a limb between contractions, if she has found this helpful during your relaxation practice.

- Use the comfort measures in this chapter and verbal reminders to help the mother relax during and between contractions. Trial and error will tell you what works best. Once you find something that works, stick with it.

- If labor becomes so intense that the mother is unable to relax *during* contractions despite your efforts, then help her relax and rest *between* contractions. Use soothing words, touch, and other comfort measures.

HYPNOSIS

Many laboring women can achieve a trance state during which they are able to remain deeply relaxed, with a reduced awareness of the pain. The use of self-hypnosis during labor requires proper training in advance. The hypnotic trance can be induced during labor by the mother herself or by her trained birth partner or doula. (Hypnotherapists do not accompany their clients during labor.)

Hypnosis classes and DVDs are popular adjuncts to conventional childbirth education. Certified hypnotherapists with special additional training work intensively with mothers and their partners, using hypnosis to reduce fear and anxiety, build confidence, and foster mastery of pain-relief techniques (see "Recommended Resources"). Five recent research studies that compared self-hypnosis with more conventional comfort techniques in labor have found less need for pain medications among women who used self-hypnosis.

ATTENTION FOCUSING

This technique diverts the mother's mind from her pain by having her concentrate on something else. During contractions the mother can focus her attention in one of several ways:

+ She can *look* at you or at a meaningful picture, figurine, flowers, or another object. One woman hung a baby's outfit on the wall, and focused on it and the fact that she soon would fill the suit with a baby. Another woman made an inspiring collage to hang on the wall in her birthing room; it included beautiful scenery and images of powerful women doing impressive physical and artistic feats. Another posted pictures of her older child's artwork. Still another hung pictures of her many pets—her horse, three dogs, and a cat. Like the woman who focused on a hole in her partner's T-shirt, all of these women used objects to ground them or inspire them. Focusing on an object can become an all-important part of a mother's ritual.

+ The mother can *listen* to your voice, to music, or to another soothing sound (see page 160). Many women like to hear rhythmic murmuring with each contraction.

+ The mother can focus on *feeling* your touch, your massage, or your caress. Try to match her rhythm with your stroking.

+ She can *concentrate* on a mantra or mental ritual, such as counting her breaths or repeating words to herself throughout each contraction. For example, she might chant, "Ooopen . . . , ooopen . . . , ooopen . . . ," say, "I think I can . . . , I think I can . . . , I thought I could . . . , I thought I could . . . . (from *The Little Engine That Could*), or repeat, as one woman did, "Be still like the mountain and flow like the river." One woman even loudly repeated the word *epidural* over and over while she swayed through the contractions. I asked her whether she wanted an epidural. She replied, "No, if I can say it, I don't need it!" Usually these rituals are unplanned and emerge spontaneously. You might join her if she is counting, chanting, or moaning aloud. Certainly, whatever you do, do not interrupt her rhythm. Help her maintain it.

VISUALIZATION

The mother can visualize something positive, pleasant, or relaxing, using her contractions, her focus, or her breathing as a cue. For example, she might visualize her exhalations or your soothing touch or massage as drawing her tension and pain away. She might imagine herself to be in a special, safe, comfortable place, where her contractions are cues to relax more deeply into the comfort of the place. She might visualize each contraction in various ways: as a wave, with herself floating over the crest, or as a mountain, which she climbs up and down as the contractions come and go. She might use the onset of the contraction as a cue to imagine herself soaring like a seagull above the waves of contractions below. Several women from my childbirth classes have told me that during labor they visualized the opening of the cervix of my knitted argyle uterus, which I use during classes to demonstrate contractions and dilation.

Some visualizations are planned; others emerge spontaneously in labor. Spontaneous visualizations are usually very creative and personally helpful.

Sometimes couples plan visualizations together during pregnancy, so the partner can guide the mother through them during labor. I recommend recalling some positive or empowering experiences that you and the woman have shared or that she has gone through herself. Following are guidelines for two personal visualizations, one for early and one for active labor.

To plan a visualization for early labor:

◆ Think of an event in which the two of you were relaxed and content together (for example, a trip you took, a beautiful afternoon, a warm conversation).

- Take a walk together, or have a delicious meal together, and recall as many details of that experience as you can.

- Then weave the details into a brief description with a beginning, a middle, and an end. During contractions you will narrate the visualization, varying the details with each contraction.

For example, one couple had taken a canoe trip early on a cold misty morning. The river was still; the mist was rising; birds were soaring overhead; a ramshackle barn was visible in the distance; a fallen tree partly blocked the river; and so on. In labor, the woman was in a large tub and a friend was pouring water over her back in rhythm with her breathing. With each contraction, her partner would tell the mother, "Now let's get in the canoe and glide over the contraction. There are the birds flying overhead; and the barn with the roof caved in. There is no one in sight. It's all so still and beautiful. And now take your rest." He varied the details but repeated them often. Later the woman said, "He took me back there. My breathing became the strokes of my paddle. The sound of the water being poured over my back became the drips off the paddle when I took it out of the water."

For active labor:

- Ask the mother to think of a time when she was challenged—physically, mentally, or artistically—and met the challenge. You may or may not not have been present during this challenging event.

- Weave the event into a brief description that can be narrated during contractions as a reminder of her ability to meet challenges.

- Plan to vary or intensify the description as labor becomes more intense.

For example, one woman recalled regularly riding her bicycle on a trail that had one very steep, long uphill stretch. For a long time she was unable to make it all the way to the top without walking her bike part way. She persisted, though, and was eventually able to pedal to the top before coasting down the other side. In active labor, she pictured each contraction as that hill and recalled the persistence that it took, with shortness of breath and aching muscles, to get to the top. Her mantra became "Keep it up. Keep it up." Her partner encouraged her by repeating her mantra and then, "Almost there—a little more—that's right. Now you're over the top. Coast your way down." She said later that each hill became higher and tougher to climb as the contractions intensified, but her memory of successfully pedaling up the hill helped her every time.

RHYTHMIC BREATHING AND MOANING

Every method of childbirth preparation has used rhythmic breathing as its mainstay. In fact, success in every demanding physical activity, or sport, as well as meditation and stress-reduction techniques, requires breath awareness and rhythm. Rhythmic breathing or moaning (which is actually vocal breathing), along with relaxation, has tremendous value because it offers the following unique pain-relieving capabilities:

- Breathing or moaning in a steady rhythm helps the mother relax, especially when she has learned to release tension each time she breathes out.

- Rhythmic breathing or moaning is calming, especially when labor seems in turmoil.

- Rhythmic breathing or moaning may let the mother know she has some measure of control over her responses to the contractions, even though her uterus, with its involuntary and all-encompassing contractions, is completely outside her conscious control.

- When institutional policy or the woman's own condition does not permit comfort measures such as a bath or shower, massage, or movement, rhythmic breathing or moaning is always available. (Many comfort measures are impossible, for example, when the mother cannot get out of bed, electronic fetal monitor belts or an intravenous line is in the way, or she has received pain medications. See "When the Mother Must Labor in Bed," page 188, for specific suggestions for such circumstances.)

The mother will be able to use breathing rhythms most effectively and with the least effort during labor if she masters them beforehand.

There are two basic rhythmic breathing patterns for the dilation (first) stage: slow breathing and light breathing. I suggest that you and the mother learn each of these, adapt their speed and rhythm so she feels comfortable with them, and then use them as you like during labor. The mother's preferences and the nature of the contractions should guide the two of you in deciding how and when to use the patterns.

Slow breathing or moaning. Because this is the easiest and most relaxing of the two patterns, I suggest beginning with it. Start when distracting activities no longer keep the mother comfortable; that is, when the contractions become so intense that they stop her in her tracks and she cannot continue walking, or talking, or whatever she is doing, right through each contraction. From this point on she should continue with slow breathing for as long as she can relax well with it, perhaps moaning or sighing audibly with each out-breath.

For slow breathing to be most relaxing and calming, the key is for the mother to breathe easily and fully, and not work to keep it slow: "Easy in, easy out." If she is working too hard, her breathing will sound tense and strained.

This is how to use slow breathing during labor:

1. When the contraction begins, the mother focuses her attention as described on pages 124 to 125.

2. She takes a big, relaxing sigh, releasing tension throughout her body and, if she wishes, making a low moaning sound as she breathes out.

3. She breathes slowly—preferably, though not necessarily, in through her nose and out through her mouth—in long breaths, with each out-breath sounding like a sigh or moan. At the end of each out-breath, she pauses and waits for a moment, rather than rushing to inhale. The rate should be somewhere between 5 and 12 breaths a minute. With each out-breath she relaxes, releasing tension all over or from a different part of her body (such as her brow, jaw, shoulders, or right or left arm).

4. When the contraction ends, she resumes normal activities and does not think about her breathing.

The mother should use slow breathing for as long as it helps her relax. Some women use only slow breathing throughout labor; others use it until the cervix opens to 6 to 8 centimeters; still others, who have very intense, close contractions, may get relief by switching to light breathing even earlier. If the mother switches to light breathing early in labor, she might be able to return to slow breathing after a while. Suggest this, because slow breathing is restful and light breathing may be tiring.

Light breathing. Mastering the light breathing rhythm takes some practice, just as it takes time to learn to breathe rhythmically while swimming the crawl stroke. And, just as rhythmic breathing when swimming enables one to swim better, the light-breathing rhythm enables the mother to better manage pain. This is how to use light breathing during labor:

1. When the contraction begins, the mother focuses her attention.
2 She begins breathing in short, light breaths through her mouth, with a silent in-breath, an audible out-breath, and a brief pause after each out-breath. The rate is about one breath every one or two seconds, or 30 to 60 breaths per minute. With each out-breath, she breathes out tension.
3. She continues at this rate until the contraction begins to subside. Then she either slows her breathing rate, if she wishes, or continues at the same rate until the contraction is over.
4. When the contraction ends, she rests or resumes whatever she was doing before it started.

Please encourage the mother to practice this rhythm enough to master it. She'll need only a few practice sessions. At first light breathing is uncomfortable (it may cause dry mouth, lightheadedness, or a feeling that she can't get enough air), but by adapting it and working with it, she can become relaxed and comfortable while doing it. Light breathing may become her best friend in labor (besides you).

Practice light breathing until the mother is able to breathe at the rate of 30 to 60 breaths per minute for a full $1^1/_2$ to 2 minutes without stopping or feeling lightheaded (from hyperventilating). If she feels lightheaded, have her slow her pace slightly, pause a bit longer at the end of each out-breath, or breathe more shallowly (so as not to move as much air in and out). The lightheadedness is harmless, although it is annoying and uncomfortable; it will not occur once she masters the technique. If she masters light breathing before labor begins, it is very unlikely that she will hyperventilate during labor.

As she practices rhythmic breathing, see that the mother relaxes all over, especially in her shoulders and trunk. If she is tense, she is more likely to hyperventilate. Remind her to relax. Pace the mother by breathing with her or by using your hand to "conduct" her breathing. Keep your hand and wrist relaxed and floppy while conducting, remembering to stop briefly at the end of each out-breath. Your own relaxation is contagious and will help her relax.

The mother should feel free to adapt these breathing rhythms during labor in whatever way makes her comfortable. She may want to combine slow and light breathing; for example, she might begin and end the contraction with slow breathing and use light breathing over the peak.

Do remember, however, that rhythmic breathing is beneficial only if the mother can use it easily—without thinking much about it, without discomfort, and without tensing. Rhythmic breathing should be relaxing; it becomes an attention-focusing aid in itself once the mother has practiced it.

PUSHING (BEARING-DOWN) TECHNIQUES

There are four techniques for handling the urge to push: One is used to *avoid forceful pushing* (or bearing down) when this would be non-productive or harmful. The others are used during the birthing stage, when the mother *should* be pushing; they are *spontaneous bearing down*, *self-directed pushing*, and *directed pushing*.

Avoiding forceful pushing. There are three occasions during labor when the mother should not push—that is, hold her breath and strain—even though she feels like doing so. These are:

◆ Before the cervix has completely dilated. A premature urge to push sometimes happens as early as 6 centimeters, if the baby's head is positioned so that it puts abnormal pressure on the vaginal wall.

◆ During transition (between 8 and 10 centimeters dilation) if there is still a firm lip, or rim, of cervix remaining (see page 84).

◆ During the birthing stage, as the baby's head crowns and emerges.

During dilation or transition, forceful pushing might increase the pressure of the baby against the cervix, cause the cervix to swell, and thus slow the progress of labor. With a strong urge to push long before the cervix dilates, changing to the open knee-chest position or side-lying position may help (see page 139). During transition, until any lip has disappeared, the mother should push only enough to satisfy her urge (see "Transition," page 84).

If the mother is told not to push because of a lip, "grunt-pushing" can help to keep her from straining too hard. Grunt-pushes are quick but gentle breath holds followed by forceful releases of air, which make a grunting sound. You might talk her through each contraction, helping her to keep breathing or doing grunt-pushes.

During the birthing stage, pushing hard might cause too rapid stretching and injury to the mother's vagina, or too rapid a delivery. The mother can avoid holding her breath at this time by raising her chin and blowing or panting lightly whenever she feels the urge to push. This is sometimes easier said than done, because the urge can be very strong. You can help by keeping eye contact and breathing with her, or nodding your head in the rhythm of her panting.

Don't expect too much from these techniques; they do not take away or diminish the mother's urge to push. All they do is help her keep from adding to the pushing that her body is already doing.

Spontaneous bearing down. Once the mother feels like pushing and her cervix is fully dilated or nearly so, her caregiver will give the go-ahead. Then the mother should push spontaneously. Spontaneous bearing down works like this:

1. The contraction begins. The mother focuses her attention as described on page 124.

2. She uses whichever breathing rhythm—slow or light—seems best, until her urge to push is so strong that she cannot resist bearing down.

3. The urge to push comes in waves or surges—three to six in each contraction. These surges of the uterus sweep the mother along into an involuntary bearing-down effort (holding her breath or grunting, moaning, or straining) that lasts five to seven seconds. Do not worry that she loses her rhythm while pushing. In the birthing stage, her urge to push guides her, and rhythm is of little importance.

4. Once each surge subsides, she breathes lightly again until the next surge. She continues in this manner until the contraction is over.

5. The contraction ends, and she rests until the next one.

Self-directed pushing. This is reserved for those times when the mother's spontaneous bearing down is ineffective. Her eyes may be clenched shut and she may be arching her back, tipping her chin up (this is sometimes referred to as "diffuse pushing"). If she is making progress while pushing this way, do not worry. But if the baby is not coming down, try this:

1. Between contractions, tell her to keep her eyes open during the next contraction.

2. If she opens her eyes for a few seconds, then shuts them again, keep reminding her to open them.

3. Ask her to look down toward where the baby will come out. This will keep her focused on the direction toward which she will be pushing. If there are visible signs of progress, you might hold a mirror where the mother can see the baby in it. (Do not be surprised if she does not want to look. This should be her choice.)

4. She should bear down spontaneously, while looking toward where her baby will emerge.

5. If she is still bearing down ineffectively, suggest a change of position. Any change of position—it almost does not matter which position she uses—may help her focus better and push more effectively.

6. If these measures do not succeed, try "Directed Pushing."

Directed pushing. Until the late 1980s, directed pushing was the only bearing-down technique used in virtually every hospital. With this technique, the woman would hold her breath and strain as hard as she could for a count of 10, then grab a breath and repeat this throughout every contraction. Research has shown that using forceful prolonged breath holding may exhaust the mother, cause distress in the baby (because the mother's breath holding decreases oxygen for the baby), and cause extreme and unrelenting stretching of the pelvic-floor muscles and the ligaments supporting the mother's bladder and uterus, which can lead to later bladder and bowel problems. Today, directed pushing is used under the following circumstances:

- When the mother has been given an epidural and cannot fully feel the urge to push, and so cannot use the spontaneous bearing-down pattern. In this case, however, she can use the modified form of directed pushing described on page 131.

- When the baby's descent is too slow with spontaneous bearing down and the caregiver is considering assisting the delivery with instruments—forceps or a vacuum extractor (see pages 234 to 236)—or episiotomy (see page 231). The mother should try directed pushing before the instruments are used.

- When directed pushing remains the routine in the institution. Ask the mother's caregiver in advance whether the staff advocates spontaneous bearing down or directed pushing.

Except when needed to avoid the use of instruments, the directed-pushing technique can be modified to resemble spontaneous bearing down as follows to reduce undesirable effects:

1. The contraction begins. The mother focuses.

2. She breathes in and out two to four times, and then she takes her next breath and holds it. She holds her breath and strains (pushes) for a count to five or six, then releases her breath. She takes several quick breaths in and out, and repeats the breath holding and straining. She continues in this way until the contraction subsides.

3. The contraction ends. She rests until the next one.

MOVEMENT AND POSITION CHANGES

When the mother is free to move and change positions:

◆ She is more comfortable, and her labor may even speed up.

◆ She finds positions or movements that feel right to her.

◆ She may stand, walk, sit, recline, squat, kneel, lie on her side, get on hands and knees, or lean on you, the wall, a birth ball, the bed, or the nightstand (see the illustrations on pages 135 to 141).

◆ She may walk, rock, or sway rhythmically.

Encourage the mother to try a change in position or movement if she is restless, discouraged, or in a lot of pain, or if labor has slowed down. A change every half hour or so may make a positive difference under these circumstances. During the birthing stage, too, the mother may use several different positions, especially if this stage takes more than an hour. Just before the actual birth of the baby, the caregiver may ask the mother to assume a position that the caregiver prefers, such as semisitting or lying flat on her back with her legs drawn up to her chest. See pages 135 to 141 for a list of useful positions and the possible benefits of each.

Most hospitals have birthing beds that can be raised or lowered and that have moving sections and add-ons that can be configured to support a woman in a variety of positions, such as semisitting, sitting upright, kneeling forward, and squatting with a bar for support. Most of these beds have electronic controls. Try pushing all the buttons to see how the bed works, and try the many possible positions.

POSITIONS AND MOVEMENTS FOR LABOR AND BIRTH

POSITION/MOVEMENT	UNIQUE CONTRIBUTIONS
Standing 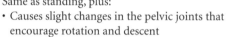	• Takes advantage of gravity during and between contractions • Makes contractions shorter and more productive • Helps position the fetus to enter the pelvis • May speed labor if the woman has been lying down • May increase the urge to push in the second stage
Walking* 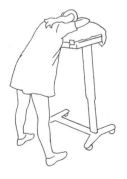	Same as standing, plus: • Causes slight changes in the pelvic joints that encourage rotation and descent
Standing and leaning forward on the partner, the bed, or a birth ball*	Same as standing, plus: • Relieves bachache • Makes it easy for the partner or doula to give a back rub • May be more restful than standing upright • Can be used with an electronic fetal monitor (the mother must stand by the bed unless wireless monitors are used)

* These positions are particularly helpful for back labor.

Positions and movements for labor and birth

POSITIONS AND MOVEMENTS FOR LABOR AND BIRTH *(continued)*

POSITION/MOVEMENT	UNIQUE CONTRIBUTIONS
Slow-dancing: The mother leans against her partner, resting her head on his or her chest or shoulder. The partner's arms are under the mother's, around her back, with fingers interlocked at her low back. She can tuck her thumbs into the partner's waistband or belt loops for comfort. They sway, perhaps to music, and breathe in rhythm.* 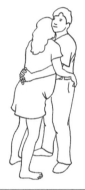	Same as standing, plus: • Causes changes in the pelvic joints that encourage rotation and descent • Being embraced by a loved one increases the mother's sense of well-being • Rhythm and music add comfort • Pressure from the partner's hands relieves back pain
Standing lunge: Standing beside a chair and facing forward, the mother places one foot on the chair seat, with her raised knee and foot turned out. Bending her raised knee and hip, she "lunges" sideways repeatedly during a contraction (either in the direction that is more comfortable, or to the right for two or three contractions, and then to the left). She holds the stretch for two to five seconds at a time. She should feel the stretch in her inner thighs. Secure the chair, and help her keep her balance.*	• Widens the side of the pelvis toward which she lunges • Gives room for the baby to change position, if necessary • May ease backache after trying this for a few contractions • Can also be done in a kneeling position 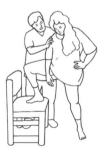

* This position is particularly helpful for back labor.

Positions and Movements for Labor and Birth *(continued)*

Position/Movement	Unique Contributions
Kneeling lunge: From starting position a, she bends her raised knee and hip and "lunges" sideways (as in b) repeatedly during a contraction in the direction that is more comfortable, or to the right for 2 or 3 contractions, then to the left for 2 or 3. She holds the stretch for 2 to 5 seconds at a time. She should feel the stretch in her inner thighs.* 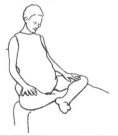 a b	• Same as standing lunge
Sitting upright 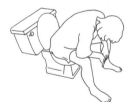	• Gives the mother a rest between contractions • Uses gravity to help the baby descend • Can be used with an electronic fetal monitor
Sitting on a toilet or commode** 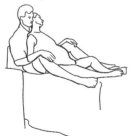	Same as sitting upright, plus: • May help relax the perineum for effective bearing down
Semisitting**	Same as sitting upright, plus: • Makes a vaginal exam possible • Easy position to get into on a bed or delivery table

 * This position is particularly helpful for back labor.
** These positions are useful during the birthing stage.

Positions and movements for labor and birth

POSITIONS AND MOVEMENTS FOR LABOR AND BIRTH (continued)

POSITION/MOVEMENT	UNIQUE CONTRIBUTIONS
Sitting and rocking in a chair or swaying on a birth ball 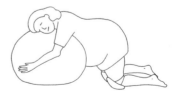	Same as sitting upright, plus: • May speed labor • Helps relax the mother's trunk and perineum
Sitting, leaning forward with support* 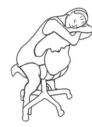	Same as sitting upright, plus: • Relieves backache • Makes it easy for the partner to give a back rub
Hands-and-knees position* ** 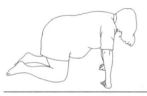	• Helps relieve backache • Assists the rotation of a baby in OP position • Allows for pelvic rocking and other body movements • Takes pressure off hemorrhoids
Kneeling, leaning forward on a chair seat, the raised head of the bed, a birth ball, or the side of a tub* 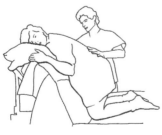	Same as hands and knees, plus: • Puts less strain on wrists and hands • Relieves back pain very effectively when done in a large tub

* These positions are particularly helpful for back labor.
** This position is useful during the birthing stage.

POSITIONS AND MOVEMENTS FOR LABOR AND BIRTH *(continued)*

POSITION/MOVEMENT	UNIQUE CONTRIBUTIONS
Open knee-chest position: The mother gets on hands and knees, then lowers her chest, spreads her elbows, and rests her head on her hands. Make sure her knees are back far enough to raise her buttocks higher than her chest. You can support her by sitting on a chair, your feet about 9 inches apart. She puts her head between your shins, and leans her shoulders against them.*	• May be helpful in pre- or early labor • Uses gravity to move baby's head (or buttocks) out of the pelvis, which may be desirable in early labor if the mother has backache or the baby is OP. Should be done for 30 to 45 minutes. • May reduce pressure on her cervix, which helps if it is swollen. (Also used for prolapsed cord; see page 256)

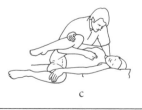

Side-lying or semiprone: In the side-lying position, the mother lies on her side with both knees flexed and a pillow between them (a). In the semiprone position, she straightens her lower leg, rolls slightly toward her front, flexes her top hip and knee, and rests the top knee on one or two pillows (b). During the birthing stage, you can hold the mother's top leg up as she pushes (c).**	• Gives the mother some rest • Makes interventions easy to perform • Helps lower elevated blood pressure • Safer than standing or the hands-and-knees position if pain medications are used • May promote the progress of labor when alternated with walking • Can slow a very rapid second stage (c) • Takes pressure off hemorrhoids • Allows relaxation between pushing efforts • Shifting between side-lying and semiprone positions, on both sides, helps change the baby's position • Works well with an epidural

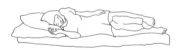

a

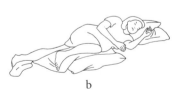

b

c

* These positions are particularly helpful for back labor.
** These positions are useful during the birthing stage.

Positions and movements for labor and birth

POSITIONS AND MOVEMENTS FOR LABOR AND BIRTH *(continued)*

POSITION/MOVEMENT	UNIQUE CONTRIBUTIONS
Squatting: The mother squats on the floor or bed, holding onto your hands (a), a railing, or a squatting bar (b) attached to the bed. Or, if you sit with your feet spread, she may stand between your knees (facing away from you) and lower herself into a squat, with her arms resting on your thighs for support (c).**	• May relieve backache • Uses gravity to help the baby descend • May aid the baby's rotation • Widens the pelvic outlet • Provides the mechanical advantage of the upper trunk pressing on the uterus • May help bring on the urge to push • Requires less bearing-down effort • Allows freedom to shift weight for comfort

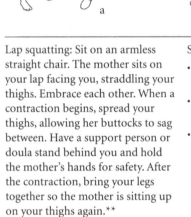

a   b   c

Lap squatting: Sit on an armless straight chair. The mother sits on your lap facing you, straddling your thighs. Embrace each other. When a contraction begins, spread your thighs, allowing her buttocks to sag between. Have a support person or doula stand behind you and hold the mother's hands for safety. After the contraction, bring your legs together so the mother is sitting up on your thighs again.**	Same as squatting, plus: • Avoids the strain on the mother's knees and ankles • Allows for more support with less effort for an exhausted mother • Enhances feelings of well-being, as the mother is held close by a loved one

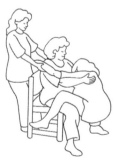

** These positions are useful during the birthing stage.

Positions and movements for labor and birth

POSITIONS AND MOVEMENTS FOR LABOR AND BIRTH *(continued)*

POSITION/MOVEMENT	UNIQUE CONTRIBUTIONS
Dangle with partner: Hold the mother under her arms as she leans with her back against you during contractions, and bear all her weight. Between contractions, she stands.** 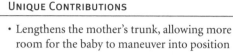	• Lengthens the mother's trunk, allowing more room for the baby to maneuver into position • Enhances pelvic joint mobility, allowing the baby to push the pelvic bones as needed to descend • Uses gravity to help the baby descend
Dangle: Sit on the edge of a high bed or counter, with each foot supported on a chair and your thighs spread. Standing, the mother backs between your legs and places her flexed arms over your thighs. During contractions she lowers herself. Grip her chest with your thighs as she lowers. You support her full weight. Between contractions, she stands.** 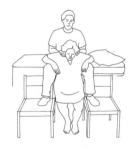	Same as dangle with partner, plus: • Puts much less strain on the partner
On back with legs drawn up: The mother lies flat on her back and holds her knees apart and draws them to her shoulders. She lowers her legs between contractions. You can help her get into the position with each contraction.** 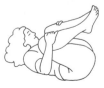	• Should not be used routinely • Tiring and works against gravity • May be helpful in prolonged second stage • Rotates pubic bone upward; may help if baby's head is not descending beneath the pubic bone, by moving pubic bone over the baby's head

** These positions are useful during the birthing stage.

Positions and movements for labor and birth

Comfort Aids and Devices

In addition to the self-help comfort techniques just described, there are also many comforting items or devices: some are built in or available in the birth setting; others are not. You may wish to bring them with you. Use the information here to explore these items and decide which you might want to use during labor. Most items are easily found in popular stores or online. If you cannot locate some, ask your childbirth educator, midwife, or doula where to get them.

BATHS AND SHOWERS (HYDROTHERAPY)

One of the safest and most effective forms of pain relief in labor is immersion in deep water or a warm shower. Hydrotherapy has been used for relaxation, healing, and pain relief for centuries, and today it is widely used in physical therapy, sports medicine, and other health disciplines. It has been used in childbirth, however, only since the 1980s. Today showers are available in most hospitals, and bathtubs (some large enough for the woman to move around in or to share with her partner!) have been installed in most modern hospitals and all birth centers. Some hospitals have tubs on wheels that can be moved from one birthing room to another. Lightweight tubs can be rented and set up temporarily in one's home for a home birth, or possibly even in a hospital, if the staff is willing and arrangements have been made in advance (see "Recommended Resources").

Most women who use water in labor use it for pain relief. As everyone knows, soaking in a tub or lingering in the shower is soothing and relaxing. Numerous studies have shown that hydrotherapy, when used correctly during labor, is safe, reduces pain, and frequently speeds labor. It has advantages over pain medications: The mother can move about normally, and she remains clear-headed.

Some women give birth in water. Unfortunately, this practice is restricted almost completely to out-of-hospital settings in North America, although it is supported in many European hospitals.

Showers and baths differ from one another in their effects on the laboring woman. While both enhance relaxation and ease (but do not eliminate) pain, the shower is simpler to use and requires fewer pre-

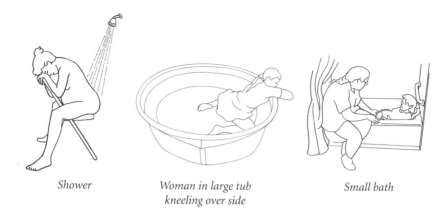

Shower *Woman in large tub kneeling over side* *Small bath*

cautions. Water temperature is less of a safety concern with the shower than the bath (see page 144). The woman can use the shower early in labor, whereas the bath is better reserved until active labor. Yet the shower is more tiring, since the woman cannot recline, and it does not have the labor-enhancing effects that immersion in deep water often has.

Water = relaxation

How does a bath reduce pain and speed labor? When a laboring woman sits in a deep, warm bath, a series of physiological changes begins immediately. These changes alter hormone production and fluid distribution throughout the body.

The laboring woman's body responds quickly to immersion:

- The warmth and buoyancy of the water cause immediate relaxation and some pain relief, which can cause a drop in stress hormones.

- Her oxytocin production increases, and often labor progress speeds up without an increase in pain.

- The oxytocin also causes feelings of calm and well-being.

These benefits last for up to two hours or so, after which changes in the woman's circulation may lead to a slowing of contractions and the return of pain. To keep labor from slowing, it is wise to ask the mother to get out after about an hour and a half if she does not think to do so herself. Once she has been out of the water for a half hour or so, she can return.

When should a woman get into the bath? Since there is a time limit for benefits from the bath, she should not get in too early unless her caregiver wants her to try to stop premature contractions or because she is having a long and tiring prelabor. Otherwise, she should try to wait until her cervix has dilated at least 4 centimeters. When she gets into the bath after this point, she is likely to experience immediate and profound pain relief, along with faster dilation. Before this point she can take a long shower, which will not slow labor.

What water temperature is best? The water temperature should be very close to body temperature, around 98.6°F or 37°C. This is very important, because if the water is too warm the mother's temperature will go up. A rise in the mother's temperature may cause the baby in the uterus to develop a fever, and fever, even when it is not caused by infection, causes the baby's heart rate to speed up too much for safety. Furthermore, the mother may lose her energy if she is in too hot a tub for too long.

Is a bath safe if the membranes have ruptured? Numerous research studies indicate that a bath in clean water does not increase the risk of infection if a woman has ruptured membranes.

Can the staff monitor the baby while the mother is in the water? Yes. Most midwives who attend water births outside of hospitals have waterproof, hand-held ultrasound stethoscopes ("Dopplers"), and some hospitals also have these. A portable telemetry fetal-monitoring unit can be used instead. There are two types of telemetry monitors: In one, a radio transmitter is wired to the sensors on the mother's

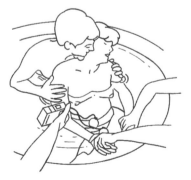

Laboring in a large bath with a partner and telemetry fetal monitoring.

abdomen. As long as the radio is held out of the water, it works well. In the other, each sensor contains its own waterproof transmitter, and the entire device is wireless. In both, the radios send information on the baby's heartbeat and the mother's contractions to the nursing station or to the monitor in the woman's room. If her caregiver has doubts about using this equipment in the shower or bath, he or she should check with the hospital's engineering department. An engineer can confirm the safety of immersing the sensing devices.

What about modesty? If the mother does not want to be naked in the water, she can wear an opaque sports bra or camisole and, until the birth becomes imminent, loose-fitting shorts. Or she can use a towel to cover exposed parts of her body. It is unlikely that she will be able to cover up completely all the time, unless she is in a conventional-sized bathtub, in which a towel will probably be adequate.

What if the baby is born in the water? This is always possible; a rapid labor is not always easy to control. If the hospital has a strong policy against birth in the water, then the woman will need to be watched closely and asked to leave the bath when she begins pushing. If the baby is born in the water, he is brought immediately to the surface and held with his head completely out of the water. His head is dried off with a towel. Mother and baby should get out of the water before the expulsion of the placenta, because the placenta causes quite a mess if expelled in the water.

Water births happen every day, and are considered a worthy option in hospitals in the United Kingdom. There, more than 4,000 water births in a 25-month period were closely studied. The outcomes were excellent, and comparable to outcomes of low-risk out-of-water births. In North America, water births take place in homes, birth centers, and a handful of hospitals.

THE BIRTH BALL

Large inflated balls made of tough polyvinyl are widely used in exercise classes and physical therapy for correcting balance problems, easing back ailments, building strength and flexibility, and aiding relaxation. In childbirth, we use such a ball as a comfort device in the following ways:

◆ The mother sits on it and sways during contractions. This helps relax her trunk and pelvic floor.

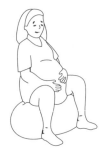

Sitting on a birth ball.

◆ The mother kneels on the floor (with padding under her knees) or on the bed and leans forward with her head, shoulders, arms, and upper chest resting on the ball. This provides the same benefits as the hands-and-knees position (for example, relief of back pain, rotation of an OP baby, and possible improvement of a baby's heart rate) but is more restful. The mother can also sway effortlessly.

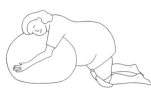

Kneeling while leaning on a birth ball.

◆ The mother stands next to a hospital birthing bed, which may be raised or lowered to a comfortable height, or a counter. The ball is placed on the bed, and she rests her head and upper body on it, swaying rhythmically and effortlessly side to side during contractions. This gives many of the same advantages of kneeling while leaning on the ball, and also uses gravity to help the baby descend.

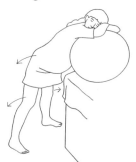

Standing, swaying with the ball.

◆ Lastly, after the baby is born, the birth ball is a great
You can almost always soothe a fussy baby quickly by
ball with the baby against your shoulder. Then you bo᷄
or vigorously—whatever works. This is a wonderful way
soothing up-and-down motion for the baby without wear᷄   ᷄r-
self out. Of course, a baby who is crying from hunger should be
fed, not bounced.

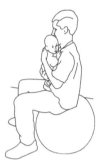

Using the ball to help soothe a crying baby.

Birth balls come in a variety of sizes and shapes. The woman of average height (5 feet 3 inches to 5 feet 10 inches) seems to benefit most from a ball with a diameter of 65 centimeters when inflated. Shorter women do well with the 55- or 65-centimeter balls, and taller women do well with the 75- or even 85-centimeter balls. The thickness and elasticity of the vinyl vary from one brand to another, and may affect whether a particular ball will actually inflate to its stated diameter. The degree of inflation can be varied to adjust the size and firmness of the ball.

Similar inflated devices come in the shapes of huge eggs and peanuts. Such shapes make swaying more difficult, although they allow some movement. Some midwives and doulas favor them because they believe a woman is less likely to fall off one of these than a round ball. I much prefer the round balls because they allow movement in all directions. I recommend that women try one out a few times before labor begins, so they will feel secure using the ball in labor. You might try the ball yourself; it can be a comfortable seat for you when the mother is not using it.

Even if your hospital has birth balls, you may want to buy your own to use to soothe your baby in the months after birth. The balls cost between $15 and $50, and are available from many toy stores, department stores, and hospital physical therapy departments. Make sure that any ball you buy is intended to hold up to 300 pounds; the box should carry this information. Less expensive balls may not be sturdy enough to hold an adult.

Your ball may come with a pump. If not, you can inflate your ball with a party balloon pump, an air mattress pump, or a service station pump. The balls bounce best when fully inflated.

Precautions with a birth ball.

- If the ball is to be used on the floor, place a clean blanket or sheet on the floor beneath to keep the ball clean.
- Place a sheet, towel, or waterproof pad over the ball before the mother uses it in labor.
- When the mother lowers herself to sit on the ball, always have her hold onto something or someone stable with one hand while holding the ball still with her other hand.
- When she sits, remind her that her feet should remain planted on the floor, in front of the ball and about 2 feet apart. She should not straddle the ball.
- Stand close by, holding her hand, until it is clear that she is completely safe and comfortable on the ball. This takes about one to two minutes with some women, longer with others.
- When she wants to get off the ball, assist her.
- The ball should be cleaned between uses if different women will use it. (Hospitals use the same cleaning compound that is used to clean a hospital bed.)
- Keep the ball away from sharp objects and heat sources.

HEAT AND COLD

Heat and cold can be used at any time during labor and afterward to relieve a number of discomforts. For example:

- Place a hot water bottle, a hot damp towel, a warm rice-filled sock, or an electric heating pad on the mother's low abdomen, back, or groin to ease pain during the dilation (first) stage. (Check with the hospital before using an electric heating pad; some hospitals do not allow this.)

◆ Use a warm blanket to relieve trembling during the transition phase.

◆ Use warm compresses on the mother's perineum (the area between her vagina and anus) during the birthing stage to relieve pain and to help her relax her birth canal.

◆ Use a cool damp washcloth to wipe the mother's neck, brow, and face between contractions.

◆ Use a cold wrap, an ice bag, a rubber glove filled with crushed ice, frozen wet washcloths, or even a bag of frozen peas to relieve low back pain. Or use an ice-filled, hollow plastic rolling pin (made by Tupperware), a can of cold juice, or a frozen, round plastic bottle of water to roll over her low back.

◆ Put frozen wet washcloths into a plastic bag, and lay the bag over her anus to relieve pain from hemorrhoids or stitches after the birth.

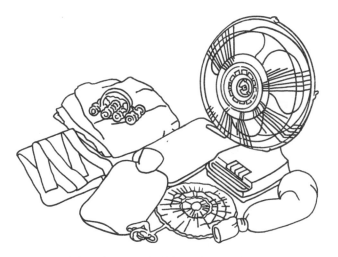

A selection of useful comfort items for labor. Clockwise from upper right: electric fan, rice-filled sock (to microwave for heat or freeze for cold), hand-held fan, hot water bottle, cold wrap to strap on lower back, fleece blanket, massage roller (on top of blanket), and foam kneeling pad.

CAUTION: Be careful not to make the packs so hot or so cold that you cause burns or frost damage to the mother's skin. The rule is this: If you can't hold it in your own hands, don't put it on her. Let the hot pack cool, if necessary, and always put one or more layers of cloth between her skin and the hot or cold pack to protect her.

TRANSCUTANEOUS ELECTRICAL NERVE STIMULATION (TENS)

TENS has been used successfully for years to treat postoperative and chronic pain. It is now also used for back pain during labor, especially early labor. Because TENS is still unknown to many obstetric caregivers, you may have to suggest it yourself if you are interested in trying it. The mother's caregiver can obtain more information about TENS from a physical therapist. Some doulas are also trained in the use of TENS in labor. A doula may be able to lend you a unit and show you how to use it.

Conventional TENS units require that someone turn two dials up and down to the same levels at the beginning and end of each contraction. Some TENS units, however, are designed specifically for use in labor. These are controlled with a single thumb switch, which the mother can use herself if she wishes. At the moment, maternity TENS units are hard to find in the United States, but they are more readily available in Canada, and they can be rented from British companies through the Internet (see "Recommended Resources"). They come with clear, simple instructions.

A TENS unit consists of four flexible, 1-by-4-inch stimulating pads connected by wires to a small, hand-held, battery-operated device that generates electrical impulses. The pads adhere to the mother's skin alongside her lower spine. You or she can turn the intensity up or down, according to her comfort level. When a contraction begins, press the thumb switch or turn the dials. She will feel a continuous vibration, or a tingling or prickling sensation, which will diminish her awareness of the pain. When the contraction ends, press the button to change the stimulation to an intermittent pattern, or turn the dials to lower the intensity.

Many women who have used TENS during labor swear it enabled them to avoid using pain-relieving medication; others report TENS was helpful in diminishing their pain, especially back pain; still others say it did little good. TENS is unlikely to help at all if begun in active labor, but starting it in pre- or early labor when the mother is having back pain may make a great difference in her ability to tolerate the back pain. As for safety, no adverse effects have been reported, except that TENS was reported to interfere with electrical signals from an electronic fetal monitor in one study. The pads should be removed if the mother wants to get into a shower or bath (they are reusable and can be reapplied later).

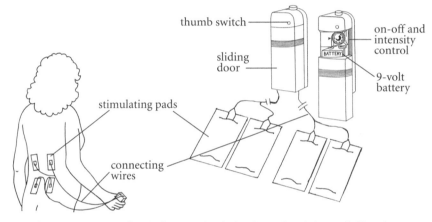

A maternity transcutaneous electrical nerve stimulation (TENS) unit in use (left) and a detailed look at the device (right).

Comforting Techniques for You to Try

In this section are some simple techniques that you can use to soothe and comfort the mother, such as touch and massage, music, and pleasing scents. Practice them with the mother and get her feedback so that you can adapt them to suit her.

TOUCH AND SIMPLE MASSAGE

Touch conveys a kind, caring, and comforting message to the laboring mother. Find out what kind of touch the mother finds soothing, and try it during labor. She may appreciate gentle, comforting, or reassuring touch—rubbing a painful spot, patting her on her back or shoulder, embracing her, holding her hand, scratching her back, stroking her hair or cheek. With your fingertips or with your full hand, you might lightly stroke the the mother's skin during contractions, on her abdomen, thighs, or wherever she wants it. Or she may prefer a real massage—a rhythmic rubbing or kneading of her back, legs, buttocks, shoulders, hands, or feet. Before beginning, pour a small amout of light massage oil into one palm, and rub your hands together briskly to warm them and the oil. Sometimes a woman finds rubbing and stroking wonderful during early labor but intolerable during transition. If this happens, you can try holding the mother's head, shoulders, hand, foot, or thigh firmly, without rubbing. A massage device—hand-held or battery-operated—may also be soothing, and may come in handy if you are not very good at massage.

How to give great mini-massages. During labor, the mother may be relaxed and soothed by brief, one- to three-minute massages of her shoulders, back, hands, or feet. Practice these ahead of time so that you can learn what she likes. Perhaps she will even reciprocate!

Follow these general guidelines:

◆ Explain what massage you would like to do, and ask for her permission ("I'd like to massage your back. Is this okay with you?").

◆ Make sure that your hands are clean and warm and that she is comfortable.

◆ Use massage oil—scented, if she likes, although you'll want to have some unscented oil on hand for labor, in case anyone in the room is sensitive to scents. Squirt a little of the oil on your hands, and rub them together briskly to cover them with the oil.

◆ Once you begin the massage, try not to remove both hands at the same time. It is unsettling to relax into a massage only to have the massager's hands vanish without warning.

◆ As you work, encourage the mother to tell you where she would like more or less rubbing or a lighter or firmer touch.

◆ When you're finished, wipe any excess oil from her skin.

Following are some of my favorite mini-massages.

Three-part shoulder mini-massage. Use this massage during or between contractions, at any phase of labor, to help the mother feel nurtured and to relax her shoulders (shoulders are one of the most common tension spots in people generally). Have the mother sit up, or she can lean forward and rest her head on her arms or a pillow. Stand behind her.

1. Place your hands comfortably on her shoulders near her neck. Stroke firmly from her neck to her shoulders and over her shoulders to her upper arms. Knead her upper arms a few times, and stroke firmly back toward her neck. Do this three or four times.

2. With your hands on her shoulders, squeeze and release her shoulder muscles as firmly as she likes for one to two minutes.

3. With the pads of the middle three fingers of one hand, do some brief, deep circle massages in small areas. Use your other hand to keep from pushing her forward. Do not move your fingertips over her skin; just move the muscles under the skin. Circle in one area for 15 to 30 seconds, and then move to another. Don't rub directly on bone. Ask her to guide you on where she would like this.

"Criss-cross" massage over the small of the back. Use this massage at any phase of labor, during or between contractions, to ease back pain or to help her relax her low back.

Have her kneel and lean over the birth ball or the seat of a chair. It will be easiest for you if she uses a ball on the bed, but you can also do this with her kneeling on the floor. She may want to wear knee pads or kneel on a foam pad like the ones sold for gardeners.

1. Facing the mother's side, place your right hand on the narrowest part of her waist on the side farthest from you, with your fingers pointing down. Place your left hand on her waist on the near side, fingers pointing up. Press her sides firmly; she should like the feeling.

2. Then, using both hands, stroke firmly up, over, and across her back. Cross one hand over the other and move to the original starting spots at her waist.

3. Maintaining the same pressure, press her sides in again, and repeat
    the crossover movement over and over as long as she wants.

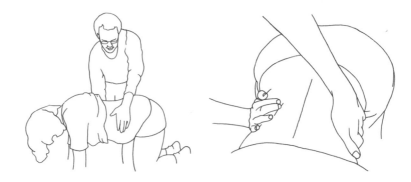

"Breaking the Popsicle" hand massage. If the mother has been
clenching her fists or gripping your hand, the bedrail, or something
else during contractions, or if she seems generally tense, this quick
massage will relax her hand and her entire arm while providing the
same pain-relieving pressure on the palm of her hand that she has
been getting from gripping things. You can do this massage during or
between contractions. Do one hand and then the other, or have
someone else do one hand while you do the other.

1. Stand or sit facing her. Ask her to relax her arm, and take her
    hand, palm down, in both of yours. Grasp her hand so that your
    thumbs touch, from their tips to their fleshy bases, on the back
    of her wrist and the pads of your fingers (not your nails) press
    into her palm.

2. Without moving your hands, increase the pressure on her palm
    gradually, and ask her to tell you when you are squeezing hard
    enough. You may be surprised at how much pressure she likes.
    When she says it is enough, maintain that pressure while slowly
    moving your thumbs and hands entirely off the back of her hand
    (see the illustrations). You are combining pressure on her palm
    and friction over the back of her hand.

3. Repeat these strokes 10 times or so. Does this massage remind
    you of how you broke apart the "Twinsicle" Popsicles when you
    were a child?

CAUTION: If her hands are very swollen, or if she has carpal tunnel syndrome (tingling or numbness in her hands that worsens with pressure), she will want very little pressure, or she will not want you to do this massage at all.

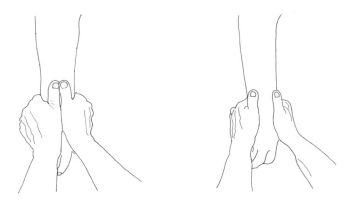

"Breaking the Popsicle" hand massage.

Three-part foot massage ("Breaking the Popsicle" with extras). If the mother complains that her feet hurt or feel tired during labor, you can use this massage to restore circulation and relieve foot aches and fatigue caused by too much standing and walking.

1. Facing the mother as she sits or lies down, ask her to relax her leg, and take her foot in both your hands. Grasp it so that your thumbs are touching each other all the way to their bases. Press the pads of your fingers (not your nails) into the sole of her foot. Squeeze until she says it is enough; you may be surprised at how much pressure she likes. Maintaining that pressure, move your thumbs apart so your hands are entirely off the top of her foot. You are combining pressure on the sole of her foot with friction over the back of her foot. Do this 10 times or so.

2. Cup the heel of her foot in your hand, and squeeze and release several times, as if you were squeezing a tennis ball. This should feel wonderful.

3. If you're massaging her left foot, hold it in your left hand; if you're working on her right foot, hold it in your right hand. With the

pads of the three middle fingers of the opposite hand, give her a deep circle massage in the "magic spot," on the top of her foot just below her ankle. The spot is slightly off the center of the foot, toward the outside. Do not move your fingers on her skin; rather, move her skin over her underlying muscles and bones. Do this for 30 to 60 seconds.

Once you have completed all three steps on one foot, repeat with her other foot. Then she will be ready to walk some more!

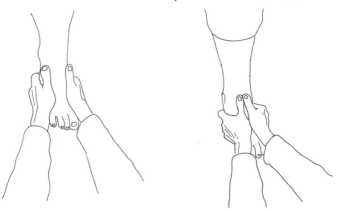

"Breaking the Popsicle" foot massage.

Acupressure. Shiatsu, or acupressure, has been practiced in Asia for many centuries. This healing art is derived from the ancient Chinese understanding of the principles of yin and yang. The body is made up of 12 meridians, along which vital forces flow; acupressure corrects imbalances in the flow of these vital forces that impair health and well-being. Acupressure uses the same points for stimulation as does acupuncture, but involves finger pressure instead of needles. The use of both acupressure and acupuncture has grown rapidly in the West, and scientific studies of their use in labor have found beneficial effects on childbirth pain. Many people successfully combine acupressure with other methods to enhance comfort and progress in labor.

By pressing with your finger or thumb at certain acupressure points, you may be able to relieve the mother's pain and speed up her labor. You may want to try this if the mother is facing induction or if her labor slows (see page 224). The two most popular points for labor are the Ho-ku point and Spleen 6. Both are sensitive spots that may hurt a bit when you press them. Your goal, however, is not to cause pain, so do not press hard enough to hurt her.

The Ho-ku point is on the back of the hand, where the bones forming the bases of the thumb and index finger come together. Press steadily into the bone at the base of the index finger with your thumb for 10 to 60 seconds, three to six times, with a rest of equal length in between. You can repeat this as often as you and the mother want.

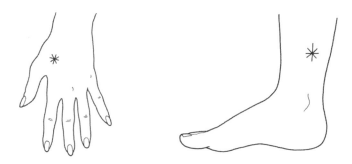

The Ho-ku point (left) and Spleen 6, four of her finger breadths above her inner ankle bone (right).

Spleen 6 is on the inner side of the lower leg about four finger breadths above the ankle. Press your thumb into the bone from slightly behind it for 10 to 60 seconds at a time, three to six times, with a rest of equal length in between. You can repeat this in labor whenever you and the mother want.

CAUTION: Experts advise against pressing these points on a pregnant woman before her due date, as they can cause contractions and increase the risk of premature labor. Find the points on yourself, but don't use them on the mother until the need arises.

Counterpressure for back pain. Try this during contractions if the mother has back pain. While the mother stands or kneels, leaning forward over a bed or birth ball, hold the front of her hip with one hand to help her maintain her balance, and, with your fist or the heel

of the other hand, press steadily and firmly in the low back or buttocks area. The right spot is usually off center, and it varies from
woman to woman and within the same labor. Try pressing in several
places, and she will tell you which feels best. Keep the pressure steady
throughout the contraction; if you release it too soon, her pain will
get worse immediately. You will probably have to press hard during
every contraction. Between contractions, you might massage the area
or use cold or hot compresses (see page 149).

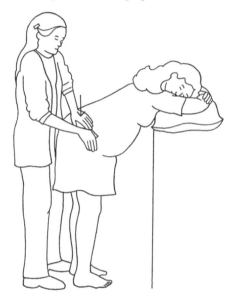

The double hip squeeze. This also helps to ease back pain. In fact, this
technique and counterpressure can often make the difference between tolerable and intolerable back pain.

The mother stands or kneels and leans forward onto a bed, birth
ball, or chair seat, or gets on her hands and knees. Her hips should
be flexed. From behind, use your fingers to locate the pelvic bones at
the sides of her hips, just below her waist. From there, move your
hands down her hips to the roundest part of her buttocks. Press on
both sides of her buttocks with your whole hands (not with the heels
of your hands—that would hurt). Push toward the center, pressing
her hips together. Experiment to find the right places to press. When

you have found the right places, press them steadily throughout each contraction. Apply as much pressure as she needs.

The Double Hip Squeeze is difficult and tiring work for one person. It is much easier with a helper. The illustration shows how two people can use this technique.

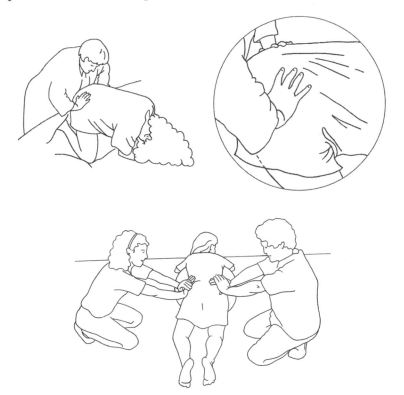

Rolling pressure over the low back. This is another helpful technique for backache. Use a rolling massager, similar to the one illustrated on page 149, a rolling pin (a hollow one that you can fill with ice is particularly useful), or a cold can of juice or soft drink (keep a six-pack in a bowl of ice so you'll always have a cold can). Since rolling pins and cans of juice are usually unavailable in hospitals (though soft drinks *are* available), you may want to bring such an object with you, especially if she has backache with contractions before you leave home. During or between contractions, roll the object, with some pressure, over the mother's low back.

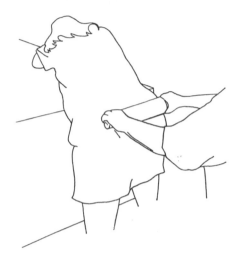

Besides the bath, shower, acupressure, massage, heat, and cold, many of the positions shown in the chart on pages 135 to 141 and indicated by an asterisk are especially helpful for back pain, as are the techniques described under "Backache in Labor" in chapter 5.

Music and Sound

Many women can relax and focus better if their favorite music, relaxation narration, or environmental sounds (ocean waves, a babbling brook, a rain shower) are played during labor. Familiar and well-loved music has been found to raise levels of endorphins (the body's own pain-relieving substances). Soothing sounds may overcome some of the beeps, pages, and other sounds that are part of any modern birthing room.

You might suggest that the mother select some of her favorite recordings to play during labor. Check on the availability of audio equipment in the hospital or bring your own player.

Aromatherapy or Pleasing Scents

Pleasant aromas create feelings of well-being and relaxation, and they cover up hospital smells. Scents such as lavender, sandalwood, citrus, and peppermint may appeal to the mother. You can purchase scented massage oil, sachets, bath beads, liquid soap, or cologne, or you can simply cut a lemon in half for her to sniff.

Because preferences for scents are very personal, ask the mother whether she would like to have them available and, if so, which ones she would like. She may want none at all, or she may pick one or two favorites to have available during labor.

Unless a trained aromatherapist prepares special mixes of essential oils for her for specific purposes, stick with store-bought lotions and oil mixes. Essential oils are very strong, and if they are too concentrated or used incorrectly, they can cause burns, allergic reactions, and other side effects.

Check with the hospital or birth-center staff before using scented products, since some people are allergic to some essential oils. See "Recommended Resources" for books on aromatherapy.

Taking Care of Yourself

Labor can be long and tiring, stressful, and demanding for the birth partner, just as it is for the mother. Losing a night's sleep is never easy. Standing for long periods, skipping meals, and offering the mother continual encouragement are tiring, especially if you are worried or overextended. To be an effective birth partner you will need to pace yourself, draw on the experience and wisdom of others, and look after your own basic needs. This cannot mean taking long breaks for naps or meals, because the mother may need you and want you to stay. She will probably depend heavily on you to help her through every contraction. There are ways you can take care of her and yourself at the same time. Here are some suggestions to help you conserve energy and get appropriate help from others:

- Be sure to have your supplies handy. Review the list of suggested items for the birth partner's use during labor (see page 14).

- Eat and drink tasty, nourishing food and beverages regularly during labor. Choose foods without strong odors (think about how they will affect your breath), and keep them with you so you do not have to leave the room to get them.

- Wear comfortable clothes, and have a change of clothes, a sweater, and slippers available.

- Rest, by making yourself comfortable near the mother. Don't stand when you can sit. If the mother is lying down and you also need some rest, you can lie down next to her if the bed is wide enough, or sit and rest your head on the bed beside her. If there is enough time between contractions, doze. You will not have trouble waking up to help her if you keep a hand on her arm or belly.

- Ask for reassurance. If you are worried about the length of labor or about the mother's pain or discouragement or fatigue, ask the caregiver or nurse whether everything is all right; express your concerns. It is best, however, to do this outside the mother's hearing.

- Ask the nurse or caregiver for ideas for comfort measures. If you are uncertain whether you are helping the mother enough, ask for suggestions.

- Make arrangements to have a doula, or at least a friend or relative, help you during labor.

A woman in labor often needs the help of two people, one in front helping her maintain her rhythm, and the other behind her, pressing on her back; or one running an errand while the other remains. A doula, with her broad perspective on childbirth and her experience, can make concrete suggestions for comfort measures, help you remember some of the things you learned in childbirth class, and remind you and the mother of her Birth Plan. Also, if you have a helper, either of you can take a break during a long labor without leaving the mother alone.

You might not need a break, however. Researchers compared the behavior of two groups of fathers during labor. In one group, the fathers were the only support persons for the mother; in the other, there was also a doula in attendance. In the group in which a doula was present, the fathers generally spent more time in the room with the mother and stayed closer to her. Because the doula takes pressure off the partner, the partner may not need to take a break as often.

For all of these reasons, you might welcome an experienced, calm, confident support person who can remain with you through the birth.

Checklist of Comfort Measures for Labor

Check the following list of comfort measures at any time during labor when you believe a change from what you are doing may be helpful.

Relaxation/Tension Release
- During or between contractions
- Aromatherapy (lotions, oils)

Rhythmic Breathing
- Slow
- Light

Bearing Down
- Avoiding bearing down
- Spontaneous bearing down
- Directed pushing

Massage/Touch
- Still touch, stroking, hand holding
- Shoulders
- Criss-cross
- Hand
- Foot
- Acupressure

Hydrotherapy
- Shower
- Bath

Attention Focusing
- Visual focus, focus on music, voice, or touch
- Mental activity
  - Visualization
  - Count breaths
  - Chant, mantra, song, prayer

Hot Packs
- To lower abdomen or groin
- To perineum during second stage
- To low back

Cold Packs
- To low back
- To perineum after birth

Positions and Movements
- Standing, leaning forward
- Walking, slow-dancing
- The lunge (standing or kneeling)
- Kneeling, leaning forward on ball or chair
- Side lying /semiprone
- Semisitting
- Flat on back (tilted slightly to side)
- Squatting
- Supported squat / dangle
- Lap squatting

Measures for Backache
- Counterpressure
- Double hip squeeze (by 1 or 2 people)
- Criss-cross
- Rolling pressure
- TENS
- Cold pack
- Hot pack
- Shower
- Large bathtub (with room to kneel and lean over the side)
- Open knee-chest position
- Abdominal lifting
- Hands-and-knees
- Kneeling, leaning forward on ball or chair
- The lunge (standing or kneeling)
- Walking, slow-dancing

Help from Birth Partner
- Suggestions, reminders
- Encouragement, reassurance
- Compliments
- Patience, confidence in mother
- Immediate response to contractions
- Undivided attention
- Aid with positions, relaxation, rhythm
- Take-Charge Routine
- Expressions of love
- Hugs and kisses

CHAPTER 5

Strategies for Challenging Variations in Normal Labor

After 14 hours of labor, Terry started to push, but her cervix swelled because of the baby's position. She needed to stop pushing until the swelling went down, but she didn't think she could stop—her urge to push was so strong. So she opted for an epidural that she hadn't wanted. It took away the pushing feeling, and three hours later it was okay to begin pushing. She watched in the mirror. When she saw her baby's head, she said, "This is surreal!" A few more contractions, and he was born and placed straight on Terry's chest. J. C. said, "Oh, oh, I can't stop crying!" to which Terry replied, "It's the only time I've seen you cry!"

—HEATHER, THEIR DOULA

Labor, even when perfectly normal, rarely follows a predictable "textbook" pattern. Variations within a range of normal are to be expected. The emotional reactions of women in labor vary, depending on the type of labor pattern they have. For example, if prelabor or early labor drags on for a long time, the mother may be challenged by exhaustion, worry, or a loss of confidence. If, instead, labor starts suddenly with long, painful contractions that threaten to overwhelm the mother, her pain and panic are the birth partner's main concerns. Women and their birth partners work best with labor when they are open and flexible, and when they are confident that they can and will (with the help of their caregivers and support team) handle whatever comes their way.

This chapter will help you deal with situations more stressful than any encountered in the average labor but still falling within the range of "normal." These situations require more intense and active support from you. Both you and the mother will need more resourcefulness, effort, decision making, patience, and reliance on the doula's and caregiver's encouragement and advice. The special situations covered here are:

> The Take-Charge Routine (for Labor's Toughest Moments)
> On-the-Spot Coaching (When You Have Had No Childbirth Classes)
> The Very Rapid Labor
> The Emergency Delivery
> When Labor Must Start (Labor-Stimulating Measures)
> The Slow-to-Start Labor
> Slow Progress in Active Labor and the Birthing Stage, with or without Back Pain
> When the Mother Must Labor in Bed
> A Breech Baby
> A Previous Disappointing or Traumatic Birth Experience
> Incompatibility with the Nurse or Caregiver

Not covered in this chapter are complications in labor—situations that are outside the limits of normal. To learn how a caregiver detects complications and treats them with medical or surgical interventions, and how you can be most helpful to the mother, read chapters 6, 7, 8, and 9.

The Take-Charge Routine

When labor becomes very intense, the mother may struggle to maintain her rhythm or lose it entirely. If this happens, she needs calm, confident, and kind but firm guidance to regain and maintain her rhythm. Reserve this routine for when the mother reacts in any of these ways:

◆ She is unable to maintain a rhythmic ritual in her breathing, moaning, or movements.

◆ She despairs, weeps, cries out, or says she cannot go on.

◆ She is very tense and cannot relax.

◆ She is in a great deal of pain.

The Take-Charge Routine is exactly that. You move in close and do all you can to help the mother until she regains her inner strength. Usually her despair is brief; with your help she can pass through it and her spirits will rise. If she planned before labor to request pain medication under these circumstances, use the Take-Charge Routine to help her until the medication can be given. Use whatever parts of this routine seem appropriate:

♦ *Remain calm.* Your touch should be firm and confident, not anxious and tense. Your voice should remain calm and encouraging. Your facial expression should reflect confidence and optimism.

♦ *Stay close.* Face her or stay right by her side, your face near hers.

♦ *Anchor her.* Hold her shoulders or her hands—gently, confidently, firmly. Do not shake her to get her attention.

♦ *Get her to look at you.* If her eyes are clenched shut, you will not be able to help her. Tell her to open her eyes and look at your face or your hand. This is all-important. Say it loudly enough for her to hear you—but calmly and kindly.

♦ *Talk to her between contractions.* Make suggestions; for example, "With the next one, let me help you more. I want you to look at me the moment it starts. I will pace you with my hand so it won't get ahead of us. Okay? Good. You're doing so well. We're really moving now."

♦ *Help her regain the rhythm she had, by moving your hand or head up and down in that rhythm.* You can combine this with "rhythm talk" (see the next item). Pause briefly after each downbeat to keep from going too fast.

I wear a ring with a blue stone on my right hand. I ask women to "follow my ring" as I "conduct" them in a breathing rhythm. I love to think of the many, many women who have let my ring guide them through some tough moments in labor. It's one reason I never take the ring off.

♦ *Use "rhythm talk" by vocally pacing the rhythm of her breathing or moaning.* Say "Breathe with me . . . BREATHE WITH ME . . . That's the way, . . . just like that . . . Good . . . Keep your rhythm . . . STAY WITH IT . . . just like that . . . LOOK AT ME . . . Keep your rhythm . . . Good for you . . . It's going away . . . Good . . . Good . . . Now just rest, that was so good." You can whisper these words or say them in a calm, rhythmic, confident, and encouraging tone of voice. If she is vocalizing, you may have to raise your voice to get her attention, but do not shout. Also, you don't need to actually breathe with the mother as you say the words; you shouldn't even try if your breath is stale or the breathing makes you lightheaded. She can breathe to the rhythm of your words as well as your hand or head movements.

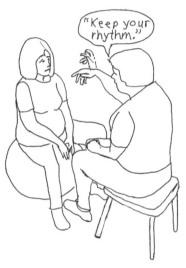

◆ *Repeat yourself.* She may not be able to continue doing what you tell her for more than a few seconds, but that's fine. Do not conclude that what you are doing does not help at all. Say the same things again and again, and help her continue.

What if the mother says she can't or won't go on? Here are some guidelines:

◆ When she is between contractions, tell her that you want her to *change the ritual she has been using during contractions*, because it is no longer working. Then suggest a different position or breathing rhythm.

◆ *Don't give up on her.* This is a difficult time for her. You cannot help her if you decide she cannot handle it. Acknowledge to her and to yourself that it is difficult, but remind yourselves that it is not impossible.

- *Ask for help and reassurance.* The nurse or caregiver can check the mother's dilation and give you advice. Perhaps the mother is in distress because labor is progressing very rapidly; just knowing this may help her. A doula or other support person can spell you, model the technique for you, suggest something new, and reassure both of you that the mother is okay and that her reactions are normal. If you're having trouble with the Take-Charge Routine, the doula might "take charge" while you hold the mother or press on her back.

- *Remind the mother of her baby.* It may seem surprising, but women can get so caught up in labor that they do not think much about the baby. It may help the mother to remember why she is going through all this, and to recognize that her baby is working with her.

What about pain medications? Should you suggest them or not? This depends on:

- The mother's prior wishes: Did she want an unmedicated birth? How strongly did she feel about it? (See the "Pain Medications Preference Scale," page 294.) Sometimes women who ask for pain medications are really saying, "I need more help."

- Her rate of progress and how far she still has to go. A couple of centimeters of dilation should be very encouraging. A complete lack of progress is very discouraging.

- How well she responds to the Take-Charge Routine or the doula's help. If the mother cannot get back into a rhythm, even with a lot of help, and she is making little progress, she may need pain medications.

- Whether she is willing to try something else, such as a bath, a change of position, a progress check, or just coping with three more contractions to see whether things get easier.

- Whether she truly wants the medications or is just agreeing to the nurse's or caregiver's suggestion.

- Whether she asks for medications *between* contractions. Many women ask for medications *during* a contraction, but do not mention them when the contraction ends.

The Take-Charge Routine

◆ Whether she uses her "code word" (see page 292).

Numerous women have said to their partners, "I never could have done it without you. If it hadn't been for you, I would have given up." By using the Take-Charge Routine, you can indeed get the mother through those desperate moments when she feels she cannot go on; you can truly ease her burden by helping her with every breath. And if you and she agree in advance on a code word she can use if she decides she wants medications, you will know that you're not forcing her to suffer.

On-the-Spot Coaching (When You Have Had No Childbirth Classes)

If the due date nears and you have taken no childbirth classes, or if you took only a very short, "crash" course, you should consider hiring a doula to help you comfort the mother and guide the two of you through labor. But what if you have no doula, and labor starts early? What if you and the mother have had no time to work together to learn the pain-relief techniques described in chapter 4? Here are some suggestions: (1) Don't try to learn everything at once while the mother is in labor; (2) use some simple breathing rhythms and a few on-the-spot comfort measures; and (3) tell the staff that you and the mother have had no classes.

RHYTHMIC BREATHING

Rhythm is everything in labor. Once the contractions become uncomfortable, the mother can use rhythmic breathing or moaning patterns through each one. She may find her own pattern, or you can show her how to breathe in a particular rhythm. Then breathe with her (make sure you do not have bad breath), verbally pace her through each breath, or conduct her breathing with rhythmic hand signals. Between contractions in early labor, work together to learn *slow breathing*, to use first, and *light breathing*, to use later, if needed. Both patterns, described on pages 128 and 129, are simple and quick to learn.

With each out-breath, encourage the mother to release tension. As she breathes out you might say, "Let go right here," and touch her shoulder, brow, or whatever part of her body is tense.

ON-THE-SPOT COMFORT MEASURES

Here are other on-the-spot comfort measures to try:

Movement and position changes (see page 134)
Counterpressure (see page 157)
Bath or shower (see page 142)
Heat or cold (see page 149)
Touch or massage (see page 151)
Relaxation (see page 121)
Attention focusing (see page 124)
The Take-Charge Routine (see page 166)

Most of these measures can be used fairly well without much preparation. In fact, you can read about them between contractions and apply them immediately.

The Very Rapid Labor

Some women have labors that start with intense, frequent, painful contractions and are over in a matter of a few hours. It seems the mother barely has time to adjust to being in labor before the baby is born.

Sometimes only the first (dilation) stage is rapid. The cervix dilates so quickly that the mother can't catch up mentally; but then, in the second (birthing) stage, the contractions space out. If this happens, the mother has to cope with the difficulties of both fast and slow labors.

It is impossible to predict which women will labor in these ways, but a rapid labor seems to be more likely if:

◆ The mother has had a rapid or quicker-than-average (less than 10-hour) labor before. A second or third labor tends to be faster than the first.

On-the-spot coaching

◆ Her cervix is very soft, thin, and already partially dilated before labor begins, and the baby is low in the mother's pelvis in a very favorable position.

◆ Her bag of waters ruptures with a gush rather than a slow leak, especially if she is also having contractions.

Few women or their birth partners are prepared for a rapid labor, especially after reading and hearing about typical labor patterns and prolonged prelabors. The mother will be caught off guard if she was expecting the early contractions to be gentle, short, and far apart, but her labor begins instead with contractions that are long, painful, and close together—almost like the contractions of the transition phase.

How Is the Mother Likely to React?

You can expect any of the following reactions from the mother if her labor begins rapidly:

◆ *Shock and disbelief.* She may not be able to respond constructively. She may not realize that this is real labor.

◆ *Fear or panic.* She may think that something is terribly wrong—that she or the baby is in danger. She may be frightened if she cannot reach you, her caregiver, or anyone else for help, and she may worry about getting to the hospital in time.

◆ *Loss of confidence.* If the mother thinks these are the "easy" contractions of early labor, she may lose all confidence that she can cope with labor once it progresses.

◆ *Dependence on you.* She may barely be able to change positions between contractions, let alone get ready to go to the hospital. She may need your constant help to cope with the contractions.

◆ *Annoyance with you or her caregivers.* If you or they do not grasp the situation. (Women tell stories of their partners going back to sleep, assuming there is a long wait ahead, and of caregivers who tell *them* to go to sleep, which is impossible, or to wait an hour and then call again.)

How Should You React?

- Believe what you see. If the mother is shaky, in pain, and having strong, fast contractions, don't assume she is overreacting to early labor. Assume she is having a hard labor, and move right into a leadership role in helping her cope.

- Don't worry about trying to help her relax. These contractions will not allow her to relax.

- Use the "Take-Charge Routine" (see page 166) if she has trouble coping with the contractions.

- Don't lose faith in her or criticize her. Give her the benefit of the doubt. Her response truly reflects that this labor is really hard.

- Call the caregiver, go to the hospital or birth center, or both. Drive carefully, but don't waste time.

The Emergency Delivery

What if the baby is coming and you and the mother are on your own—in your car or at home? You will know that it is too late to go to the hospital if (1) the mother says she can feel the baby coming out; (2) you can see the baby's head at her vaginal opening; or (3) she is pushing and grunting forcibly and cannot stop.

If all of this happens at home, stay where you are, and call 911 for an emergency vehicle with a paramedical team. You may also call the hospital; the hospital may send an emergency team, or a nurse may stay on the phone with you to tell you what to do.

If all this happens in the car, pull over to the side of the road, put on your flasher lights, and tend to the mother's needs. If the weather is cold, leave the motor running and the heater on.

Basic Rules for an Emergency Delivery

Before the birth, this is what you do:

- Believe the mother if she says the baby is coming.
- Remain calm (at least try to act calm!).

- Get help—from paramedics, friends or neighbors, even children.
- Turn up the heat in the car or at home.
- Gather blankets, towels, or warm clothing to wrap the baby in.
- Find newspapers, a bowl, paper towels, or a plastic bag to hold the placenta.
- Reassure the mother.
- Help the mother avoid pushing. To slow the delivery, she should pant or blow lightly with her chin up when her body starts to push.
- Help the mother lie down on her side or recline in a semisitting position. This may slow the delivery slightly, and it will ensure a safe landing place for the baby.
- Wash your hands thoroughly, if possible, unless the mother needs you to stay with her or if the baby is coming out.
- Get ready to catch the baby. Have something ready to dry and cover the baby immediately (towels, blanket, your shirt or jacket).
- Keep your hands on the baby so he does not fall out. If the mother is standing or squatting, or if there is no soft place for the baby to land, place your body so that he will land on you if you don't catch him.

    As the baby comes out, this is what you do:

- Help the mother to pant, not push.
- Wipe the baby's face and head when they emerge. If the membranes cover the baby's face, tear them with your fingernail or pull them away so the baby can breathe.
- Catch the baby or guide her to a soft place.

    As soon as the baby is out, do the following:

- Watch the baby's chest and listen to check the baby's breathing. Babies normally begin breathing or crying within seconds after birth.
- Dry the baby, and wipe away any mucus, blood, or vernix from her nostrils or mouth.
- If the baby doesn't begin breathing right away, rub her head, back, or chest briskly, or slap the soles of her feet. She might sputter and choke out some mucus or fluid from her airway.

- Place the baby naked on her side or stomach on her mother's naked abdomen. Cover them both to keep the baby dry and warm, but keep the baby's face exposed so you can monitor her condition.

- In the unlikely possibility that the baby does not breathe within two minutes, and you know how to do infant CPR, do it now. Otherwise, get to the hospital as quickly as possible. Don't worry about tying or cutting the cord, and don't wait for the placenta.

- If the placenta comes immediately, try to catch it in a bowl or wrap it in something. Then feel the mother's uterus by pressing below her navel. The uterus should be hard and firm, like a large grapefruit. If you cannot feel the uterus, it is too relaxed and may bleed too much. Rub her lower belly very firmly in a small circle (you should feel the uterus tighten as you do so), then have her do this until the paramedics arrive or you get her to the hospital.

- If the placenta comes while you are driving and the hospital is still 20 minutes or more away, it might be wise to pull over and check the mother's uterus as just described.

- If the mother is bleeding, place the baby at her breast; her sucking or even nuzzling at the breast will help contract the uterus and slow the bleeding. If the baby is not ready to suck, the mother should roll one nipple between her fingers while massaging her uterus.

The emergency delivery

When Labor Must Start
(Labor-Stimulating Measures)

Under some circumstances, the caregiver recognizes that delaying or awaiting the baby's birth for much longer carries unacceptable risks to mother or baby. The caregiver will suggest labor induction—starting labor by giving drugs, breaking the bag of waters, or other means (see "Induction or Augmentation of Labor," page 224). Under some of these circumstances, the caregiver may believe that a medical induction should be done immediately (see page 227), but more often the need is not urgent and the mother has an opportunity to try self-induction methods. If she is successful, she can avoid medical induction, which carries some risk and is invasive (see "Disadvantages of Induction for Medical Reasons," page 227).

Many doctors offer induction routinely at 39, 40, or 41 weeks, for no medical reason. This is called elective induction. See pages 227 to 231 for a discussion of medical and nonmedical reasons for induction, and use the "Key Questions for Informed Decision Making" (see page 202) to recognize whether induction is "medically indicated" or not. It is usually safer, especially for the first-time mother, to wait for labor to begin spontaneously than to have an elective medical induction or to try self-induction.

Why might a woman try the self-induction methods? Probably the most compelling reason is that medical induction is considered to be indicated if the woman goes two weeks beyond her due date. If she wishes to avoid a medical induction and is at 41$^1/_2$ weeks, she may want to start trying to get herself into labor. Another reason could be that her blood pressure is slowly rising, in which case her doctor may advise induction in a few days.

Self-induction may or may not succeed. If it does not succeed, the mother will end up with a medical induction anyway. Some women feel it is worth trying to get into labor on their own; others do not. That the methods are easy to use and carry little risk (but see the following sections for precautions) persuades some to try them. Chances of success depend on the mother's readiness for labor (she must have a ripe, thin cervix) and the techniques she chooses.

SELF-INDUCTION METHODS

Before using these techniques to start labor, make sure the mother discusses them with her caregiver. She should ask the caregiver whether there is any reason that she should not try to start contractions, using the methods described here. If there is none, you and she can get started.

Nipple stimulation. Stimulating the mother's nipples causes the release of oxytocin, a hormone that contracts the uterus. Taking advantage of this physiological connection between breast and uterus may start labor or at least cause some contractions. Nipple stimulation probably will not work, however, if the mother is currently breastfeeding a toddler, in which case her body has adapted to increased levels of oxytocin, or if her cervix has not ripened or thinned significantly. Her caregiver can tell her how ready her cervix is after a vaginal exam.

Either you or the mother can stimulate her nipples, in one or more of the following ways, to bring on or intensify contractions:

◆ Lightly stroke, roll, or brush one or both nipples with the fingertips. Or you can caress, lick, or suck her nipples. Often, within a few minutes the mother will have stronger contractions. You or she may need to continue this stimulation intermittently for hours to keep the contractions coming.

◆ Massage the breasts gently with warm, moist towels for an hour at a time, three times a day.

◆ Use a gentle but powerful electric breast pump with double-pumping capability (which allows you to pump both breasts at once). A manual or battery-operated breast pump is less likely to work as well as one with a wall plug. Pump one breast for a half hour three to five times per day, pausing when a contraction begins and resuming when it stops. If no contractions occur within about 10 minutes, try pumping both breasts, pausing with each contraction. If necessary to increase the intensity or frequency of the contractions, continue pumping during as well as between contractions.

With all these methods, start with one nipple. If stimulating only one nipple does not initiate contractions in a reasonable length of time, or if the contractions the mother is already having do not increase in frequency, length, or strength, try stimulating both breasts at once, between contractions at first, and then, if necessary, continuously. If there are no contractions, after an hour or two, wait a half day before trying again, or try some of the other methods.

Precautions when using nipple stimulation. Many caregivers are very comfortable with their clients' use of nipple stimulation to bring on labor, but others are wary, because stimulating the nipples sometimes causes excessively long or strong contractions. These caregivers worry that strong contractions may stress the fetus, especially if the mother is at high risk for complications. Before approving the use of nipple stimulation, the caregiver may want to check the baby's response to such stimulation by having the mother try it first during electronic fetal monitoring in the hospital or office.

To help avoid excessively strong or long contractions, it is wise to time the length and assess the intensity of all contractions resulting from nipple stimulation. Stop stimulating the breasts if contractions become painful or long (more than 60 seconds).

Walking. Although effective in speeding a slow labor, walking is unlikely to get labor started. If you want to try anyway, take the mother for a fairly brisk walk, but don't go too far away from home or the labor room. If nothing else, walking is a pleasant distraction before labor.

Acupressure and acupuncture. Certain acupressure (shiatsu) points can be activated to stimulate contractions. See pages 156 to 157.

Acupuncture is the use of fine needles (sometimes combined with heat or electrical stimulation) to painlessly stimulate specific points along the 12 meridians along which vital forces (called chi) flow. The purpose is to remove any blockage in energy flow that may impair bodily functions. Acupuncture is becoming increasingly available for all sorts of health purposes, including many related to pregnancy and childbirth. Among them is the need to start labor.

Although acupuncture is not a method of self-induction, it is usually arranged by the baby's parents, with the knowledge and approval of the mother's caregiver. If the mother is interested in trying acupuncture, check with her midwife, doctor, doula, or childbirth educator for names of licensed acupuncturists who work with childbearing women. Treatment varies depending on the acupuncturist's training and the perceived cause of the problem.

Sexual stimulation. Sexual intercourse with orgasm is the most effective form of sexual stimulation in starting labor. Orgasm causes the release of oxytocin and contractions of the uterus, and it may also cause the release of prostaglandins, hormone-like substances that soften the cervix. Semen also contains prostaglandins.

Clitoral stimulation by hand or mouth, even without orgasm or intercourse, may also be somewhat effective in bringing on contractions.

If you choose one of these methods of stimulation, make them as pleasant as possible. Try to forget your goal of starting labor, and free yourselves to enjoy the sexual experience—more than once, if needed.

There are a few precautions to follow when using these methods:

◆ Avoid placing anything within the vagina if the membranes have ruptured, because doing so would increase the risk of infection.

◆ Do not blow into the vagina.

Modify or avoid these methods if either of you has any sores that could spread or if the mother has an uncomfortable vaginal condition.

Bowel stimulation with castor oil. The mother may be able to start labor by taking castor oil to stimulate and empty her bowels. A laxative, castor oil may cause powerful contractions of the bowels and diarrhea (reactions vary, but the effects can be quite unpleasant for a few hours). The oil has been used for generations to induce labor, with some success. Taking castor oil may increase the mother's level of prostaglandins, which are produced when the bowels contract. Prostaglandins, again, cause the cervix to soften and thin.

Make sure the mother checks with her caregiver before using castor oil. If the caregiver approves, follow these guidelines:

1. Give the mother 4 tablespoons (2 ounces) of unflavored castor oil to start. The oil is more palatable if you mix it with an equal amount of orange juice and a teaspoonful of baking soda; stir the mixture, and tell the mother to drink it quickly. Or try scrambling the oil with two eggs or mixing it with root beer in an ice cream float.

2. A half hour later, if she has had little or no reaction, the mother may take 2 tablespoons (1 ounce) more of the oil in any of the same ways.

3. After another half hour, she may take 2 tablespoons (1 ounce) more. She should take no more than three doses, totaling 4 ounces.

Contractions may come immediately, but usually they don't. When the method works, contractions pick up within half a day. Sometimes castor oil fails to get labor started but does improve the readiness of the cervix to dilate, and labor is started the next day through nipple stimulation or another method.

Enemas, previously used for starting labor, have been found ineffective for this purpose, even though they do help to empty the bowels.

Teas, tinctures, herbs, and homeopathic remedies. Some midwives and physicians use certain herbal teas or tinctures, such as blue and black cohosh tea and evening primrose oil, or homeopathic remedies, such as caulophyllum, to bring on or speed up contractions. Use these teas or tinctures only with the approval of the mother's caregiver and the guidance of an experienced herbalist or homeopath who knows about appropriate dosages and potential side effects.

The Slow-to-Start Labor

Besides the very rapid labor and the one that does not begin spontaneously, another challenging sort of labor is the one that is slow to start. In this case, contractions, sometimes painful, go on for hours or days before the cervix finally begins to dilate. We don't know exactly why this happens to some women and not to others, but if the following conditions are present, a woman is more likely to have a slow-to-start labor:

+ The mother's cervix is still long (or thick), firm, and posterior when contractions begin (see "Labor Progresses in Six Ways," page 52).

+ Her cervix is scarred from previous surgery or injury. A scarred cervix may resist thinning, and so may require more time and more intense contractions to overcome this resistance. Once thinning has occurred, labor usually progresses normally.

+ Her uterus is contracting in an uncoordinated fashion, so that the contractions do not open the cervix. The reason this sometimes happens is not understood, but the condition often resolves with time, rest, or medications to promote sleep or to induce labor. See pages 224 to 226.

+ The baby's head is high in the pelvis (see page 54) or OP (occiput posterior; see page 45). The problem most often will correct itself with time and strong contractions.

◆ The mother is very anxious and tense about the labor or the baby. Increased production of stress hormones (such as adrenaline) in early labor can interfere with labor progress.

Unknown conditions may also play a role. Most slow-to-start labors eventually hit their stride and proceed normally after the initial long prelabor period. Some slow-to-start labors, however, are part of a generally prolonged labor, in which all phases proceed, but at a very slow pace. When a labor begins slowly, you cannot know in advance just when it will speed up; only time will tell. Fatigue and discouragement can present a serious challenge in this type of labor, and medical interventions may be required. Your role as birth partner will be to maintain the mother's morale and help her pace herself mentally and physically. If interventions are being considered by her caregiver, you can also help her to be well informed about the options. See pages 221 to 231.

STRATEGIES FOR A SLOW-TO-START LABOR

If the mother's long prelabor is tiring and discouraging, though not necessarily painful, the following measures will help:

◆ Be patient and confident. This labor will *not* go on forever, and your positive attitude will help the mother keep her spirits up.

◆ If she is worried, remind her that *a long prelabor does not necessarily mean that anything is wrong* with her or the baby. Her cervix simply needs more time before it thins and begins opening. The two of you need to find ways to wait without worrying.

◆ Call her friends, family, caregiver, or doula for encouragement and morale boosting. Do not call anyone who is going to make you worry more. A doula, with her confidence, experience, and perspective, can be a great help in such labors.

◆ Try not to become preoccupied with the labor or to overreact to every contraction. This will only make the labor seem longer.

◆ Encourage the mother to eat and drink high-carbohydrate, easily digested foods (for example, toast with jam, cereals, pancakes, pasta, fruit juice, tea with sugar or honey, sorbet, or gelatin desserts).

◆ Create a clean, tidy environment with whatever makes the mother comfortable—music, a fire in the fireplace, flowers, favorite scents, and so on.

Additionally, you can help her pass the time by rotating among distracting, restful, and labor-stimulating activities. Here are some suggestions:

1. During the day, try distracting activities. Encourage the mother to get out of the house. If she is willing, she can visit friends, go for a walk, get a massage, go to work (let her decide whether she can), or go to a movie, the mall, or a restaurant (you can hope you'll have to leave before you finish your meal!). You'll find that when she is out of the house she will try to minimize her reactions to the contractions, and thus avoid overreacting to them. This is easier for her to do when she is among other people than when she's alone at home.

   At home you can try these distracting activities: watch TV programs or movies that *she* likes; dance; clean; pay bills; play games; start a time-consuming project, such as baking bread or a birthday cake (she will almost hope that labor doesn't start until the project is finished!); wash and put away the baby's clothes; arrange or file photos; fix and freeze meals for after the baby is born; have friends over, especially to relieve you if you are tired.

2. Help her rest or sleep at night, or nap during the day. If she is tired but cannot sleep, try the following:

   ◆ Suggest a bath. Fill the tub with warm (not hot) water; provide an inflatable bathtub pillow or folded towels for a headrest. She should plan to stay in the tub for a long time; you may have to add hot water from time to time to keep it warm enough. Rest and sleep may come more easily in a warm bath. Keep an eye on her; make sure she doesn't slip down so her head goes under the water. Remember that a bath tends to slow contractions in early labor, and should be used then only when a woman needs a rest.

   ◆ If no bath is available, encourage the mother to try a long shower. You might need to turn up the water heater.

- ◆ Play some soothing music.
- ◆ Rub her back.
- ◆ Give her a relaxing beverage (warm milk, herbal tea).
- ◆ Use relaxation techniques and slow breathing during contractions. See page 128.

3. Try labor-stimulating measures for periods of one to two hours at a time to initiate stronger, more frequent contractions. Follow the guidelines in "When Labor Must Start," page 175, noting the precautions for these procedures.

4. If the mother is not only sleepless but also in pain, long baths, relaxation, massage, and slow breathing will help. See "Self-Help Comfort Measures," page 121, for ideas.

5. Try different positions and movements. The following positions and movements sometimes stimulate labor, by taking advantage of gravity, changing the shape of the mother's pelvis, or encouraging the baby to wiggle into a better position, while relieving backache if she has it.

    - ◆ *The open knee-chest position* (see page 139).
    - ◆ *Hands and knees, with or without pelvic rocking* (see page 138).
    - ◆ *Walking and slow-dancing* (see page 136).
    - ◆ *Abdominal lifting.* While standing, the mother interlocks her fingers and places them against her pubic bone. During contractions, she lifts her abdomen up and slightly in, while bending her knees. This often relieves back pain while improving the position of a baby in the pelvis. You can help her by standing behind her, placing a long woven shawl, folded to about 5 inches wide, around her trunk and below her abdomen, and lifting her abdomen as shown in the illustration. Loosen it when the contraction is over. If you have a nurse or midwife with you, it is a good idea to ask her to listen to the baby's heartbeat during a contraction while the mother does the abdominal lift, just to be sure that the umbilical cord isn't in a place where it can be pressed.

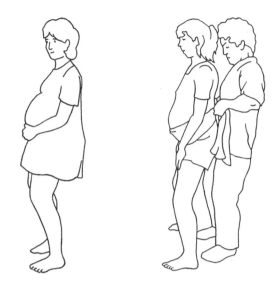

She can alternate these positions and movements with rest.

If these strategies are not enough to get her through a long prelabor, her caregiver may suggest an alcoholic beverage, morphine, or another drug (see page 296).

If the two of you are worried that the mother won't have the stamina to cope with "real" labor after this prolonged prelabor, remind yourself—and her—that she is well equipped at this time in her life to cope with a long period without sleep. Although she feels tired and discouraged, once she begins to make progress her energy level and her spirits will probably rise, allowing her to continue without distress.

Slow Progress in Active Labor and the Birthing Stage, with or without Back Pain

Sometimes labor begins with good progress, but slows down once the woman gets into active labor (after 5 centimeters or so). The delay in progress may be temporary, or it may continue until the birth. This delay is sometimes associated with back pain, sometimes not.

RELIEVING BACK PAIN IN LABOR

One in three women has back pain during active labor, or "back labor." One possible cause is a poor fit between the baby's head and the mother's pelvis. The actual size of the baby's head is less often a problem than is its position in the pelvis. The most favorable head position is occiput anterior, or OA (where the back of the baby's head is toward the mother's front), with the baby's chin tucked to his chest. If instead the back of the baby's head is toward the mother's back (OP, occiput posterior), or the baby's head is tightly positioned sideways (OT, occiput transverse) or tipped back or to one side, then a larger diameter of the baby's head is pressing down into the pelvis. The baby's hand placed next to his face as he enters the pelvis can also cause back pain, and so can variations in the mother's pelvic and spinal anatomy. All these factors and others may cause a delay in labor as well as back pain. Reducing this pain and repositioning the baby are a major focus for the mother and her support team.

Comfort measures for backache during labor. Relaxation and breathing are usually not enough to cope with the pain. Try one or more of the following comfort measures, described in chapter 4: counterpressure, criss-cross massage, the double hip squeeze, rolling pressure over the low back, heat and cold, baths and showers, and transcutaneous electrical nerve stimulation (TENS).

Problems that cause both back pain and a delay in active labor usually resolve spontaneously, but this is likely to happen more quickly if the mother is active and if she tries ways to help the baby change his position.

ENCOURAGING THE BABY TO CHANGE POSITION

It is not always easy to identify the position of the baby in the pelvis; even the most experienced nurses, midwives, and doctors have trouble doing this sometimes. (To learn more about a baby's position in labor and the many ways to identify it, consult www.spinningbabies.com and *The Labor Progress Handbook*; see "Recommended Resources".) But you do not need to know the baby's position before trying some of the measures described in this and the preceding chapter. If there

Slow progress in active labor and the birthing stage, with or without back pain

is a delay in active labor, whether or not the mother has back pain, you should assume there is a need to change the baby's position. Help the mother use the following positions and movements to encourage the baby to change position. Some of these techniques may also relieve back pain.

♦ *Pelvic rocking* (see page 138).

♦ *Slow-dancing* (see page 136).

♦ *Abdominal lifting* (see page 183).

♦ *The lunge* (see page 136), during contractions. Have her try lunging in each direction and then continue with the direction that is the most comfortable for her, for five or six contractions. Help the mother with her balance, and keep the chair from sliding. The lunge is not easy to do, but it may very well correct the problem.

♦ *Side lying.* The mother lies on her side with both hips and knees flexed, and a pillow between her knees. If the nurse or midwife is quite sure the baby's back is toward the left side of the mother's back (left occiput posterior, or LOP), the mother lies on her left side; if she believes the baby is ROP, the mother lies on her right side. If you are not sure of the baby's position, have the mother turn from one side to the other every 20 to 30 minutes.

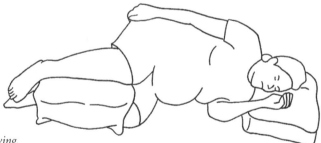

Side lying.

♦ *Lying semiprone.* If the nurse or midwife thinks the baby's back is toward the left side of the mother's back (LOP), the mother lies in the right semiprone position—on her right side with her lower leg out straight. She flexes her upper hip and knee, rests her knee on a doubled-up pillow, and rolls toward her front. If the baby's back is toward the right side of her back, she lies the same way on her left side. If you are not sure of the baby's position, have the mother change sides every 20 to 30 minutes. (The semiprone position is quite different in its gravity effects than the side-lying position, so instructions regarding which side to lie on are different for the two positions.)

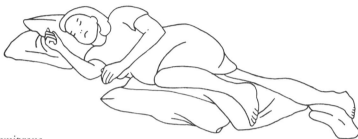

Semiprone.

- *Kneeling and leaning forward.* The mother rests her upper body on a chair or a birth ball (see page 138). Some special hospital beds, called birthing beds, can be adjusted to support this position.
- *Standing and walking.* These take advantage of gravity in encouraging the descent of the baby. In addition, the alignment of the baby within the pelvis is thought to be most favorable when the mother is upright. Also, walking allows some movement within the pelvic joints, which may encourage the baby's rotation.

PROMOTING THE BABY'S DESCENT IN THE BIRTHING STAGE

If there is a delay in descent during the birthing stage, it is important that the mother change position. She can try shifting from semi-sitting to side lying to squatting to sitting on the toilet. She can try unconventional positions such as the dangle, lap squatting, and lying on her back while lifting her head and drawing her knees up toward her armpits. All these positions are described and illustrated on pages 135 to 141.

NOTE: The positions that require the mother to get out of bed are next to impossible if she has been given an epidural. See pages 137 and 139 for positions to use with an epidural.

Also, the dangle and lap squatting require practice ahead of time, and they may not be acceptable to the hospital staff. If you and the mother think these positions are ones that you might want to try, discuss this with her caregiver ahead of time.

Occasionally a baby does not reposition herself, despite the mother's efforts, especially if the baby is large. If so, the baby may be born facing forward ("sunny-side up"), though such a birth is rare. Otherwise, medical or surgical interventions are probably needed to deliver the baby. Possibilities include pain medications (usually an epidural); intravenous Pitocin to strengthen the mother's contractions (see page 226); delivery with forceps or a vacuum extractor (see pages 234 to 236); or, if nothing else works, a cesarean delivery (see pages 305 to 321). It's wise to read about these procedures ahead of time.

You can help the mother deal with a delay in labor by (1) maintaining patience and optimism, (2) helping her change position so the baby can change position and descend, (3) using the techniques described in chapter 4 to relieve any back pain, and, if necessary, (4) helping her ask the "Key Questions for Informed Decision Making" (see page 202). The caregiver's role in this situation is described on page 254 in chapter 7.

When the Mother Must Labor in Bed

Sometimes a woman must remain in bed for labor and birth. These are the most common reasons:

- The mother has high blood pressure. A woman's blood pressure tends to drop when she lies on her left side.

- The mother has used pain medications. If a woman is sleepy or groggy, or if half her body is numb with an epidural, she is able to move in bed but cannot safely get out of bed.

- The mother needs to use equipment that attaches her to machines. Intravenous lines, electronic fetal monitors, bladder catheters, and other devices all tend to make it difficult or impossible for the woman to move out of bed.

- Keeping laboring women in bed is the hospital's custom. Unfortunately, in many hospitals even women with normal labors are routinely discouraged from leaving their beds. There is no medical reason for such a practice.

Being restricted to bed may not distress the mother, especially if it does not add to her pain, or if she had not expected to do otherwise. Many women, however, find lying down to be most uncomfortable in labor. Some women become very restless and are unable to stay down. A woman who had planned to use movement and positioning for comfort or to help her labor progress will be disappointed and will want her caregiver's permission to get out of bed.

Sometimes restricting a woman to bed slows her labor and increases the pain from contractions. She is also prevented from doing many of the things that speed labor and increase comfort.

Here are some things you should do if the mother does not have an epidural and is confined to bed:

1. Find out why. You and she may be able to persuade her caregiver to change the orders if there is no compelling medical reason for the mother to remain in bed. If bed rest is medically necessary, you will both be better able to accept it and cooperate if you understand why.

2. Find out how strict the order is. The mother may be told not to leave the bed, or she may be told not to turn from her left side at all. She may be allowed up for short periods or to go to the bathroom. She may be able to take a bath, which could be as effective for lowering blood pressure as lying on her left side.

3. Ask about alternatives. The mother may be able to use a telemetry unit (see page 219) for electronic fetal monitoring and an IV pole on wheels. These would allow her to be out of bed and walking. Even if she is connected to many machines and containers, she may be able to stand or to sit in a rocker beside the bed.

4. Help her focus on the many pain-coping techniques and comfort measures she can use while in bed, without dwelling too much on what she cannot do. Try relaxation (see page 121), rhythmic breathing (see page 127), attention focusing (see page 124), spontaneous rituals (see page 119), counterpressure and other techniques for relieving back pain (see page 157), massage and

acupressure (see pages 152 to 157), heat and cold (see pages 148 to 150), transcutaneous electrical nerve stimulation (TENS; see page 150), hypnosis (learned ahead of time, see page 123), or the Take-Charge Routine (see page 166).

Although remaining in bed may add to the mother's stress, with your help she can handle this challenge. The key is to understand and accept the reasons she must remain in bed, to focus on the comfort techniques she can still use, and to make sure to give her excellent support.

A Breech Baby

In late pregnancy, about 1 in 30 babies is in a breech presentation, with head up and buttocks or feet, or both, down at the mother's cervix. Many breech babies turn spontaneously to a head-down position, but as the birth approaches they are less likely to do so, because there is less space for large movements like a somersault. There are three types of breech presentation: the *frank* breech, with the buttocks down at the cervix; the *complete* breech, with the knees bent so that both buttocks and feet are down at the cervix; and the *footling* breech, with one or both feet down at the cervix.

Although most breech babies can be born safely, the breech presentation presents some special problems, particularly if the baby is premature or very large. If the bag of waters breaks with a gush, the cord is more likely to prolapse (see page 256), especially with a footling or complete breech presentation. Other difficulties are due mostly to the fact that the head is born last. Sometimes there is a delay in the birth of the head, because it is the largest part of the baby. Sometimes the baby inhales amniotic fluid and vaginal secretions, which can interfere with breathing after birth. Also, when the head is still inside, it can pinch the cord while the baby still depends on it for oxygen.

These risks are reduced when an experienced, skilled caregiver attends the birth. There are few doctors with the necessary skills, however, since obstetric training programs have stopped teaching how to assist at breech births. Doctors who have the necessary skills are unwilling to use them, because the standard of care today requires that all breeches be delivered by cesarean.

If the baby is breech near the mother's due date, a cesarean will probably be scheduled before her due date. Some mothers ask to have their cesareans after labor has started spontaneously, to reduce the odds that their babies will be born prematurely. The option of planning a cesarean after the onset of labor is less available today than in the recent past, because our high cesarean rate means that operating rooms are busier than ever before. Scheduling a cesarean to occur before labor begins increases the efficient use of the surgical facilities.

If the mother wants a vaginal birth, the best bet is to try to turn the baby to a head-down position before labor. Between 32 and 35 weeks' gestation, the mother can try to turn her baby by using one or more of the following techniques: the breech-tilt position, musical or vocal stimulation, or an acupuncturist's technique called moxibustion. Of these techniques, however, only moxibustion has shown some success in scientific studies. Still, these techniques seem generally harmless, and they may help in some cases.

Breech tilt. Three times a day, when her stomach is not full and her baby is active, the mother should either get into the open knee-chest position (see page 139) or lie on the floor or bed on her back with her knees bent and feet flat. While she lifts her hips 12 to 18 inches, slide firm cushions beneath her hips to hold her in the tilted position. She remains in the position for 10 to 15 minutes (less if she is uncomfortable), while she consciously releases tension in her abdomen and trunk and visualizes her baby's head pressing "down" against the top of the uterus and the baby trying to get her head "up" again. *Either breech-tilt position should be avoided if the mother finds it very uncomfortable.*

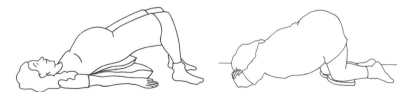

The breech tilt position, done two ways.

Recorded music and your voice. Place stereo headphones low on the mother's abdomen and play rhythmic music at a normal volume. Some people believe babies particularly like baroque or classical music. The idea is that the baby may try to move her head closer so she can hear the music better. You might combine this technique with either breech-tilt position.

You might also try lying with your head in the mother's lap, facing her abdomen, and calling the baby. At a normal voice level, tell her to come down so she can hear you better. Who knows—she just may flip so that she can better hear your voice, with which she is already familiar.

Moxibustion. With this technique, a smoldering stick of a dried herb (mugwort) is held about $1/4$ inch away from the lower outside corner of the nail of each small toe for 15 to 20 minutes two or three times per day. Many acupuncturists teach women and their partners how to do this treatment themselves. It is thought to work by increasing the baby's physical activity.

If this technique appeals to you and the mother, ask your midwife or doctor, childbirth educator, doula, or yoga instructor for a referral to an acupuncturist who is experienced with it. Be sure your caregiver is aware that you want to do this.

BREECH VERSION

If the baby is still breech at 36 to 38 weeks' gestation, the mother and her caregiver may decide to try an *external version*, a procedure for turning a breech baby. Versions have been done for generations in many cultures. This is how they are done today in a medical setting:

1. The mother goes to the doctor's office or hospital, preferably with her partner or a doula to help her relax. An ultrasound scan is performed to confirm the breech presentation and to assess the baby's size, the location of the placenta, the amount of amniotic fluid, and other conditions. An electronic fetal monitor is used to perform a nonstress test to assess the baby's well-being (see page 216).

2. The mother may be given an injection of terbutaline, which relaxes the uterus. A few doctors also give an epidural, to relax the

mother's abdominal muscles and prevent pain from the procedure. Most doctors don't do this, however, because it is too complex, time-consuming, and expensive for such a brief procedure. It is not known whether an epidural improves the chances of a successful version.

3. The mother lies on her back and relaxes.

4. The doctor rubs a lubricant on the mother's abdomen and, with the guidance of ultrasound, presses on her abdomen to lift the baby out of the pelvis and gradually turn the baby around so the head is down. If unsuccessful at first, the doctor may try once or twice more, but usually not more than that.

5. The mother remains as relaxed as possible; the procedure is sometimes quite uncomfortable. You can help by guiding her in light rhythmic breathing, using eye contact, and "conducting," with your hand or head movements, as in the Take-Charge Routine (see page 166). The more relaxed the mother is, and the more tolerant she is of the pressing on her abdomen, the more likely the procedure is to succeed.

6. The baby is checked with ultrasound throughout the procedure. If at any time the baby appears not to be tolerating the procedure, the doctor stops.

7. After the procedure, the mother undergoes another nonstress test to see that the baby has tolerated the procedure well.

After the initial preparation, the version procedure takes only 5 to 20 minutes. Although breech version as practiced today has many built-in safeguards, it also has some slight risks, including fetal distress and bleeding by the mother. These complications are usually identified before they are serious, but, to be safest, most caregivers notify the hospital's labor-and-delivery unit that they are doing a breech version, so that if a serious problem should arise, a cesarean can be performed at once.

Versions are successful 60 to 70 percent of the time. Most of the women who undergo versions give birth vaginally to healthy babies. (Some have cesareans for unrelated reasons that arise during labor; see page 306.)

When a version is unsuccessful, a cesarean delivery is usually planned. If this happens, see pages 318 to 321 for ways to make the cesarean birth special.

A Previous Disappointing or Traumatic Birth Experience

Many women who have gone through labor have some doubts about whether they can "do it again." For those whose previous birth experiences were normal and satisfying, confidence and optimism tend to outweigh apprehension or doubt. But, for the mother who has had an unexpected and scary cesarean birth; a difficult, exhausting, frightening, or traumatic labor; a premature, sick, disabled, or stillborn baby; or a labor in which she felt unsupported or helpless, the memories of these past difficulties may keep coming up. You may also have sadness and self-doubt left over from such an experience. As you both anticipate the upcoming labor and birth, you may be haunted by various doubts and anxieties. The mother may not feel confident about being able to cope with childbirth again; she may be anxious about her own safety, especially if her previous labor ended with a cesarean or with a difficult forceps or vacuum delivery; or she may be worried about the baby, especially if her last baby did not survive or was very ill. You may feel guilty that you did not do enough to help the mother or prevent her disappointment, and you may want to find a way to help her more with the coming birth.

The mother will benefit from special preparation for labor and special understanding and support during labor. The following suggestions should help you to help her:

◆ Look for books about giving birth after a previous cesarean, recovery from a traumatic birth experience, or pregnancy after the loss of a baby (see "Recommended Resources"). You both should read these books.

◆ Look for a support group or a class that helps women and their partners prepare for labor after a previous disappointing birth experience. ICAN (International Cesarean Awareness Network) support groups, VBAC (vaginal birth after cesarean) classes, postpartum depression groups, and Pregnancy After Loss meetings may all be available in your area. These programs help the mother realize that she is not the only woman troubled by a previous difficult birth and that she *can* cope. They also teach the birth partner how to be especially helpful during labor. Ask your caregiver, doula, or childbirth educator for the names of instructors or leaders of these classes and groups.

◆ Browse Web sites and join e-mail groups that focus on difficult childbirths (see "Recommended Resources").

◆ Consider having a doula. As an on-site guide who knows the stress you are under, the doula can advise and assist you to make this birth more satisfying than the previous one.

◆ If either or both of you are very troubled, consider requesting counseling from a seasoned doula or childbirth educator, or a psychotherapist with an understanding of birth-related disappointment or trauma.

◆ Consider the unlikely possibility that the mother's upcoming labor might be similar to the preceding one. Which of the controllable factors would she want to be different this time? For example, if her labor stalled for seven hours last time, would she want earlier intervention if labor should stall again? If she had an induction, or a cesarean that she felt was unwarranted, would she want more of a say in the decision, and a clearer explanation of the reasons, if her caregiver felt such an intervention were needed this time? Does she want to make a different plan this time for the use of pain medication? By facing the possibility that a similar labor could occur, and knowing that it will be handled differently, she will be freed of much of her fear and will be able to look forward to a better experience.

◆ Encourage her to discuss her distress and her wishes with her caregiver, and note her previous experience and her worries in her Birth Plan.

You should also anticipate the mother's unique emotional needs. Besides the typical emotional responses to labor (see chapters 2 and 3), there are some additional emotional hurdles that the woman who has had a disappointing past experience may have to overcome during labor. They are described here, along with suggestions about how you can help:

- *Early labor.* As she gets into labor, the mother may suddenly lose heart. This is her "moment of truth," and she may be flooded with self-doubt. Encourage her to talk about her feelings, and then remind her that such feelings are normal under the circumstances. This will help her to carry on and avoid overreacting to her contractions out of fear. Review chapter 2, "Getting into Labor," and "The Slow-to-Start Labor," page 180, for ideas about helping the mother accept rather than dread her labor.

- *Flashbacks to the previous labor.* At times, the mother may not be able to escape the feeling that her labor is "just like last time." You can help by acknowledging the similarities in the two labors, by discussing the mother's feelings, and, most important, by reminding her that this is not "last time" but a completely new labor that she must deal with as such.

- *Reaching the point in labor at which she had the cesarean or other difficulty in the last labor.* Some women feel a great deal of apprehension before they reach this critical point, and are relieved only after it has passed. Try to help the mother with distraction and stress-reduction measures (see chapter 4, "Comfort Measures for Labor"), and then rejoice with her when she has passed beyond her critical point.

A great potential for healing and growth exists when a woman confronts her difficult memories and deals constructively with them. With preparation beforehand and sensitive, capable support during labor—from you, a doula, and a caring, understanding staff—the mother's experience of birth is almost certain to be far more satisfying and fulfilling than her previous experience was.

Incompatibility with the Nurse or Caregiver

One shortcoming of the North American system of maternity care is that the mother is usually cared for by people she has never met. She hardly ever knows her nurses; she scarcely knows her doctor, whom she may have met briefly no more than eight times during her pregnancy. And if her own doctor is not on call when she goes into labor, she is assisted by a substitute doctor who may be a complete stranger. Spending time getting to know the mother is one of the features of good midwifery, but some overworked midwives' practices today have the same shortcomings as doctors' typically do.

Most of the time no serious problems arise in the birth room; the mother, her partner, her caregiver, and the nurses get along quite well. What do you do, though, if one or both of you is uncomfortable with the nurse or caregiver? Differences in attitudes toward childbirth, in personality, or in perceptions of each other's roles sometimes become obvious during labor. Discomfort or friction may arise. This *never* works in the mother's best interests. She needs to be surrounded by kind people who she believes will encourage and support her.

If, before labor, you or the mother anticipates problems, be sure to prepare and discuss a Birth Plan with her caregiver (see page 26). Also, consider hiring a doula to work with the two of you, ahead of time and during labor, to help smooth relations with the staff and to help you and the mother advocate for yourselves.

Usually, problems with the staff are not serious and can easily be resolved. Following are some suggestions for avoiding, minimizing, or solving conflicts:

◆ Do not be the cause of any friction yourself. By your attitude and your behavior, show that you are friendly, respectful, and polite, that you expect to work well with the staff, and that you appreciate their experience and the contributions they can make to the mother's comfort and well-being. If you appear suspicious, frightened, or hostile, the staff might react defensively.

◆ Make an effort to communicate any of the mother's special concerns—for example, a desire for natural childbirth, a fear of needles or blood, and so forth.

◆ Have a copy of the mother's Birth Plan at hand for the nurse to read. If there is time, discuss the Birth Plan with the nurse or caregiver, and ask for help in following the plan as closely as possible. If a staff member has any concerns about the Birth Plan, it is better to discuss these concerns than to ignore them. Differences can usually be resolved easily.

◆ Call the nurse or caregiver by name.

If there are differences between you or the mother and the nurse, try one or more of the following tactics:

◆ Deal with the nurse politely. Say, for example, "I cannot talk with you during contractions because I need to help [the mother] breathe and relax," or "I think there is a misunderstanding. Our doctor said it would be fine for [the mother] to walk around and use the shower. Would you please check with her doctor?"

◆ Talk to the head nurse. In a nonaccusatory way, explain any differences you and your assigned nurse have, and ask the head nurse to assign another nurse or to help mediate the problem.

◆ Talk directly to the mother's caregiver (by phone, if necessary). If there is an apparent misunderstanding over the nurse's management of labor, ask the caregiver to deal with it.

If the problem is with the doctor or midwife (especially if this is someone the mother has never met before), you can try to discuss it directly. If this doesn't solve the problem, ask the nurse to intervene on the mother's behalf and advocate for her. Or, if the problem involves a clinical decision, ask for a thorough explanation, using the "Key Questions for Informed Decision Making" (see page 202), or ask for a second opinion.

How can a doula help you? The doula has no authority to intervene with the staff on your behalf. She cannot be your voice or the mother's. She is, however, likely to recognize when a particular action or intervention may lead to a significant departure from your Birth Plan. She can cue you to ask the Key Questions for Informed Decision Making,

Incompatibility with the nurse or caregiver

or suggest that you ask for more time before agreeing to an intervention that you had hoped to avoid. This will help ensure that you and the mother will participate in decisions, and will not be rushed.

Sometimes the best interests of the mother are served by avoiding conflict rather than by resolving it. In other words, to avoid a stressful confrontation, you may have to accept a less-than-ideal arrangement and work with it.

If you are in the unlikely position of being stuck with a nurse or caregiver with whom you are incompatible and who will not yield, accept the situation for the moment and focus your energies on helping the mother cope. You may feel powerless and frustrated under these circumstances, but you cannot stop labor while the problem gets settled. And trying to resolve a disagreement in the midst of labor might make the labor harder and more stressful for the mother. After the baby is born, you can pursue the matter, by discussing the situation with the caregiver or a counselor, or both, and writing a letter to those responsible for patient care. Although this effort will probably not benefit you, the mother, or the baby, your efforts may help prevent similar difficulties for another laboring woman in the future.

Incompatibility with the nurse or caregiver

PART THREE

The Medical Side of Childbirth

The caregiver's primary role in childbirth is to safeguard the health of mother and child. Throughout pregnancy, the caregiver relies on a wide assortment of tests, technologies, and procedures to detect and treat problems before they become serious. Similar tests, technologies, and procedures (often referred to as "interventions") are available during childbirth.

Caregivers differ among themselves regarding what should constitute routine basic care during childbirth. Some caregivers feel birth is so unpredictable that it is safest to use many medical procedures in every labor, whether they are needed or not. Others believe that childbirth is essentially a normal physiological process, and use medical or surgical interventions only when problems are suspected or detected. Pregnant women differ among themselves over the same issues. Some are fearful and feel more secure with a highly medical approach, while others perceive birth as normal and are wary of excessive interventions. They place more trust in their bodies and their inner resources than in technology.

Research has shown that, for a healthy woman, labor proceeds normally and without hazard most of the time, and that careful observation is all that is necessary to detect problems in time to take medical action. Actually, one way to *avoid* problems is to be cautious about using optional procedures and medications; these can sometimes *cause* problems. For example, any procedure that restricts the mother's freedom to move might slow labor or increase her pain, thus making further interventions more likely and actually increasing her risk of developing other problems. For these reasons, technology, medications, and procedures are appropriate and necessary only when problems already exist or are very likely to occur.

Tests and interventions always involve tradeoffs. The mother needs to know what she gives up and what she gains before deciding whether to accept a nonemergency intervention. When considering interventions, discuss the following questions with each other and with the caregiver.

Key Questions for Informed Decision Making

When a test is suggested, ask:

◆ What is the reason for the test? What questions will it answer?

◆ How is the test done?

◆ How accurate or reliable are the results? Is there a margin of error? In other words, might the test miss a problem that exists, or indicate a problem that does not exist?

◆ If the test detects a problem, what happens next (for example, further testing or immediate treatment)?

◆ If the test does not detect a problem, what happens next (for example, a repeat test in a day or two, other tests, or no further concern about the problem)?

◆ What will this test cost the mother, if anything?

When a treatment is suggested, ask:

- What is the problem, and how serious is it?
- How urgent is the need to begin treatment?
- What is the treatment, and how is it done?
- How likely is it to solve the problem?
- If the treatment fails, what are the next steps?
- Are there any side effects to the treatment?
- Are there any alternatives (including waiting, doing nothing, or other treatments)?

If an alternative is suggested, again ask how it is done, how likely it is to work, what its side effects are, and what happens if the alternative treatment fails.

In most situations, there is plenty of time to discuss these questions. In an emergency, however, there may not be time. The caregiver should tell you how serious and urgent the situation is. If it is urgent, you must trust the caregiver and help the mother accept the interventions. A full explanation may have to wait until the emergency is over. In this case, simply ask, "Will this intervention improve the odds of a healthy mother and baby?"

Chapters 6 through 9 discuss the tests, technologies, interventions (including cesarean birth), and medications commonly used in childbirth, along with the problems they are designed to detect and treat.

CHAPTER 6

Tests, Technologies, Interventions, and Procedures

She was now a full-on tube-o-saurus—the IV and Pitocin tube in her vein, the epidural tube in her back, the urine catheter, baby heartbeat and contraction monitors up inside her, and a mask to super-oxygenate her blood so the baby could get more oxygen. The nurse checked her cervix and said she was now at 4 centimeters—she had been at 3 centimeters six hours earlier. I said, "All that crap for 1 centimeter?"

—KEVIN, FIRST-TIME FATHER

During the last month of pregnancy, women usually see their caregivers once a week. This is a time when problems that can affect labor may surface for the first time, and their detection now may help the caregiver plan how to care for the mother during labor. Following are descriptions of some common late-pregnancy tests and why and how they are done. This information cannot substitute for discussing the Key Questions (see page 202) with her caregiver but may provide background on which to base your questions. Omitted here are routine tests given in early pregnancy or at every prenatal checkup.

Late-Pregnancy Tests

During the final weeks or months of pregnancy, the mother's caregiver watches closely for conditions in the mother or baby that might affect the outcome of the birth. Results of the tests described here guide her caregiver in planning the clinical management of the birth.

GROUP B STREP (GBS) SCREENING

This is a test for the presence in the mother of particular bacteria, called Group B streptococci. Offered at 35 to 37 weeks of pregnancy, the test involves culturing a sample of secretions from her vagina or rectum. Results are usually available in about two days, although a rapid test, which gives results within minutes, is being developed.

One in every three to four pregnant women is a "carrier" of GBS, which means that the bacteria are present in her bodily fluids but she shows no signs of infection. Approximately 1 percent of babies born to these women acquire a GBS infection, which can cause serious illnesses in the newborn, such as pneumonia, sepsis (infection in the blood), and meningitis. GBS infections in newborns can be almost entirely prevented by giving intravenous antibiotics to every mother who has tested positive for Group B strep, after her membranes rupture or when she goes into labor. The antibiotics, which reach the baby via the placenta, lower the risk of newborn infection to 1 in 2,000 to 4,000. The antibiotics also lower the mother's risk of developing an active GBS infection, which may cause fever, uterine or urinary-tract infection, and abdominal pain.

If a GBS carrier gives birth before she has received sufficient antibiotics, her baby is observed for symptoms of infection, tested for Group B strep, or both. The tests used vary among caregivers. Some rely on only a blood culture; others also culture the baby's urine and spinal fluid. Some caregivers treat all these babies with intravenous antibiotics and observe them closely for signs of infection for two to three days, until the tests are complete. Others watch the babies closely and treat only if the baby shows signs of infection before the test results come back. If Group B strep bacteria are present in the cultures, the antibiotic treatment continues for many days, during which the baby must remain in the hospital.

The main disadvantage of GBS screening is that, if a woman is found to be a carrier, she not only must take antibiotics but will probably also have labor induced if her membranes rupture without contractions. Several doses of antibiotics may be given during the waiting period. A common practice is to give a maximum of four doses, and to plan induction if the mother does not go into labor within 24 hours. Some caregivers are more patient than others under these circumstances, as are some women. Either choice—large amounts of antibiotics over time, or induction—has disadvantages (see page 229).

Many women are happy to learn that the antibiotics, although given intravenously, are administered only every four to six hours, depending on the antibiotic. Between doses, the IV line can be plugged and disconnected. Women planning an out-of-hospital birth do not have to switch to a hospital birth because of Group B strep, but they do have to visit their midwife every four to six hours for the antibiotics.

ULTRASONOGRAPHY

This complex technology involves the transmission of high-frequency ("ultrasound") sound waves through a hand-held "probe" into the woman's uterus from outside her abdomen or within her vagina. This allows for a detailed see-through picture of the baby (brain, heart, other organs, facial features, limbs, genitals—everything), placenta, umbilical cord, cervix, and other structures. The picture appears on a video screen that you and the mother can see along with the technician.

Ultrasonography is used for numerous purposes throughout pregnancy. In late pregnancy, it is used mostly to identify the baby's presentation when a breech or other difficult presentation is suspected, to estimate the baby's growth and weight, and to measure the volume of amniotic fluid. A decrease may indicate that the placenta is no longer functioning very well; an increase may indicate a problem with the mother's fluid regulation or the baby's kidneys. Unfortunately, the margin of error with these estimates can be considerable.

Ultrasonography is done this way: The mother lies in a dimly lit room, and the ultrasonographer lubricates her abdomen and slides the probe over her belly. Photographs are taken and measurements made at different depths of the mother's and baby's tissues. The whole scan may take up to 30 minutes.

Then a radiologist analyzes the ultrasonographer's report for the obstetrician or midwife, who makes recommendations, such as continuing the pregnancy without concern, administering more tests, inducing labor, delivering the baby by cesarean, or trying a breech version.

If during labor the baby is suspected to be OP, a brief ultrasound scan may be done to determine the baby's position (see page 45).

Nonstress Test

This test assesses the baby's well-being by measuring heart-rate changes that occur when the baby moves in the uterus. The nonstress test is recommended when the mother notices a slowing of the baby's movements (see "How to Count Fetal Movements," page 23), when the caregiver feels the baby's growth may be less than expected, or when the mother is overdue or has high blood pressure, diabetes, or another medical condition.

Using an external electronic fetal monitor (see page 216), the mother presses a button when she feels her baby move. If the baby's heart rate speeds up, this is a good sign; the heart rate is said to be "reactive." If the rate stays the same or slows—if it is "nonreactive"—this may indicate that the baby is stressed, and further tests or corrective action may be necessary.

The nonstress test is not wholly accurate. When the test indicates that a baby is doing well, this is usually so. When it indicates that a baby is not doing well, however, the results are often wrong. Further testing is usually a good idea under these circumstances. Combining ultrasonography with the nonstress test (in what is called the Fetal Biophysical Profile) seems to give a more complete picture of a baby's well-being.

Essential Observations During Labor

What constitutes basic care during the labor of the low-risk mother—that is, the mother who is in good general health, who has experienced a normal pregnancy, and whose baby is in a favorable position within the uterus? By making certain simple observations regularly during the labor, the skilled caregiver or nurse can accurately assess whether the mother and baby are fine or whether closer observation or treatment is needed.

Basic care includes the following essential observations of the mother, the progress of labor, the amniotic fluid (the water in the bag of waters), the fetus, and the newborn.

The caregiver or nurse makes these observations of the mother:

- Her behavior, activity, and emotional state during and between contractions and after the birth.
- Her basic body functions: eating, drinking, urination, bowel movements.
- Her contractions: their frequency, intensity, and duration.
- The tone of the uterus between contractions.
- The location and nature of labor pain (in her abdomen, back, or both, and whether the pain is continuous or intermittent).
- Her rating of her pain (on a scale of 0 to 10). Most hospitals, by policy, assess every patient's level of pain and offer pain medication if the pain is increasing or if it is distressing to the patient.
- Her vaginal secretions.
- The progress of labor (determined by the pattern of contractions, her behavior, and occasional vaginal exams).
- Her vital signs: temperature, pulse, and respiration.
- Her blood pressure.
- The tone of her uterus after childbirth.
- The amount of bleeding after childbirth.

When the mother's bag of waters breaks, the caregiver or nurse makes these observations of her amniotic fluid:

◆ The color. If the fluid is clear, the baby has probably not been stressed. A brown or green color indicates a fetal bowel movement (meconium), which means the baby has been stressed.

◆ The amount (a leak or a gush). Losing a large amount of fluid increases the likelihood of pressure on the umbilical cord during contractions, which could cause stress to the baby.

◆ The odor. A foul smell indicates infection.

The caregiver or nurse makes these observations of the fetus:

◆ The heartbeat, monitored by frequent listening with an ultrasound device or a stethoscope.

◆ The size (approximate weight).

Immediately after birth, the caregiver or nurse makes these observations of the newborn:

◆ The Apgar score at 1, 5, and perhaps 10 minutes after birth.

◆ The baby's temperature, respiration, and pulse.

◆ The baby's general behavior and state of alertness.

◆ The baby's physical appearance.

THE APGAR SCORE

SIGN	0 POINTS	1 POINT	2 POINTS
Heart rate	Absent	Below 100 per minute	Over 100 per minute
Breathing	Absent	Slow, irregular	Good, crying
Muscle tone	Limp	Arms and legs close to body	Active, moving
Reflex irritability	No response to suctioning	Grimace	Struggle, cough, or sneeze
Color	Blue-gray	Body pink or ruddy, fingers and toes blue	All pink or ruddy

These simple observations, if made frequently by a caregiver or nurse who is with the mother continuously or nearly so, give a very good idea of both the mother's condition and the baby's. As long as they indicate normal conditions, these observations are all that are truly needed. One-to-one care of the mother by the caregiver or nurse, and the continuous presence of the birth partner, doula, or another supporter, allows for strong emotional support and help with pain-relieving measures at all times. Being with the mother continuously also allows the caregiver or nurse to make other important but less tangible observations about the labor, the mother, or the baby.

In many busy hospitals, continuous one-to-one care from a nurse is impossible. Instead, each nurse cares for two or three laboring women at a time. Each mother has periodic contact with a variety of nurses and doctors, and there is greater reliance on technological substitutes (electronic fetal monitors that transmit data to the nurses' station, intravenous fluid pumps, and pain medications) that allow the nurses to care for more women simultaneously.

The two approaches result in about the same proportion of healthy mothers and babies. The difference lies more in how these outcomes are achieved. The two approaches can be combined, of course: Continuous nursing and emotional support can be offered along with technology and interventions. This combination is the safest and most effective way to care for mothers who are at moderate or high risk for having problems during labor.

Conditions Influencing the Amount of Intervention

Beyond the essential observations, many tests, procedures, and medications constitute the medical side of childbirth. These include the use of highly specialized equipment, a variety of drugs, and surgery. How and when they are used depends on a number of considerations:

◆ *The medical condition of the mother.* As I have already noted, there is less need for intervention when the mother has had a healthy pregnancy and labor is progressing well.

- *The apparent well-being of the fetus.* If the fetus is fully developed and mature, of normal size, and apparently unstressed, most interventions are not needed.

- *The training and philosophy of the caregiver.* Some caregivers routinely use more interventions than others, preferring to treat problems before they arise. Although this practice often results in unnecessary treatment, these caregivers feel that the overtreatment is harmless, and that without it they would miss problems. Better safe than sorry, they believe. Other caregivers are comfortable watching the mother, baby, and labor progress, and using treatment only if a problem arises; they believe that unnecessary treatment can cause problems. The scientific literature supports the latter approach.

- *The usual practices or policies of the institution and nursing staff.* These practices or policies are determined by current standards of care, nurses' training, the size and competence of the staff, customs, legal concerns, financial constraints, and other factors. There is much variation in usual practices among hospitals, even in the same geographical area. In one hospital, for example, women may be encouraged to be out of bed and moving about or using the bath in labor. In another hospital nearby, they may be discouraged from doing these things. Rates of labor induction, epidural analgesia, and cesarean delivery also vary widely among hospitals.

- *The preferences of the mother.* Within each institution and within each caregiver's practice, there is room for choice. Make sure the caregiver knows the mother's preferences (see "Prepare and Review the Mother's Birth Plan," page 26); try to ensure that her preferences are considered in all of the decisions that are made.

Common Obstetric Interventions

Following are descriptions of many common obstetric procedures and their purposes, disadvantages, and possible alternatives. These are usually unnecessary when labor is normal, but they may become necessary if problems arise. Chapter 7, "Complications in Late Pregnancy, Labor, or Afterward," discusses the circumstances under which these procedures are necessary for medical reasons.

As her birth partner, you will be the liaison between the mother and the hospital staff. A doula can advise you in this role. It is important for you to be familiar with common obstetric interventions so that you can inform the staff about the mother's preferences, help the mother make decisions about optional procedures, and help her handle any additional discomfort—emotional or physical—that may arise from the interventions. It is also important for you to make sure the mother understands any changes in her labor that make particular interventions necessary for safety.

INTRAVENOUS (IV) FLUIDS

An intravenous drip is a plastic bag of liquids that include water and electrolytes, dextrose, or medications. The bag hangs from a pole attached to the bed or a pole on wheels; the latter allows the mother to walk. A tube extending from the bag is inserted into a vein in the mother's hand or arm. The liquid drips into the vein.

Purposes of giving IV fluids. Intravenous fluids may be given (1) to provide the mother liquids, calories, or both, instead of having her take them by mouth; (2) to administer medications; (3) with an epidural, to increase her blood volume to protect against a drop in blood pressure; or (4) to keep a vein open, just in case the mother requires medications later on.

Many caregivers give intravenous fluids to all their patients in labor, because they do not want the women to eat or drink anything. They feel an empty stomach is best. Their reason dates from the time when most women gave birth while unconscious under general anesthesia. It was dangerous for a woman to have a full stomach while under general anesthesia, because she might vomit and breathe in the vomited material. General anesthesia is now rarely used for childbirth and, when it is, better techniques help protect the patient from this complication. Still, many caregivers today continue the out-of-date and unnecessary policy of giving all mothers IVs.

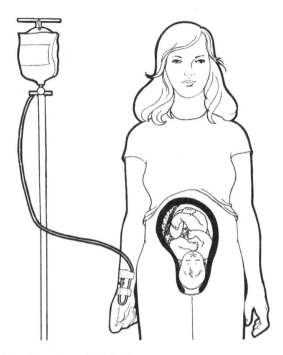

A woman receiving intravenous (IV) fluids.

Some caregivers have a less positive attitude toward intravenous fluids. They believe intravenous fluids are problematic much of the time, and they encourage mothers to meet their need for fluids by drinking enough to satisfy their thirst. Intravenous fluids are reserved for times when they are "medically indicated"—that is, when they are necessary or desirable because of the medical condition of the mother or baby.

When are IV fluids medically indicated?

- When labor is very long.

- When the mother has continuous nausea and vomiting.

- When she will receive local or general anesthesia (see pages 288 to 290).

- When she needs certain IV medications—to stop preterm labor, to induce or augment labor, to control blood pressure, to reduce pain, or for another reason.

- When she has a condition that might require immediate medical action.

Disadvantages of giving IV fluids. These are:

- IV fluids in large amounts may cause temporary low blood sugar in the mother and baby after birth (if the fluids contain dextrose, a type of sugar), or electrolyte imbalance (if the fluids contain electrolytes) in the baby soon after birth.

- Large amounts of IV fluids cause fluid retention in the mother, especially in her legs and breasts. This takes days to disappear, and the increase in breast engorgement makes breastfeeding more difficult during the first week. Rarely, excess fluid accumulates in the mother's lungs (this is called pulmonary edema).

- An IV line is inconvenient and somewhat stressful for the mother, who must make sure it is out of the way as she rolls over or gets out of bed.

- IV lines sometimes "infiltrate," that is, they poke through the vein. The fluids then go directly into the mother's tissue, causing pain and swelling. If the fluids contain medications, they do no good, since they do not get into her bloodstream.

IV fluids are unnecessary if the mother drinks enough liquid and does not need IV medications. She requires about $1/4$ cup liquid per hour, or somewhat more if she is sweating a lot or doing mostly light breathing. The best policy is usually to encourage her to drink when she feels thirsty, or to offer liquids after every contraction or two for her to take or not, as she wishes.

Alternatives to consider. You and the mother can discuss the following alternatives to an IV with the mother's caregiver:

- If labor is proceeding rapidly, give the mother no IV fluids; she may get along well without any fluids, by vein or by mouth.

- Offer the mother fluids to drink, such as water, fruit juice, or sports beverages (with their added electrolytes), or frozen juice bars to eat. It is a good idea for her to drink a little after each contraction or two.

♦ Keep a vein open so the caregiver can give intravenous medications very quickly if the need arises. The caregiver or nurse places a short, flexible tube in a vein in the mother's arm above her wrist, but then plugs it instead of connecting it to an intravenous line. This procedure (called a *heparin lock* or *saline flush*) allows the mother more freedom to move around than does an intravenous line.

ELECTRONIC FETAL MONITORING (EFM)

There are two methods of electronic fetal monitoring (EFM): external and internal.

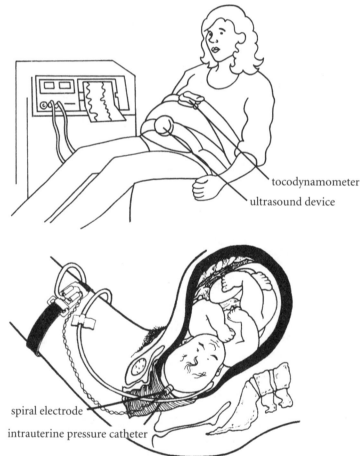

Electronic fetal monitoring (EFM): external (above) and internal (below).

With external monitoring, the nurse or caregiver places two stretchy belts around the mother's abdomen. One belt, placed low on the woman's abdomen, holds an ultrasound device that detects the fetal heartbeat. The other, placed higher, holds a device (a *tocodynamometer*) that detects contractions.

With internal fetal monitoring, a thin, spiral wire electrode is placed in the skin of the baby's scalp to detect the fetal heart rate electronically, and a fluid-filled tube (an *intrauterine pressure catheter*) is placed within the mother's uterus to measure the intensity of the contractions. When the uterus contracts, fluid is squeezed out of the tube, and a gauge precisely measures the strength of the contraction.

Both external and internal monitoring devices are connected by wires to a calibrating and recording machine that flashes numbers every second on a digital display, indicating both the fetal heart rate and the tone of the uterus. These readings are continuously printed out on paper in graph form. Some women and their partners find the contraction monitor a helpful guide to when to begin rhythmic breathing and relaxation for each contraction.

External monitoring is easier to apply, less invasive, and much more widely used than internal monitoring, but the latter is more accurate. Internal monitoring is reserved for times when external monitoring is not tracking the fetal heartbeat or the contractions accurately enough (as with an obese mother, contractions of questionable intensity, and other situations).

Purposes of EFM during labor. EFM is used to help the caregiver or nurse assess the baby's response to labor and tell when the woman has contractions (as if she does not know!), and to record the length, frequency, and (with internal monitoring) intensity of the contractions.

When is EFM medically indicated during labor?

◆ When labor is prolonged and the caregiver is considering speeding progress by administering Pitocin (see page 226). The length and frequency of the contractions can be assessed with the external tocodynamometer. If the caregiver needs an accurate measurement of the intensity of the contractions, the intrauterine pressure catheter is used.

- When a nurse or a midwife cannot be with the mother continuously or frequently.

- When the mother receives Pitocin or other medications that make the contractions too intense for the fetus.

- When there are doubts during labor about the fetus's well-being (because of prematurity, small size, meconium-stained amniotic fluid, or possible lack of oxygen).

- When the mother is considered to be at high risk for complications.

Disadvantages of EFM. These are:

- The mother's movements are restricted, although she can change position in bed and sometimes even stand by the bed or sit in a chair. Internal monitoring is less restrictive than external monitoring.

- Sometimes more attention is paid to the machine than to the mother. As her birth partner, do not allow yourself to fall into this trap.

- Interpretation of the monitor printouts ("tracings") is extremely complex, and experts even disagree about what different heart-rate patterns really mean and when intervention is necessary.

- Internal monitoring requires breaking both the bag of waters and the skin of the fetal scalp. These procedures slightly increase the risk of infection to mother and baby, especially if the mother has an infection or sore in her vagina. Also, breaking the bag of waters may cause additional stress to the fetus by removing the cushion of fluid that protects the head and cord.

- EFM measures only the fetal pulse, not actual fetal distress—that is, a shortage of oxygen. When a cesarean is done solely because of EFM tracings, the baby may show no signs of having suffered fetal distress. For this reason, other tests have been tried to confirm the findings of EFM (see "Fetal Scalp Stimulation Test," page 220, and "Fetal Pulse Oximetry," page 220).

Alternatives to consider. Before labor, you and the mother can discuss the following alternatives to EFM and then state your preferences in your Birth Plan:

- Have a nurse or the caregiver listen frequently to fetal heart tones with an ultrasound stethoscope or a fetal stethoscope, for 1 to 2 minutes at a time during and after a contraction. Many studies have compared this method of monitoring with continuous EFM, and all have found that listening to heart tones intermittently results in equally healthy babies and fewer cesareans. This method, called *auscultation*, requires that the nurse have good listening skills and be available for about 5 minutes out of every 15 in active labor, and continuously during the birthing stage.

◆ Use external EFM intermittently for 10 to 15 minutes each hour. This enables the mother to move around the rest of the time.

◆ Use a portable radio-transmission (telemetry) EFM unit. There are two types: In one, the woman wears a radio transmitter around her neck; the transmitter is connected by wires to the sensors in the belts. The other, newer version is wireless. The radio transmitters are located within each sensor, and the sensors are waterproof. Either type allows the mother to move about freely (within about 200 feet of the nurses' station) while information is radioed back to a central monitor and the monitor in her room. Find out whether the hospital has telemetry units available.

◆ Use a hand-held waterproof ultrasound stethoscope or the waterproof telemetry units for listening to the baby when the mother is in the bath.

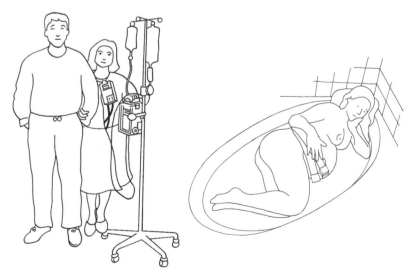

Portable telemetry units: wired (left) and wireless (right), with woman in the bath.

FETAL SCALP STIMULATION TEST

The caregiver performs this simple test by pressing or scratching the baby's scalp during a vaginal exam. If the baby is in good condition, his heart rate will speed up with such stimulation. If the baby is distressed (that is, short of oxygen), the heart rate will not speed up. The results of this test have been found to correlate well with the actual condition of the fetus.

Purposes of the fetal scalp stimulation test. This test is performed to check whether the baby is truly in distress when EFM or monitoring by stethoscope suggests that he may be. The test is medically indicated at any time fetal distress is suspected, and certainly before a cesarean is performed for fetal distress. It can be performed any number of times during labor.

Disadvantages of the fetal scalp stimulation test. A vaginal exam is required every time the test is performed. It is reliable in detecting the baby's condition at the moment, but it is not predictive; that is why it may need to be repeated.

Alternatives to consider. The alternatives to performing the fetal scalp stimulation test include the following: (1) relying on EFM alone; (2) relying on frequent listening to the fetal heart rate alone; or (3) relying on EFM plus fetal pulse oximetry (see the discussion that follows). None of these provides an advantage over the fetal stimulation test; the first two result in more false diagnoses and unnecessary treatment of fetal distress, and the last is far more expensive and cumbersome, and far less effective.

You and the mother can ask for the fetal scalp stimulation test whenever fetal distress is suspected. Discuss it with her caregiver in advance, and state your preference for it in her Birth Plan (see page 26).

FETAL PULSE OXIMETRY (FPO)

In some large teaching hospitals, this procedure may be used with electronic fetal monitoring when EFM indicates that the fetal heart-rate pattern is "nonreassuring" or that the baby may not be getting enough oxygen. FPO involves the insertion of a Band-Aid-sized sensor through the cervix. Connected by a wire to the monitor console, the sensor is placed alongside the baby's cheek, where it detects the amount of oxygen in the baby's blood.

An advantage over the fetal scalp stimulation test is that FPO provides a continuous rather than periodic record of the oxygen level in the baby's blood.

Purposes of FPO. As a more direct measure of fetal well-being than electronic fetal monitoring alone, FPO has been thought to identify which babies with "nonreassuring" heart-rate patterns are actually suffering from a lack of oxygen, and which are not. When first introduced in the early 2000s, FPO was believed capable of sparing women from cesareans for misdiagnosed fetal distress. Unfortunately, large scientific trials have found that FPO does not lower either the total cesarean rate or the cesarean rate for fetal distress. Furthermore, there have been no improvements in outcomes for the newborns in the studies. For these reasons, FPO is unlikely to be adopted into widespread use.

Disadvantages of FPO. These are:

◆ FPO is very expensive compared to the fetal scalp stimulation test, which costs nothing. Each single-use sensor costs $100 to $200, and if it is placed incorrectly or it becomes covered with the baby's vernix (a creamy coating on the skin), it has to be discarded and replaced.

◆ The sensor must be placed flat against the baby's cheek, which is challenging because it must be done by feel. A doctor's skill at this improves with experience, however.

◆ Before FPO can be used, the membranes must be ruptured and the cervix partially dilated. If the membranes have not ruptured spontaneously, the caregiver ruptures them artificially (see below).

◆ FPO is not helpful in reducing the risk of a cesarean for misdiagnosed fetal distress.

ARTIFICIAL RUPTURE OF THE MEMBRANES (AROM)

To rupture the membranes, or "break the bag of waters," the caregiver inserts a long, thin instrument (an *amnihook*) into the vagina and through the cervix, and painlessly tears the sac holding the amniotic fluid, which comes streaming out. Sometimes, following AROM, the woman's contractions suddenly increase in intensity; this is usually the aim of the procedure.

In the past, women were warned against taking baths after their membranes were ruptured, but scientific trials have found that bathing in a clean tub after AROM does not increase the chance of infection in mother or baby.

Purposes of AROM. AROM is done:

+ To speed labor. If timed correctly, AROM shortens labor by an average of 40 minutes. If the baby is malpositioned, however, the procedure may actually lengthen labor. This may be because rupturing the membranes removes the cushion of fluid around the baby's head, causing the head to be wedged more firmly into the pelvis, and lessening the chances that the baby's position will improve. It cannot always be predicted which labors will be shortened by AROM and which will not. But the gamble may be worth taking if labor progress is poor, because other interventions to speed labor are more complex and potentially risky.

+ To induce labor with or without other methods, such as prostaglandins or oxytocin (see pages 225 to 226). AROM alone is not likely to induce labor unless the cervix is very soft and thin.

+ To check the amniotic fluid for a fetal bowel movement (that is, for the presence of meconium, which signals fetal stress), for infection, for bleeding, or for other signs of problems.

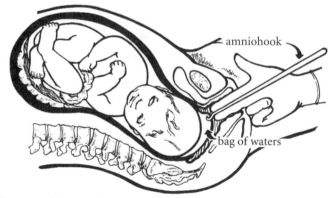

Artificial rupture of the membranes.

◆ To apply the electrode and catheter for internal EFM (see page 218) or the sensor for FPO (see page 220).

When is AROM medically indicated? This question is controversial. The frequency with which caregivers use AROM, especially in early labor, varies widely. Some believe it is innocuous and use it for most of their patients in labor. Others believe its advantages rarely outweigh its disadvantages; they reserve it for situations in which they feel they must intervene. Otherwise, they prefer to leave the membranes intact.

Disadvantages of AROM. These are:

◆ Frequently, it does not speed labor.

◆ The chances of the mother or baby getting an infection increase with the passage of time after the bag of waters is broken, and with the number of vaginal exams performed.

◆ Removing the protective cushion of fluid from around the baby's head may increase pressure on the head during contractions and cause fetal distress.

◆ If the baby's head is malpositioned, removing the fluid surrounding her head may take away her "wiggle room" and thereby decrease the chance that she will be able to reposition herself.

◆ AROM increases the risk that the umbilical cord will be compressed during contractions, and this compression could cause a lack of oxygen for the baby.

◆ If the baby's head (or buttocks, if the baby is breech) is high when AROM is done, the danger of a prolapsed cord (see page 256) increases.

Alternatives to consider. The caregiver can:

◆ Refrain from breaking the bag of waters to speed labor, and suggest that the mother try self-help methods to stimulate contractions (see pages 176 to 180).

◆ Use other methods to check for fetal distress (see "Electronic Fetal Monitoring," page 216, and "Fetal Scalp Stimulation Test," page 220) or to induce labor.

AMNIOINFUSION

In this painless procedure, saline solution (salty water) is sent into the uterus via a plastic tube, the same kind used in internal EFM to assess the intensity of contractions (see page 217). Amnioinfusion is done after the bag of waters has broken, if the baby's umbilical cord is being compressed during contractions.

Purposes of amnioinfusion. The added fluid helps to cushion the cord and may protect against fetal distress. The procedure also is helpful if the baby has passed meconium in the uterus. The fluid dilutes the meconium to protect against problems that would occur if the baby were to inhale thick meconium during birth. Although the injected fluid gradually runs out of the uterus, the procedure can be repeated as necessary to maintain a sufficient volume. This simple technique, which is extremely low in cost, sometimes makes it possible to safely avoid a cesarean for fetal distress.

Disadvantages of amnioinfusion. These are:

◆ Amnioinfusion is invasive and can increase the chance of uterine infection.

◆ The mother must remain flat in bed during and after the procedure, or the fluid will run out quickly.

Alternatives to consider. Instead of trying to relieve the fetal distress with amnioinfusion, the caregiver can go straight to a cesarean if and when fetal distress warrants quick delivery.

INDUCTION OR AUGMENTATION OF LABOR

Sometimes labor is started artifically *(induced)*; at other times a labor that has slowed down is speeded up *(augmented)*. There are several ways labor can be induced or augmented:

1. Self-help methods (see pages 176 to 180).

2. "Stripping" the membranes to begin labor induction. The caregiver inserts a finger into the cervix and circles around the inside to separate the membranes from the lower segment of the uterus.

This is usually painful for the mother—it feels like a very vigorous vaginal exam—and it sometimes results in inadvertent rupture of the membranes. Stripping the membranes usually does not actually start labor, but it may hasten ripening and thinning of the cervix to make it more ready for dilation (see "Labor Progresses in Six Ways," page 52). The procedure cannot be done if the cervical opening is hard to reach because it is very posterior (pointing toward the mother's back) instead of anterior (in the center of her vagina), or if it is tightly closed.

3. Artificial rupture of the membranes (AROM). This sometimes speeds or augments labor, if it is timed correctly (see the preceding discussion).

4. Prostaglandin gels, suppositories, or tablets. Prostaglandins are hormone-like substances produced by the body and also synthesized. Like the prostaglandins that a woman produces herself, prostaglandins in drug form promote the softening, thinning, and, sometimes, dilation of the cervix. They are used when labor must be induced before the cervix has naturally softened or thinned. Prostaglandins come in these forms:

   ◆ A water-soluble gel containing prostaglandin (Prepidil). The gel is applied to the inside or the outside of the cervix through a syringe. More may be applied after 6 hours or so.

   ◆ A tampon-like device that contains prostaglandin (Cervidil). Placed in the vagina behind the cervix, the device gradually releases prostaglandin over about 12 hours.

   ◆ A tiny tablet containing another synthetic prostaglandin, misoprostol (Cytotec). The tablet is either placed in the mother's vagina, behind her cervix, or given to the mother by mouth. Tablets are given by mouth when a mother's membranes have ruptured, since placing anything in her vagina would add to the risk of infection. A second tablet may be administered after 4 to 6 hours. Cytotec in low doses (25 micrograms vaginally or 50 micrograms orally) usually acts gradually, like Prepidil and Cervidil do. Often with higher doses (50 micrograms vaginally or 100 micrograms orally) and sometimes even with the low doses, Cytotec causes sudden, very intense contractions and fetal distress. This is less likely to happen with the other prostaglandin agents.

Dosages and treatment schedules vary depending on the caregiver's preferences, the woman's preferences, and the state of her cervix. Lower doses are generally safer.

5. Intravenous administration of a synthetic form of the hormone oxytocin (also called Pitocin). This can start or speed up labor. Pitocin is mixed with intravenous fluids in a continuous drip. By regulating the dose, the caregiver can usually control the intensity and frequency of the contractions quite well. Electronic fetal monitoring is required, along with a nurse's close observation, to detect and correct excessively strong or long contractions.

   Attempts to start labor with Pitocin often fail when the cervix is firm and thick. If prostaglandin is used before Pitocin, this problem is often avoided.

   If an induction is done for medical reasons and fails, cesarean delivery is the only remaining option. If an induction is done for convenience and fails, the mother may be sent home to await spontaneous labor, but this rarely happens today. Usually, the baby is delivered by cesarean.

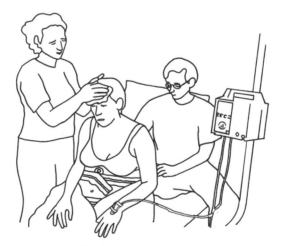

The mother is having her labor induced with Pitocin. Her contractions and the fetal heart rate are being monitored electronically.

Purposes of induction or augmentation of labor. Induction or augmentation of labor is medically indicated:

♦ When pregnancy is prolonged. Caregivers disagree about when pregnancy has gone on too long. Some offer induction at 39, 40, or 41 weeks, but most agree that, statistically, the risks to the baby of waiting beyond 42 weeks are greater than the risks of inducing before that time. After 42 weeks, the rates of stillbirth and postmaturity increase. (A baby who is postmature shows signs of placental insufficiency—peeling skin on hands and feet, and intrauterine weight loss.)

♦ When medical problems are such that continuing the pregnancy might harm the mother or the baby (for example, when the mother has high blood pressure or diabetes).

♦ When the baby is not thriving in the uterus.

♦ When the bag of waters has been broken for a long time and labor has not started spontaneously, or the mother has tested positive for Group B strep (see page 206).

♦ When the mother has frequent herpes outbreaks and wants to avoid a cesarean. A cesarean is done if a woman has a herpes sore in or near her vagina when she goes into labor (see page 247).

♦ When the mother is having a prolonged prelabor and her cervix is firm, in which case the use of prostaglandins may be appropriate (see "Prelabor," page 63, and "The Slow-to-Start Labor," page 180).

♦ When contractions in the active phase slow down and decrease in intensity, causing a delay in progress. In this case, augmentation with intravenous Pitocin may be appropriate.

Disadvantages of induction for medical reasons. These include:

♦ Medical induction usually includes more interventions for safety than does spontaneous onset of labor; such interventions include continuous electronic fetal monitoring, IV fluids, and others.

♦ Because the woman is hospitalized before her first contraction— possibly hours before—she becomes tired and hungry, and may become discouraged and even begin to perceive that her labor is very long and that something is wrong.

Sometimes labor is induced out of fear that the baby is becoming too big. The reasoning is that inducing labor before the baby grows too much will make the birth easier and prevent complications and possibly a cesarean. Although this seems to make sense, studies have shown that:

◆ It is not possible to accurately assess an unborn baby's size. Estimates are often wrong by 10 percent or more, even when ultrasound is used.

◆ When babies are thought to be large, cesareans are actually more likely if labor is induced than if labor begins spontaneously, and induction in these cases produces no improvements in the babies' health and well-being.

◆ Although the odds of a difficult labor increase when the baby's weight exceeds 8$^1/_2$ pounds, inducing labor does not prevent a difficult labor or a cesarean birth.

◆ Seventy percent of cases of shoulder dystocia (in which a baby gets stuck after her head is out) happen in average-sized babies, and this problem cannot be predicted. When this serious complication occurs, doctors and midwives use well-practiced techniques to resolve it.

Nonmedical reasons for induction. By far, most inductions done today are "elective"; that is, they are done not for medical safety but for such reasons as these:

◆ Convenience for the mother, her caregiver, or both. An elective induction may be scheduled to occur when the caregiver is on call or when the mother has household help.

◆ Routine procedure, whenever a mother reaches her fortieth week. Many caregivers see no reason not to induce labor at this point, and they are not concerned about the increase in likelihood of a cesarean (see disadvantages, below).

◆ The mother's discomfort. Swelling, backache, or fatigue makes some women want to end their pregnancies as soon as safety allows.

◆ Avoiding the stress of going to the hospital in labor, especially if the mother lives far from the hospital or has had a previous rapid labor.

It can be very appealing for the mother to be able to plan when the baby will be born. As her birth partner, you might also appreciate knowing the date and being able to plan your schedule around it. Inductions proceed more successfully if done when the cervix has already ripened (softened and thinned) considerably.

Disadvantages of nonmedical induction. Because induction is not an innocuous procedure, you and the mother should carefully consider the benefits and risks of an elective induction before making a decision. There are many potential disadvantages:

1. Inductions sometimes proceed very slowly, especially if the mother's cervix has not undergone some of the pre-dilation changes (see "Labor Progresses in Six Ways," page 52). Days may pass before the baby is born, so the induction procedures are carried out during the day and stopped at night to allow the woman to eat and get some rest. The reason for allowing plenty of time for the process is to try to avoid a cesarean; however, a slow induction can be exhausting and demoralizing for both the mother and the birth partner. (If the bag of waters has broken, the caregiver usually intervenes with a cesarean earlier.) Some caregivers are reluctant to put the woman through a long induction or to wait several days for the birth, and so they decide on a cesarean after 12 hours or so, although labor may not have even begun in this much time.

2. The timing of an elective induction may not be best for the baby, who might benefit from another few days in the uterus. Most babies continue to mature and develop greater strength and other capabilities until labor begins spontaneously. Normally the baby, when mature enough, starts the labor process, by secreting the hormones that initiate labor (although 12 to 13 percent of babies born in the United States are premature, and some, without induction by 42 weeks, would be postmature). If the mother's due date is uncertain and labor is induced, the baby might be born prematurely.

3. Prostaglandins sometimes cause nausea in the mother and rapid changes in her blood pressure.

4. The chances of a cesarean increase by two to four times in first-time mothers who have elective inductions, when compared to first-time mothers who have labors that begin spontaneously.

5. Sometimes, even though the induction date is planned, the hospital is too busy or lacking an available bed when the day comes. The mother may be told not to come in, or she may even be turned away when she arrives. She may be asked to call the hospital every few hours until a bed becomes available. This can be frustrating and worrisome, especially if she has not been warned in advance that this could happen, or if she thinks the induction was suggested for medical reasons.

6. Induced labors may cause contractions that are too long or too strong for the baby (or the mother) to tolerate. To detect such a problem, the mother must have continuous electronic fetal monitoring (see page 216). When Cytotec (misoprostol) was introduced in the late 1990s, the doses were too high, and the drug was dangerous and difficult to control; with it, the contractions sometimes suddenly became overwhelming, causing fetal distress, bleeding, and psychological trauma for the mother. High doses are no longer the norm in most hospitals, but you can ask the staff to try to avoid the sudden onset of painful contractions by starting with low doses of medication and increasing them gradually.

   If the mother's contractions are too strong for the baby to tolerate well, the nurse takes measures to stop the contractions. If the mother is receiving intravenous Pitocin, the nurse can turn it off or turn it down; the contractions usually quickly subside. If the mother has had prostaglandin placed in her vagina, the nurse either removes the insert (Cervidil) or gives a douche to wash out the gel (Prepidil) or the tablet (Cytotec). If the mother has swallowed a Cytotec tablet, another drug, such as Terbutaline, may be given to slow the contractions.

7. Use of pain medications early in the dilation process is more likely with induction, for several reasons:

   ◆ The mother may be restricted from using comfort measures such as position changes, movements, and massage by the intravenous line and the belts and cords of the electronic fetal monitor.

♦ Fatigue and discouragement over a slow onset of labor may lower the mother's motivation to deal with her contractions. She also may feel hungry, since she will probably not be allowed to eat while the Pitocin is being given.

♦ With induced labor, the contractions, especially those of early labor (to 4 or 5 centimeters), tend to come closer and last longer than they would if labor began spontaneously.

♦ If the mother is hospitalized before contractions start, the labor seems much longer and slower than it would if labor began at home, where she could keep busy with normal activities.

Although medically indicated induction has some of the same disadvantages, knowing there is a good reason for the induction makes these disadvantages more acceptable.

Alternatives to consider. If there is no medical reason for induction, you and the mother can:

♦ Wait for spontaneous labor. If the mother asks about postponing an elective induction, she will probably find that her caregiver is willing to wait for labor to start on its own, at least until she is one to two weeks past her due date—as long as there is careful surveillance of the mother's and baby's well-being.

♦ Try the nonmedical methods for stimulating labor contractions described on pages 175 to 180, "When Labor Must Start."

EPISIOTOMY

An episiotomy is a surgical cut, made with scissors, from the vagina toward the anus. It is sometimes done shortly before delivery. Anesthesia may be given before the procedure, although even if the episiotomy is done without anesthesia, the mother is hardly aware of it. Rather than feeling pain, she is aware of a relief from pressure when the episiotomy is performed. Local anesthesia is given after the birth to relieve pain that occurs when the episiotomy is stitched. The incision usually heals within one or two weeks, although pain at the site may linger, especially during intercourse, for months. If she still has pain after a few weeks, however, the mother should consult her caregiver.

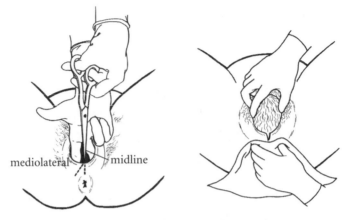

Episiotomy. The midline incision is most common in the United States.

Once routine, episiotomies are rarely performed by midwives, and physicians are doing many fewer than they were in the early and mid-nineties. The main reason for doing episiotomies was to avoid a tear in the perineum (the area between the vagina and the anus) or in the front of the vagina. Episiotomies became less common when scientific evidence showed that this rationale was unsupportable (see "Disadvantages of Episiotomy," below).

Purposes of episiotomy. These are:

◆ To speed delivery by 5 to 10 minutes if the baby appears to be distressed.

◆ To reduce pressure on the baby's head if the baby is premature or has other problems.

◆ To enlarge a very tight vaginal opening when necessary to allow delivery. It is very rare that the vagina will not stretch adequately.

◆ To allow easier placement of forceps.

Disadvantages of episiotomy. An episiotomy will *definitely* damage the mother's perineum; she will have a cut, stitches, a healing period, and some discomfort or pain. If no episiotomy is done, however, there is only about a 30 to 60 percent chance that the mother's perineum will tear. Research indicates that tears are almost always smaller and quicker to heal than the average episiotomy.

In addition, episiotomies sometimes *extend*—that is, after the cut is made, the pressure of the baby's head can enlarge the incision. This happens in approximately 1 woman in 20. Spontaneous tears are rarely (fewer than 1 in 100) as large as extended episiotomies. In other words, the chance of a serious tear is greater with an episiotomy than without.

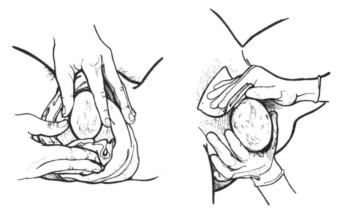

Normal delivery without episiotomy with the woman on her side. Left: The caregiver uses warm compresses to promote relaxation and circulation, and gently supports the perineum. Right: With the mother rolled toward her side, the caregiver provides slight counterpressure as the baby's head emerges.

Alternatives to consider. The caregiver can simply forego an episiotomy, even if it appears that the mother may tear. She may incur no injury, one or several small tears, or, rarely, a large tear.

The caregiver can protect the perineum from tearing seriously—for example, by placing warm compresses on the perineum, controlling the birth of the head and shoulders, suggesting positions that facilitate the baby's descent, and allowing spontaneous rather than directed bearing down (see "The Crowning and Birth Phase," page 100, and "Spontaneous Bearing Down," page 131).

You and the mother can improve her chance of an intact perineum after birth by doing prenatal perineal massage (see page 20).

Whether or not a woman ends up with a perineal tear or an episiotomy, exercising her pelvic floor muscles after birth seems to be very important to the recovery of pelvic floor tone. See page 19 for a discussion of the Kegel exercise.

VACUUM EXTRACTION

Vacuum extraction is used during the birthing (second) stage of labor. A plastic suction cup (about 3 inches in diameter) is placed on the baby's head; the suction cup is connected to handles and to a pump that creates a safe level of suction. The caregiver pulls on the device attached to the baby's head while the uterus contracts and the mother pushes. The suction cup disengages if the caregiver pulls too hard, thus protecting the baby's head.

Purposes of vacuum extraction. Vacuum extraction is done to assist or hasten delivery after the baby's head is in the birth canal. This procedure is medically indicated if:

- The birthing (second) stage of labor is prolonged because fatigue or anesthesia have made the mother unable to push effectively.

- The birthing stage is prolonged because the baby's head is slightly angled so that it doesn't fit through the pelvis, and the mother's efforts need assistance.

- There is last-minute fetal distress.

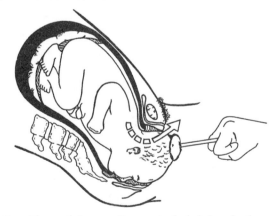

Vacuum extraction. After applying a suction cup to the baby's scalp, the caregiver pulls as the mother pushes and the uterus contracts.

Compared with forceps (see below), vacuum extraction less often requires an episiotomy, may cause less damage to the woman's vagina, can be used when the baby is higher in the birth canal, and appears to be about equally safe for the baby.

Disadvantages of vacuum extraction. These are:

◆ Vacuum extraction frequently causes a fluid-filled lump and a bruise or abrasion on the baby's head where the suction cup was. It may take days or weeks for the lump to disappear.

◆ Serious injury to the baby's head is possible, though very unlikely when the vacuum extractor is used properly, according to guidelines set by the obstetric profession.

◆ If the suction cup pops off during use, both the birth partner and the mother may be alarmed. Remember that it pops off to protect the baby from excessive strain.

Alternatives to consider. These are:

◆ The mother can bear down (push) in different positions, such as squatting or standing. See "Positions and Movements for Labor and Birth," pages 135 to 141.

◆ Forceps can be used for delivery (see "Forceps Delivery," below).

◆ A cesarean section can be performed (see chapter 9).

FORCEPS DELIVERY

Forceps are used during the birthing stage. Two steel instruments, like spoons or salad tongs, are placed within the vagina on either side of the baby's head. They are then locked together into position so they cannot squeeze the baby's head, no matter how hard the doctor grips the handles. This protects the baby's head from undue pressure. The doctor pulls during contractions while the mother pushes. Sometimes forceps are used to rotate the baby's head.

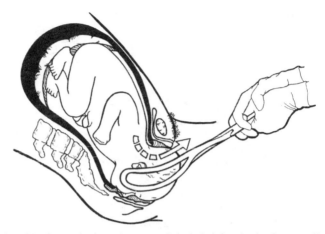

Forceps are placed in the mother's vagina around the baby's head. The doctor pulls while the mother pushes and the uterus contracts.

Purposes of forceps delivery. The doctor uses forceps to deliver the baby more quickly. A forceps delivery is medically indicated when birth is delayed because (1) the mother is not able to push effectively, (2) there is a decrease in uterine contractions, or (3) the baby is large or poorly positioned.

Forceps are also medically indicated if the baby is distressed when low in the birth canal. If the baby is high in the birth canal, either a vacuum extraction or, most likely, a cesarean delivery (see chapter 9) is a safer choice than forceps.

If a forceps delivery appears difficult, the attempt is abandoned, and a cesarean is performed.

Disadvantages of forceps delivery. These are:

- A forceps delivery usually requires an episiotomy and anesthesia.
- Forceps may bruise the baby's face or the side of his head.
- Though this happens rarely, forceps may injure the baby's head or neck, especially if used with excessive force and contrary to the professional guidelines for the safe use of forceps.
- Forceps may injure the mother's vagina.

Alternatives to consider. These are:

◆ The mother can use directed pushing in positions that enlarge the pelvis, such as squatting with or without support, the dangle, or lying flat on her back and pulling her knees up toward her shoulders. See "Positions and Movements for Labor and Birth," page 135, and "Directed Pushing," page 133.

◆ The caregiver can monitor the baby and the mother, and, if both are doing well, give the labor more time.

◆ The caregiver can use vacuum extraction (see page 234). The choice between forceps and vacuum extraction is best made by the doctor, according to his or her training and expertise.

◆ The caregiver can attempt a forceps delivery once or twice, but, if it appears that the baby is not moving, he or she can remove the forceps and prepare for a cesarean.

◆ The doctor can perform a cesarean delivery. This is the only alternative if vacuum extraction does not work and a forceps delivery would be difficult.

In summary, the purpose of medical interventions is to improve birth outcomes for mother and baby. Most interventions carry some risks or disadvantages along with benefits. Except in emergency circumstances, there is usually more than one way to accomplish the intended purpose of any proposed intervention. For this reason, you and the mother will want to be prepared to make informed choices about what interventions might be used and when.

CHAPTER 7

Complications in
Late Pregnancy, Labor,
or Afterward

*The labor went really well. I was so proud of Bess. As she
held sweet little Todd, though, her bleeding got worse. She
lost a lot of blood. We're so thankful that the doctor took
care of it quickly, and that both Bess and Todd are fine. But
I'm pregnant now, and that scary time haunts me.*

—MAUREEN, FIRST-TIME CO-MOTHER

This chapter discusses a number of complications that may arise before, during, or after labor, how they are treated, and how you can help
the mother if they occur. More serious than the difficulties discussed
in chapter 5, these complications require hospitalization and medical
assistance for a good outcome. They fall into four major categories:
problems with the mother; problems with the labor; problems with the
fetus; and problems with the newborn.

As you would imagine, the mother will be upset—worried, shocked,
stunned, frightened, anxious, or even suspicious—if serious problems
arise. You both may have difficulty accepting that there is a problem,
especially if she feels normal, as is often the case with gestational diabetes, high blood pressure, or threatened preterm labor (when contractions often feel quite mild; see page 47). It is awfully hard to cope with
much more than labor itself, and she may rely on you to assume some of
the responsibility for decision making.

As the birth partner, you can help in the following ways:

◆ Learn what is happening, why it is a problem, how serious it is, and
  the rationale for and the expected results of any corrective action to

be taken. Ask the mother's caregiver the Key Questions on page 202, adding this final one: "Will this action improve the chances of a healthy mother and healthy baby?" Help the mother understand the answers.

♦ Remain assertive and cooperative with her caregiver. Inform the staff of the mother's wishes, and learn of any alternative ways of handling the problem. Use her Birth Plan (see page 26) as your guide.

♦ Recognize the need to accept the caregiver's judgment without discussion in true emergencies, when time is of the utmost importance.

♦ Help the mother adjust to the need for a change in management. If her Birth Plan is written to reflect her understanding that complications sometimes arise unexpectedly, she will realize that a departure from some of her preferences is warranted to ensure a good outcome for herself and her baby. A doula can help you both adjust to the change in management and maintain perspective.

♦ Remain with the mother throughout. When things go wrong, she needs your help and support more than ever.

♦ Afterward, allow her time to recover emotionally. You will also need time to recover.

Complications for the Mother

This section includes explanations of complications and why they are problematic; descriptions of the ways each might be managed; how the mother may react; and how you can help. If complications arise, this information may be useful as the two of you discuss them with your caregiver.

PREMATURE LABOR

If a woman begins labor before 37 weeks of pregnancy, the labor is considered premature (see "Signs of Labor," page 47, for an explanation of signs of premature labor). Babies born prematurely are at greater risk for a number of medical problems, such as breathing difficulties, jaundice, infection, difficulty maintaining body temperature, and feeding problems.

Management of premature labor. This depends on the baby's gestational age, well-being, and stage of development. Measures may include the following:

- A vaginal exam to determine how much the cervix has dilated.

- Assessment of contractions (how long, strong, and frequent they are).

- Attempts to stop labor through the use of bed rest and medications such as terbutaline, magnesium sulfate, ritodrine, or nifedipine. Treatment is more likely to be effective if the woman's cervix has not dilated beyond 2 centimeters.

- Amniocentesis and testing of the amniotic fluid to indicate whether the baby's lungs are mature, that is, capable of breathing without difficulty after birth. This helps the caregiver determine how aggressively to try to stop the labor.

- Medications (corticosteroids) given to the mother via injection to hasten the maturation of the baby's lungs, if birth cannot be postponed and the baby's lungs are immature.

- Electronic fetal monitoring to detect contractions and to watch the baby's condition.

- A test for infections that sometimes cause premature labor (including, among other organisms, Group B strep, described on page 206). The mother is treated with antibiotics if the test is positive.

- If delivery cannot be postponed, transport of the mother to a hospital with an intensive-care nursery, especially if the baby will be born very early (at less than 33 weeks gestation).

- Summoning of a pediatrician or neonatologist to care for the baby immediately after the delivery.

- If delivery is successfully postponed, the mother may be sent home on medication and asked to reduce her activity or remain on bed rest until 36 weeks or so.

Mother's reactions. The mother will be anxious to do all she can to help the baby get a healthy start in life, but she may feel guilty if she believes that she in some way caused the contractions or if bed rest prevents her from doing her share of housework and meal preparation. She may feel concerned over adding pressure on you. She may worry how a lengthy period of bed rest will affect her strength and fitness (if so, her caregivers may be able to recommend a physical therapist who can visit her and teach her some safe in-bed exercises). She may become bored lying around all the time.

How you can help. Try not to add to her feelings of guilt. Take on added responsibilities cheerfully; consider them as your contribution to your baby's health and well-being. Ease your burden by getting household help, if possible. Encourage the mother to shop for the baby by catalog or Internet. She might communicate with others on bed rest via the Internet, too (see "Recommended Resources"). This is also a good time for her to read books and watch videos on baby care and feeding. Her childbirth educator or public library may have such videos available.

HIGH BLOOD PRESSURE

About 5 percent of pregnant women have chronic high blood pressure, or hypertension, that begins either before or soon after they become pregnant. This condition needs to be monitored carefully throughout pregnancy. Medications may be necessary, and they may need occasional adjustment.

Five to 8 percent of pregnant women develop high blood pressure (over 140/90) during late pregnancy. They are said to have gestational, or pregnancy-induced, hypertension (PIH), which is usually mild. Mild PIH may be accompanied by swelling in the legs, hands, and face, and protein in the urine. The condition usually goes away after birth, but sometimes it becomes more severe during labor.

More severe PIH or chronic hypertension can be scary. In addition to the swelling and protein in her urine, the mother may have blurring or spots in her vision, upper abdominal pain, headaches, increased reflexes (that is, when her knee is tapped, the mother's foot jerks more than usual), and liver and kidney problems (the last are detected by a blood test). The function of her placenta may be impaired, and this may slow the baby's growth. If the PIH is very severe, the mother may experience convulsions. Very rarely, women die from this condition. The complications arising from severe PIH are referred to by the terms preeclampsia, eclampsia, toxemia, and HELLP syndrome. HELLP stands for hemolysis (breakdown of red blood cells), elevated liver enzymes, and low platelets (which interferes with the body's ability to clot blood).

Management of high blood pressure during pregnancy. Measures may include:

♦ Reduction of activity (i.e., quitting work or reducing work hours) or bed rest, preferably on the mother's left side. The number of hours of bed rest each day depends on the severity of the PIH and the caregiver's belief in the value of bed rest. Opinions vary quite a lot.

♦ Medications to lower blood pressure, magnesium sulfate to prevent convulsions, or both. Hospitalization may be required. Some of the medications used to control chronic hypertension are unsafe for the unborn baby, so the caregiver may switch the mother to another that is safer.

♦ Close monitoring of the mother's blood pressure and other signs of worsening PIH (through blood and urine tests, checking of reflexes, tests of fetal growth and well-being, and weight checks).

♦ Induction of labor or even a cesarean if her condition worsens.

Management of high blood pressure during labor. Measures may include:

♦ Restriction to left-sided bed rest. Some caregivers allow a warm shower or bath from time to time during labor, as these also lower blood pressure.

♦ Continuous electronic fetal monitoring and intravenous fluids.

♦ Frequent blood-pressure checks.

♦ Medications to lower blood pressure and magnesium sulfate to prevent convulsions, if the condition is severe.

♦ Intravenous Pitocin (see page 226), if magnesium sulfate is used, since the latter drug slows labor. Pitocin also may be used to induce labor.

Mother's reactions. During pregnancy she may feel:

◆ Disbelief, since many women with mild or moderate PIH feel fine. She may not want to comply with orders to stay in bed. She may feel the doctor is overreacting.

◆ Relief, if she can quit or cut down at work, especially if it has become tiring or stressful.

◆ Worried, when she learns some of the possible serious consequences for her and the baby if her condition cannot be controlled.

During labor, she may feel:

◆ Disappointment over the required interventions, especially induction of labor (see page 224), restriction to bed, and electronic fetal monitoring (see page 216).

◆ Discomfort from the effects of medications, especially magnesium sulfate, which may make her twitch, sweat, and feel hot, flushed, and nervous. Blood-pressure medications may also have uncomfortable side effects—headaches, nausea, drowsiness, shortness of breath, and trouble urinating.

How you can help. You can sympathize with her, but help her focus on what she must do, for her own welfare and the baby's. Remind her of the comfort measures she still can use (see "When the Mother Must Labor in Bed," page 188).

GESTATIONAL DIABETES

This condition occurs in 3 to 5 percent of pregnant women. A two-step test detects gestational diabetes (also called "glucose intolerance of pregnancy"). At 26 to 28 weeks, most pregnant women take the diabetes screening test; they drink a sugary beverage, and their blood is drawn and assessed for blood sugar. Women whose blood sugar is high then take the more accurate three-hour glucose tolerance test; they have their blood drawn, drink the same sugary beverage, and have their blood drawn three more times over the next three hours. If their blood sugar is high at these readings, they have gestational diabetes. (Note that 85 percent of women who have high blood sugar on the screening test do *not* have high readings in the glucose tolerance test.) The mainstay of treatment is a very healthy, individual-ized, and tightly controlled low-sugar and low-carbohydrate diet combined with regular exercise. This may be all that is necessary to keep blood sugar levels normal. If not, the woman may also need to take insulin.

Management of gestational diabetes during pregnancy. Besides the diet and exercise already mentioned, the caregiver may recommend these measures:

- Frequent blood-sugar testing with a special glucose meter by the mother, who reports high readings to her caregiver.
- Consultations with a dietician for guidance and support in the special diet.
- Fetal movement counting (see page 22).
- Close monitoring of fetal growth and well-being with ultrasound, nonstress tests, and other tests.
- Self-administered insulin injections, if necessary, to control blood sugar levels.

Concerns for the baby. Especially if the mother's blood sugar is not well controlled, her baby is at increased risk for uneven development of her organ systems because of inadequate insulin production. Effects may include:

- Large size (because of excess glucose crossing the placenta to the baby) and associated increased risk of birth trauma.
- Low blood sugar at birth, due to the sudden drop in glucose from the mother that occurs at birth.
- Prolonged jaundice, possibly due to liver immaturity at birth.
- Respiratory problems, due to developmental immaturity of the lungs, despite the baby's large size.

Gestational diabetes is managed with the goal of preventing these complications. A neonatologist or pediatrician is usually present at the birth to observe and care for the newborn. The prognosis for the baby is very good when the mother's diabetes is well controlled.

Management of gestational diabetes during labor and afterward. Measures may include:

◆ Induction of labor at 38 or 39 weeks, or earlier if blood sugar is not well controlled.

◆ Greater likelihood of a cesarean, especially if the baby seems to be very large.

◆ Frequent checks of the mother's blood sugar during labor.

◆ Intravenous administration of glucose or insulin, depending on whether the mother's blood sugar is high from too little insulin or low from too much. Insulin levels are sometimes challenging to control.

◆ Frequent checks of the newborn's blood sugar until levels are normal.

◆ Management of low blood sugar in the mother or baby after birth.

◆ Treatment of respiratory problems, jaundice, and other problems in the baby that result from gestational diabetes.

◆ Subsequent checks of the mother's blood sugar, because women who have had gestational diabetes are at increased risk of developing Type II diabetes at a later age.

Mother's reactions. During labor, she may feel:

◆ Discouraged over the added interventions, especially if she feels fine.

◆ Worried about her baby.

◆ Helpless or unable to understand the complexities of her treatment.

How you can help. You can:

◆ Help her learn about gestational diabetes and any options she may have (see "Recommended Resources").

◆ Encourage her to ask the "Key Questions for Informed Decision Making" (see page 202).

◆ Help her understand and adjust to the demands of her diet and blood-sugar testing regime, and to the necessary interventions that she will experience during labor.

◆ Try to emphasize the things she can do to help herself in labor, rather than dwelling on all the things she cannot do.

HERPES LESION

If the mother has or has ever had genital herpes, which causes sores to appear in the genital area, she should be sure to report this to her caregiver. If the virus is active when she goes into labor, the baby could contract the virus during vaginal birth. Herpes in the newborn is very serious; it frequently causes brain damage and death. If the mother has had herpes for a long time, the risk that a sore during labor could give the baby herpes is about 1 to 3 percent. The risk is much higher if the mother has recently acquired herpes.

In an effort to prevent herpes outbreaks in late pregnancy, many caregivers offer anti-herpes medication (such as acyclovir) during the last weeks of pregnancy to all women who have ever had herpes sores. A woman who has not had an outbreak in years may reasonably refuse the medication, but a woman who has had one or more recent outbreaks may be wise to accept it.

Complementary measures that may reduce the incidence of symptoms include reducing stress, maintaining a balanced diet, and wearing underpants with a cotton crotch to avoid the moisture buildup that can come with nylon or other man-made fibers.

If a woman has a herpes outbreak at or near term, her caregiver will recommend that she take acyclovir, which can shorten the duration and severity of the outbreak (and perhaps provide protection for her baby). The caregiver may also offer to induce labor at a time when no sore is present.

Management during labor for the woman with a history of herpes. At the hospital, the caregiver may:

◆ Carefully inspect the genital area for the presence of a sore.

◆ Culture the mother's vaginal secretions for asymptomatic presence of the virus.

◆ Perform a cesarean to prevent the baby from coming into contact with a sore, if one is present.

If no sore is visible but the culture later indicates that the herpes virus was present, the baby will be treated with acyclovir. Or the baby may be tested for herpes and treated only if the test indicates that the baby is infected.

Mother's reactions. The mother will probably be disappointed, shocked, angry, or depressed when she learns she has an active herpes lesion, especially if she didn't expect it. If you were the source of her herpes, you may be the target of some of her anger. Expect her to need time, support, and perhaps counseling afterward to deal with her disappointment over any changes in plans for the birth or any problems in the baby caused by the herpes.

How you can help. Here's what you can do:

+ Give her an opportunity to express her anger or disappointment.

+ Give her time to adjust to the need to take medications.

+ Try not to become defensive if you were the source of her herpes. Your defensiveness will prolong her anger and postpone her adjustment to the cesarean.

+ Explore ways to make the cesarean more satisfying (see page 318).

EXCESSIVE BLEEDING DURING LABOR

Most bleeding during labor comes from the site of the placenta, when it begins to separate from the uterine wall. The amount of visible bleeding and the seriousness of the problem depend on where and how extensive the separation is and whether the bleeding is concealed, that is, blood does not flow out. If the placenta is very low in the uterus (this condition is called placenta previa), blood comes out of the vagina. If the placenta is high in the uterus when it begins to separate (this condition is called placental abruption), the uterus may become very firm between contractions, and the mother is in constant pain (rather than the intermittent pain that normally comes with contractions). In either case, both mother and baby are in danger; this is potentially an acute emergency.

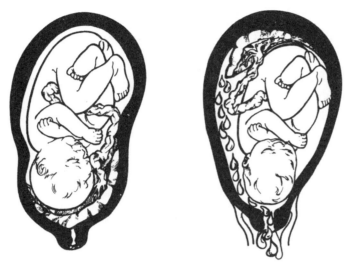

Left, placenta previa; right, placental abruption.

Management of bleeding during labor. This complication is managed in the following ways:

- If severe bleeding begins early in labor, or before labor begins, a cesarean delivery is probable. The mother may receive a general anesthetic if the blood loss is rapid; the anesthetic quickly puts the mother to sleep for the surgery. If there is time, a spinal block, which allows the mother to remain conscious, will be used.

- If severe bleeding begins late in labor, or if bleeding begins in early labor but is not severe, and the baby is not in distress, the doctor or midwife may monitor the baby's heart rate continuously and wait. If the baby's heart rate remains normal, a vaginal birth may be possible.

Mother's reactions. During labor the mother may:

- Be caught off-guard.
- Be frightened for herself and her baby over abnormal bleeding. Her fear makes other priorities irrelevant.
- Feel very nervous about waiting, and preoccupied with the baby's condition.
- Wonder whether the caregiver is overreacting.

How you can help. You can:

- Remain well informed about the severity of the bleeding and the baby's condition. Share the information with the mother.

- Continue supporting the mother during contractions, and remind her to deal with each contraction as it comes, not to fret about what may happen.

- Be prepared to comply with changes in management, and help the mother comply, if the baby shows signs of distress.

EXCESSIVE BLEEDING AFTER BIRTH (POSTPARTUM HEMORRHAGE)

Some bleeding immediately after birth is normal; it comes from the area in the uterus where the placenta was attached. The uterus usually contracts vigorously after birth, causing the bleeding to subside. You may be surprised, though, at how much blood there seems to be even under normal circumstances. Losing as much as a cup of blood is considered normal.

Postpartum hemorrhage, or excessive bleeding immediately after birth, usually occurs for one of three reasons: relaxation of the uterus, a retained placenta or fragments of placenta, or lacerations in the vagina or cervix. The loss of blood may cause the mother's blood pressure to drop; her skin may become clammy, and she may feel faint. To remedy her low blood pressure, the mother will be asked to lie flat, with her head low, and she will be given intravenous fluids, possibly containing a drug to raise her blood pressure.

For a few weeks after birth a mother normally experiences a dwindling discharge, called lochia. This fluid is composed of blood and some of the tissue that lined the uterus during pregnancy. Lochia is like a longer-than-usual menstrual period.

Management of bleeding after birth. If the uterus relaxes after the birth, it leaves the blood vessels open at the placental site. When the uterus is made to contract, it will squeeze these vessels closed and the bleeding will stop.

- To make the uterus contract, the caregiver may vigorously massage the mother's low abdomen. The massage is painful for the mother, but it is the quickest way to get the uterus to contract.

- The caregiver injects a drug that contracts the uterus—Pitocin or Methergine—into the mother's thigh, gives Pitocin intravenously, or has you or the nurse stimulate the mother's nipples to increase the body's secretion of oxytocin.

- If the placenta or parts of it are retained, the caregiver manually removes the placenta or the placental fragments. Since this is very painful, intravenous narcotics or an inhaled anethetic gas may be given first, but if the procedure will be quick the mother may be given the option of going without pain medication to save time. If manual removal fails, surgery is required to clean out the uterus and close off the large blood vessels, or, in very serious, life-threatening cases, to remove the uterus.

- If there are lacerations in the vagina or cervix, the lacerations are sutured.

- If the mother has lost a significant amount of blood, she may receive transfusions of blood or other fluids to restore her blood volume.

Mother's reactions. She may:

- Fail to realize at first how serious the blood loss is.

- Feel weak or faint if she loses a large amount of blood.

- Become frightened if bleeding continues and urgent measures are taken to stop it.

How you can help. Do whatever you are told. A hemorrhage is an emergency, and quick action is essential. There is little time for explanations. If possible, remain with the mother and help her to cooperate in whatever she is asked to do.

The Breech Presentation

See page 190 for a discussion of management of the breech presentation.

Complications with Labor Progress

The caregiver or the nurse regularly observes and records the progress of labor. He or she performs vaginal exams to determine changes in the cervix and in the position and station of the fetus. The caregiver or nurse also observes the quality of the contractions (frequency, duration, and intensity) and the mother's reactions to them. Two situations that may signal problems are very rapid progress and slow progress.

VERY RAPID PROGRESS

When contractions are exceptionally efficient or unusually powerful, or when the cervix is exceptionally yielding, labor may progress rapidly. Although not usually considered a complication, a fast labor may present clinical challenges and be extremely painful and frightening for the mother.

Main concerns of the caregiver. These are:

◆ Getting the mother to the hospital in time (or, in the case of a home birth, getting the caregiver to the home in time) to care for her adequately.

◆ How well the fetus tolerates the powerful, frequent contractions.

◆ Possible damage to the mother's perineum during a rapid birth.

◆ The newborn's adjustment afterward. Breathing problems and head trauma may be more likely as a result of this kind of birth.

Management of the very rapid labor. This involves:

◆ Supporting and reassuring the mother.

◆ Monitoring the response of the fetal heart to contractions and, possibly, using interventions (changing the mother's position, having her breathe oxygen) to improve oxygenation.

◆ Attempting to control the speed of delivery by coaching the mother not to bear down and by applying manual pressure against the rapidly emerging head.

How you can help. See "The Very Rapid Labor," pages 171 to 173.

ARREST OF ACTIVE LABOR (DYSTOCIA)

By the time the cervix has dilated to 4 or 5 centimeters, the cervix is usually quite thin and ready to open more easily. So, even if it has taken many hours or even a day or two to reach this point (see "The Slow-to-Start Labor," page 180), dilation now usually speeds up. Sometimes, though, it does not. Dilation may be very slow (this is called *protracted labor*) or it may seem to stop for two or more hours (this is called *arrested labor*).

The reasons for a delay in the active phase are more likely to be serious than are the reasons for a slow prelabor or a slow latent phase. It is not always possible to determine why labor is delayed, nor is it possible to know just how serious the delay is until time has passed. Slow progress is not necessarily a problem, but an arrest of labor is a concern for the mother's caregiver as well as for the mother and her partner. The doctor or midwife begins to worry that the mother is becoming exhausted, especially if she has tried everything (see pages 184 to 187) and there is no end in sight. At some point the caregiver begins to think that the labor should be hastened. This is when the mother crosses the line from having a "difficult labor," as described in chapter 5, to having a "complicated labor," one requiring medical intervention.

Causes of arrest in active labor. The delay may be due to one or a combination of causes:

◆ A poor fit between the baby's head and the mother's pelvis. This condition is sometimes called cephalo-pelvic disproportion, or CPD. Cephalo means head, and in the case of CPD the baby's head will not fit through the pelvis, despite the measures suggested on page 183 in chapter 5.

◆ Inadequate contractions. They lose intensity, slow down, or become shorter in duration. Or they stay the same—too weak, too infrequent, or both.

◆ Exhaustion, dehydration, excessive fear, or tension in the mother.

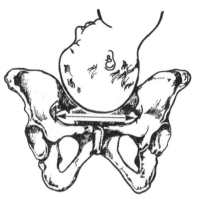

A poor fit between the baby's head and the mother's pelvis.

Management of delay in labor. The caregiver tries to determine the cause or causes of the delay by assessing the mother's contractions, her cervix, the size and position of the baby, and the mother's physical and emotional state.

Many things can be done to speed a prolonged labor and to support the woman undergoing it. Some of these things you and the mother can do (see pages 176 to 180); others must be done by the nurses and caregiver.

During the prolonged labor, the caregiver may:

♦ Monitor the fetal heart rate more often, or continuously, to help determine whether the baby is tolerating the delay.

♦ Offer the woman a narcotic or an epidural to reduce pain and help her relax, especially if she is exhausted. With an epidural or, to a lesser extent, with a narcotic, she may be able to sleep, and after a while progress may resume.

♦ Start intravenous fluids in the hope that improved hydration and some calories might reenergize the uterus.

♦ Rupture the mother's membranes in hopes of speeding labor (see page 221).

♦ Use intravenous Oxytocin (Pitocin) to stimulate contractions, if they appear to be decreasing or inadequate to change the cervix or the baby's position (see page 226).

- Use an intrauterine pressure catheter (internal electronic fetal monitoring) to find out just how strong the contractions are or whether Pitocin improves them.

- Use forceps or a vacuum extractor (see pages 234 to 237) if the delay occurs in the birthing (second) stage.

- Recommend a cesarean delivery if there is no progress even with the passage of considerable time and after efforts have been made to correct the problem (see chapter 9).

Mother's reactions. She may:

- Be willing to try suggested measures to improve progress for a while.

- Feel exhausted and discouraged, if nothing seems to work.

- Want a break, and ask for an epidural, even if she had originally wanted to avoid the epidural.

- Need acknowledgment of her great efforts, and validation that this labor is unusually difficult.

- Fear that something is wrong with her body or uterus.

- Be ready for Pitocin, a cesarean, or anything that will end her labor and bring the baby.

How you can help. You can help the mother during an arrest of labor in these ways:

- Confer with the doula or nurse on ways to help the mother.

- If the mother hasn't tried them yet, suggest the measures discussed in chapter 5 under "Slow Progress in Active Labor and the Birthing Stage," pages 184 to 187, and "Nipple Stimulation," pages 176 to 178. She may not have thought of the bath, changing positions, or labor-stimulating measures.

- If she is tired and discouraged, the mother may be reluctant to do things to make her contractions more intense. Consider her prior preferences regarding the use of pain medications (see pages 294 to 295). An epidural under these circumstances may allow her to sleep while her contractions intensify and (one hopes) progress to vaginal birth.

- Be attentive and understanding of the mother's emotional state during an exhausting labor. If she feels ignored when she expresses discouragement, she may later feel she was alone or unheard by you or others. (See "A Previous Disappointing or Traumatic Birth Experience," page 194.)

- Try to take care of your needs. Eat, rest, and refresh yourself by washing your face and brushing your teeth, but do not leave the mother unless someone else (a doula, a friend, or a relative) is there to help her.

Complications with the Fetus

The ability of the fetus to tolerate labor varies. Usually, labor benefits the baby by facilitating alertness, respiration, temperature regulation, and suckling. Sometimes, however, conditions that existed prior to labor interfere with the fetus's or newborn's well-being. The woman's caregiver watches for signs that the fetus is not tolerating labor well and that interventions may be needed.

PROLAPSED CORD

On very rare occasions, the umbilical cord prolapses—that is, it slips below the baby, into or through the cervix. This can occur before or during labor, and it is a true obstetric emergency that can result in the baby's death if it is not promptly and correctly managed. The danger is this: If the cord prolapses, it can be pinched by the baby's head at the cervix. This obstructs blood flow through the cord and deprives the baby of oxygen. The baby can survive only a few minutes without oxygen.

Signs to recognize. A prolapsed cord is rare under any circumstances, but it is most likely to happen if two conditions are present: (1) The baby is in a breech presentation (buttocks or feet down), or the head is high or off the cervix; *and* (2) the bag of waters suddenly breaks

CAUTION: *In late pregnancy, the mother should ask her caregiver at each appointment whether the baby is high and floating, low in the pelvis, or pressed against her cervix.* She should also ask, "If my bag of waters should break with a gush with my baby at this level of descent, should I be concerned about a prolapsed cord?" Then, if her caregiver says yes, and her bag of waters later does break with a gush of fluid, you and she should take the following measures just in case the cord has prolapsed:

◆ You or she should call the caregiver and the hospital. If you or someone else can't drive her to the hospital immediately, she should call 911 and say that she is pregnant and that her bag of waters has broken. To ensure a rapid response, she should say that she thinks she has a prolapsed cord (even though she is unlikely to know this).

◆ With your help, she should get onto her hands and knees, and then drop her chest down to the floor or bed. This open knee-chest position uses gravity to move the baby away from the cervix and off the cord.

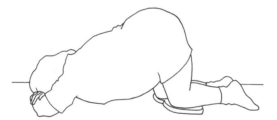

◆ She should go immediately to the hospital. Before she stands up to walk, however, move the car close to the door of the house, move the front seat forward, and open the back door of the car for her.

◆ She should ride in the back seat of the car or in the ambulance in the open knee-chest position, with her buttocks high.

Drive carefully, but waste no time. Drive to the hospital emergency entrance. Leave the mother in the car in the knee-chest position. Go in and tell the person on duty that your wife or friend is pregnant, her bag of waters broke, and you think she has a prolapsed cord. The mother should remain in the knee-chest position on a stretcher until a doctor or nurse can listen to the fetal heart rate. If the heart rate is normal, as it most likely will be, you can all relax and rejoice.

Prolapsed cord

with a gush, either spontaneously or because the caregiver has ruptured it. With this combination of circumstances, the cord may slip out around the baby's head or buttocks as the fluid escapes; then the baby, who has been "floating," presses down upon the cord.

A cord prolapse is extremely unlikely when the baby is already low in the pelvis and the head or buttocks are already pressing against the cervix.

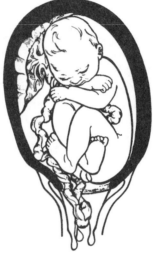

Prolapsed cord with a breech baby.

Management of a prolapsed cord. The caregiver gets the mother into the knee-chest position and places a hand in her vagina to hold the baby off the cord. A cesarean section is performed as soon as possible. With this rapid action, the baby will probably be born in good health.

Mother's reactions. She may:

- Feel excited that her bag of waters has broken, since this is a sign of labor.

- Feel reluctant to get into the open knee-chest position for the ride to the hospital, thinking she is being overly dramatic.

- Be willing to go straight to the hospital, but insist on sitting up for the ride.

- Feel frightened that her baby may be in danger, and willing to do whatever will improve the odds for the baby.

Prolapsed cord

◆ Feel she knows just what to do because she had asked her caregiver whether her baby was high or low in her pelvis, and whether she should be concerned about a prolapsed cord if her bag of waters should break with a gush before labor.

How you can help. As scary as all this is, the odds of a prolapsed cord even if the baby is high or breech and the bag of waters breaks with a gush are low—perhaps 1 in 100. In the event of a cord prolapse, however, your actions and the mother's will be most important, since time and her position are the crucial factors in the baby's well-being. Cooperate with the hospital staff in whatever way possible.

FETAL DISTRESS

Although a healthy baby has a remarkable ability to compensate for temporary oxygen deficits during labor, brain damage can occur if oxygen deprivation is severe and continues for too long, or if the baby has another problem that reduces his ability to compensate. *Fetal distress* means that the unborn baby is receiving less oxygen than normal and is showing signs of having to adjust physiologically.

How fetal distress is diagnosed. At present, the two main indicators of fetal distress are the fetal heart rate and the presence of meconium in the amniotic fluid. They are assessed in the following ways:

◆ A nurse or midwife listens to the fetal heart rate with a fetal stethoscope or an ultrasound fetoscope at frequent intervals during labor (see page 218). This requires that the nurse or midwife remain by the bedside much of the time.

◆ The caregiver or nurse monitors the fetal heart rate, as well as the strength of the mother's contractions, with an electronic fetal monitor (see page 216). The nurse observes the monitor tracings in the mother's room or, possibly, at the nurses' station.

◆ If the bag of waters breaks spontaneously or is broken by the caregiver (see page 221), the amniotic fluid is examined for the presence of meconium, which would indicate fetal distress.

Remember: If EFM indicates fetal distress, this does not necessarily mean that the baby is definitely in trouble. It may mean only that

Prolapsed cord

the baby is compensating for a temporary oxygen deficiency by slowing her heart rate to spare oxygen use. In other words, she may be in trouble, or she may be adjusting very well to the decrease in oxygen.

To find out whether the baby really is in trouble, the caregiver needs to rely on more than EFM. Tests such as the fetal scalp stimulation test (see page 220) and fetal pulse oximetry, or FPO (see page 220), are used to reduce the likelihood of unnecessary treatment for fetal distress. As stated earlier, however, scientific studies have not found FPO to be useful for this purpose.

Management of fetal distress. If monitoring indicates that the fetus may be in distress, the nurse or caregiver may do any or all of the following:

- Try to correct the fetal distress by having the mother breathe extra oxygen through a mask. The oxygen is carried via her bloodstream to the placenta and through the cord to the baby.

- Have the mother change her position to relieve pressure on the umbilical cord, which may be causing the fetal distress.

- Discontinue any drugs that might be causing the distress, such as high doses of Pitocin, which can cause contractions that are too long or too strong. During such contractions, oxygen flow through the placenta may be reduced.

- Give a drug to slow contractions (see page 296).

- Call for further testing: a change from external to internal monitoring (the latter is more accurate), the fetal scalp stimulation test, or fetal pulse oximetry.

- If the fetal distress appears to be severe, immediately deliver the baby vaginally, with forceps or vacuum extraction (possibly with an episiotomy), or by cesarean. The choice of delivery method depends on how close the mother is to giving birth.

Because EFM by itself does not always indicate true fetal distress, cesareans are sometimes done unnecessarily. You might ask ahead of time what tests the mother's caregiver uses to confirm fetal distress before performing a cesarean. But, except for the fetal scalp stimulation test (which takes only a few seconds or minutes), tests and corrective measures take time, and, depending on how the EFM tracing looks, the caregiver may be too anxious about the baby's condition to wait for results. The truth of the matter is that there is no technology that can give us a clear and accurate indication of how well a baby is doing or is likely to be doing in the next hours. In a risky situation, most caregivers are less inclined to be patient and "wait and see" whether the baby will remain stable and healthy. They are more inclined to act quickly before the condition becomes an emergency.

Mother's reactions. The mother is likely to react in these ways:

- She will probably be very frightened and shocked when told that her baby shows signs of fetal distress.

- She will probably not question the caregiver's decisions under these circumstances.

- After the delivery, especially if it was sudden and frightening, the mother may have very mixed feelings: relief and joy that the baby is all right, confusion about all that has happened, and regrets or doubts about the cesarean and about her own behavior or decisions.

How you can help. You can help the mother in the following ways:

- Try to keep abreast of what is going on and what the staff is thinking.

- Ask questions, but do not keep the caregiver from doing what is necessary if the baby seems to be in danger.

- Ask for the quickly performed fetal scalp stimulation test to confirm the diagnosis of fetal distress.

- Follow the suggestions near the beginning of this chapter, pages 239 to 240, keeping in mind that if the situation is urgent, there will not be time for discussion.

Complications with the Newborn

The newborn baby is assessed immediately after birth. If all is normal, the baby is usually placed in the mother's arms for cuddling and suckling. If there are problems, the baby will probably go to the nursery for special care.

If the baby has problems, try to take part in the decision making about appropriate care. The "Key Questions for Informed Decision Making" (see page 202) will help. The mother may be unable to think clearly right after the birth because of the excitement and the effects of drugs, exhaustion, or problems of her own. Provided that you are legal next of kin, it may fall upon you to agree to the course of treatment. (If you have no legal or biological tie to the baby—if you are, for example, a lesbian co-parent—make arrangements ahead of time whereby you may make decisions about the baby if the biological mother cannot.)

If the baby must remain in the special-care nursery for several days or more, you will need to be his advocate, despite your distress. When a baby is hospitalized, many caregivers (for example, pediatricians, neonatologists, other physician specialists, nurses, laboratory personnel, X-ray and ultrasound technicians, respiratory or physical therapists, and social workers) are usually involved. They come and go, each providing care and information according to their roles and responsibilities. Keeping track of everything can be most confusing and may seem next to impossible. Parents and their partners often feel helpless, depressed, and either distrustful of the baby's caregivers or resigned to accepting whatever they say. Good communication and record keeping are ways to prevent these feelings of helplessness.

You should remain with the baby as much as possible. The baby needs someone who loves him close by, to hold him (if his condition permits), to stroke and talk to him, and to keep track of what is going on.

When you need to leave, ask a relative or friend to stay with the baby at least some of the time you are gone. The point is to remain informed as the various professionals participate in the baby's care. Keep a written log of each visit, including the date, the time, the professional's name and specialty, the purpose of the visit, and a summary of any communication regarding the baby's condition, plans for testing, medications, and so on. Keep all the records in one notebook, not on scraps of paper; this will make it easier for you to locate the items you want to ask about. Also, write down your questions so you will not forget to ask them. Above all, you should know who is coordinating the baby's care, and how to reach that doctor or, when he or she is off duty, a substitute.

The mother should remain with the baby as much as she is able. Try to make sure that there is a comfortable chair or bed for her, and that she has access to nourishing food. If the baby cannot breastfeed, the mother should be provided with a breast pump and instructions for using it. Pumped breast milk can usually be fed by bottle; if the baby cannot yet take a bottle, a stomach tube is used. Even if the mother is not planning to breastfeed, the pediatrician may ask her to provide her own milk until the baby can take formula well, since breast milk helps protect the baby from infection during this vulnerable time. Formula cannot do this.

Kangaroo care. Studies have shown that being held skin to skin against a parent's chest and covered with a blanket keeps a baby warmer than does a heated baby bed. The baby benefits not only from the parent's warmth but also from his or her movements, soothing voice, touch, and even heartbeat sounds. Both parent and baby are more content when they spend some hours each day in this "Kangaroo Care." Babies who have been "kangarooed" gain weight faster, suckle better, cry less, and are discharged from the hospital sooner. Kangaroo Care has been done even with babies who are receiving oxygen or tube feedings or who are very premature or sick. Ask the baby's caregiver or nurse about Kangaroo Care, and see "Recommended Resources" for more information on this subject.

Detailed descriptions of all possible newborn problems are beyond the scope of this book, but following are some fairly common problems that might arise shortly after birth.

BREATHING PROBLEMS

A newborn may have difficulty breathing because of fluid in the lungs, meconium aspiration (see "Suctioning the Baby's Nose and Mouth," page 332), narcotic drugs that were given to the mother at the wrong time (see chapter 8), infection, immature lungs, or congenital abnormalities. A baby who is slow to breathe on her own, or who breathes very fast and grunts as she breathes, may need medications, intravenous feeding, an incubator, deep suctioning, resuscitation, mechanical assistance with breathing, extra oxygen, or other help.

Low Body Temperature

A baby whose body temperature drops below normal uses up oxygen and energy to bring her temperature up. It is important to keep the baby warm. See "Kangaroo Care," page 263, and "Warming Unit," page 336.

Infection

A newborn sometimes acquires an infection while in the uterus or soon after birth. Depending on the organism causing it, the infection may be very serious (see "Group B Strep Screening," page 206). Prompt diagnosis and treatment with antibiotics or other medications, along with special care in the nursery (intravenous feeding, an incubator, and close observation) are needed.

Since infection in a newborn can become very serious very quickly, painful interventions may be necessary. These may include tests of various body fluids, obtained by heel sticks, spinal taps, bladder taps; scalp-vein intravenous lines; nasogastric tubes; and many other complex procedures. You and the mother will find all this confusing and frightening. Try to keep informed so you can understand what is done and why, and follow your baby's progress.

Birth Trauma or Injury

Some babies are injured during the birth process, especially if the birth is difficult. A very rapid birth or a difficult forceps, vacuum, or cesarean delivery can cause bruises, a broken collarbone, cuts, or nerve damage. Although wise management reduces the chances of such injuries, they can occur even with the most skilled caregivers.

For some vulnerable babies (for example, premature babies, babies with birth defects, and babies with genetic or other preexisting problems), even the normal birth process is too much. Some very large babies also suffer, if great effort by the caregiver is required to deliver them. Vulnerable babies can usually, but not always, be identified before labor, and plans can be made in advance for their special care.

Sometimes, even with the best of care, a baby is unexpectedly born with serious problems requiring emergency treatment or long-term care. This possibility haunts parents and professionals alike, and motivates attempts to develop better diagnostic and treatment methods.

DRUG EFFECTS

Improvements in pain medications and other drugs used during labor, and in the ways these drugs are given, have reduced the severity of side effects. Still, if a baby is born with a drug in his system, the drug may subtly or noticeably affect his behavior. Depending on the drug and the amount used, he may show some degree of sleepiness, poor suckling and breathing, lack of muscle tone, irritability, jitteriness, jaundice, or sluggishness of some reflex behaviors; or he may show other atypical signs. When the drug wears off, the baby behaves more normally. Sometimes other drugs (such as narcotic antagonists, which counteract some narcotic effects) or treatments (such as phototherapy for jaundice) hasten the baby's recovery.

LOW BLOOD SUGAR

Low blood sugar is rather common in (1) babies of diabetic mothers, (2) very large, small, or premature babies, (3) babies whose mothers received large amounts of intravenous dextrose or glucose solution during labor, (4) babies born after prolonged labors, and (5) babies born under certain other conditions. Symptoms of low blood sugar in the baby include jitteriness, irritability, breathing problems, temperature problems, and others. The diagnosis of low blood sugar is made by drawing blood from the baby's heel and analyzing it. Treatment usually consists of giving the baby some glucose water, formula, or colostrum and rechecking blood-sugar levels. The problem usually resolves itself quickly. See page 336 in chapter 10.

JAUNDICE

If the baby's skin or the whites of her eyes become yellowish, the baby is jaundiced. Usually harmless, physiologic jaundice is caused by elevated levels of bilirubin, a yellow pigment that results when red blood cells break down as part of their normal life cycle. Physiologic jaundice goes away on its own, usually in a few days, but high levels of bilirubin in some vulnerable babies may cause brain damage. Premature babies, babies who had particular difficulties during birth, and those with blood types incompatible with their mothers' are more vulnerable to brain damage from high bilirubin levels.

Jaundice is diagnosed by measuring bilirubin in the baby's blood, a sample of which is taken through a heel stick. Further tests of blood type, liver function, and bowel function help determine the cause of jaundice.

Jaundice is treated with phototherapy, which consists of exposing the baby's skin to special bright light almost constantly for a few days. Light breaks down (photo-oxidizes) bilirubin as it circulates through the blood vessels in the baby's skin and thus lowers total bilirubin levels. Portable phototherapy units are available for treatment at home. These are blankets or sleeping bags containing fiberoptic light filaments; these blankets can be wrapped around the baby to expose large areas of her skin to the light. Prolonged exposure to indirect sunlight (through a window) helps, but less reliably than artificial light. Frequent nursing (more than eight times per day) also helps relieve jaundice.

If the bilirubin levels are very high or if the baby is premature, jaundice is more serious, and a complete exchange transfusion of the baby's blood may be done.

PREMATURITY OR LOW BIRTH WEIGHT

The premature infant (born before 37 weeks' gestation) or the low-birth-weight infant (weighing less than $5\frac{1}{2}$ pounds) is more susceptible to all the newborn problems described here than is the full-term, average-sized baby. Premature babies are therefore watched more closely and receive more aggressive treatment. As they approach average size and weight, their vulnerability to problems decreases.

DEATH OF A BABY

Rarely, a baby dies during or around the time of birth. Words cannot describe the shock and grief felt by the parents and their loved ones. Of course, nothing can bring the baby back to life, but memories can be created that will have great meaning as time passes.

As difficult as it is to think through the possibility that your baby could die, it is a good idea to find out the kinds of things that can be done to bring some positive meaning to such a tragedy. Please see pages 29 to 30 for some suggestions. Decision making is very difficult when one is grieving intensely, but parents may later feel regret if they did not say goodbye in the way they would have chosen. See "Recommended Resources" for more helpful information.

Many hospitals have sensitive and compassionate staff members who will do all they can to create a meaningful opportunity for parents to be alone with their baby. Staff members may also provide referrals for support groups and grief counseling. Please make a plan, and then put it aside, with the peace of mind that you have it in case you need it. Now focus on a healthy outcome and a beautiful baby.

After It Is All Over

Any complication during labor or the early postpartum period, whether in the mother or in the baby, presents a challenge to all of you—to the mother, to the caregiver, to the baby, to the doula, and to you, the birth partner.

Each complication requires quick acceptance of a change in plans and expectations, often without a complete understanding of the situation. You do what has to be done, even if you are almost in a state of shock. But afterward, as you and the mother look back over the events, the feelings hit. Even if both the mother and the baby have come through alive and healthy, the emotional impact can be great. Unanswered questions and feelings of guilt, anger, or disappointment may arise, especially if everything happened too quickly for either or both of you to grasp, or if you, the mother, or the baby was treated unkindly or disrespectfully.

It may take time, especially for the mother, to come to terms with unrealized expectations. She will benefit from your patience and acceptance of what is, in reality, a grieving process. For both of you, a conference with the mother's caregiver may fill gaps in your understanding of the events and answer your questions. Sometimes consulting with a childbirth educator, trauma counselor, or psychotherapist helps either or both parents sort out feelings and gain a healthy perspective on a physically or emotionally traumatic birth experience. Please see page 318, "Your Role During and After a Cesarean Birth," for further discussion of emotional reactions following a difficult birth.

In the end, with the birth behind her, let us hope that the mother recognizes the courage and grace she displayed as she dealt with the unexpected challenges posed by a complicated labor.

CHAPTER 8

Medications for Pain During Labor

We both thought it would be great to make it through without an epidural, but labor went on and on and the pain got worse, and she (and I) got really tired. Every contraction was like this huge ordeal. She asked for an epidural. It went in smoothly and her pain was gone. She didn't even know when she was having a contraction! We both slept. It was almost hard to believe she was in labor.

—JOHN, FIRST-TIME FATHER

She had wanted an unmedicated birth this time, but she also knew she couldn't count on it because of all the unknowns of labor. I didn't know why it mattered so much to her. In labor, though, I really got into it. We were a real team. I loved working with her. But after a long time, with no end in sight, we ran out of gas. The epidural really helped. She feels she used it just the way she planned and feels great about the birth.

—ANDY, SECOND-TIME FATHER

Next to the health of mother and baby, the major concern of everyone—the caregiver, the mother, and her support team—is the mother's comfort during labor. Although the pain of labor is very intense, it does not have to be overwhelming (see the discussion of pain and suffering on page 112). There is much the mother can do to keep the pain manageable; she can learn and rehearse many effective comfort measures (see chapter 4, "Comfort Measures for Labor"). As you know, however, she will need help—from you, your doula or other supporters, and the staff—in using these comfort measures. Labor is simply too demanding for most women to manage without help.

In hospital births, drugs can also be used to relieve labor pain (only non-drug remedies are used in home and birth-center births). To a great extent, drugs for pain are optional; the mother can decide whether and when to use them. Because they are readily available in a variety of forms, and because they can have profound effects besides pain relief, they require precautions and extra procedures for safety. The mother should learn from her doctor, midwife, or childbirth classes about the pain relief methods that will be available to her, and decide how she feels about using them during labor. You should also be prepared. Are your feelings about her use of pain medications compatible with the mother's? Can you agree? Plan to support her in accomplishing what she wants.

It may seem somewhat foolish for a woman to plan whether or not to use pain medications in advance, since she has no idea how much pain she will feel or how she will react. Although this is true, she does know some things about herself that may help her decide: For example, does she prefer to feel as little pain or other sensation as possible? Or does she want to experience the labor, and deal with the pain using non-drug approaches as much as she can? Using the information in this chapter, you and the mother can make a plan that will guide you both as you encounter the pain of labor together.

Management of Normal Labor without Pain Medications

The pain of normal labor, though severe, can be successfully managed without the use of pain medications if:

◆ *The mother wants to avoid pain medications.* She should decide not only whether she wants to avoid pain medications but also how strongly she feels about this. See page 293.

◆ *She knows about the birth process and ways to relieve pain without medications.* If the mother wants to avoid pain medications, you both need to know the comfort measures described in chapter 4. It helps if you have rehearsed these together and adapted them to feel right to her. She will also cope better if she has access to such aids as a bath, a shower, a rocking chair, a birth ball, hot packs, cold packs, a squatting bar (as pictured on page 140), and music. (See chapter 4, "Comfort Measures for Labor.")

◆ *She has emotional support and assistance.* The mother needs competent, caring support from you—someone who loves her, who knows her well, who wants to share the birth, and who wants to help her accomplish her wishes. The continuous help of a doula improves a woman's chances of using less pain medication or avoiding it altogether, if that is what she wants. The doula accomplishes this with encouragement, reassurance, information, and guidance in the use of techniques that lessen pain and help labor progress. If a woman decides she wants pain medications, a doula helps her get them.

The mother also needs the support of the professional staff. A woman in labor is vulnerable to both positive and negative suggestions, especially from the experts—nurses, midwives, and physicians. If they believe in her and encourage her, she is more likely to carry on; if they pity or ignore her or discourage her from using her comfort measures, she is more likely to give up.

◆ *She has a reasonably normal labor.* This is partly a matter of luck. It must be a labor that does not include problems requiring many painful interventions, and that does not thoroughly exhaust and discourage her. This does not mean labor has to be short or painless. If the first three conditions are present, a woman can handle more challenges without pain medications, but you and she must realize and accept that in some labors pain medications are required.

If the mother prefers to cope without medications, prepare yourself for an active support role.

What You Need to Know about Pain Medications

To make an informed decision about pain medications, you and the mother both need some information:

◆ What is the drug? How does it work? How effective is it in relieving pain? What other effects does it have—on the mother, on the progress of labor, on the fetus, and on the newborn?

◆ What precautions or added interventions are needed to ensure safety?

◆ How does one support the woman who has taken pain medications?

Do not wait until the mother is in labor to get this information. When she is in pain and asking for medication, it is too late to try to learn all about the drugs.

Remember that, although various drugs are available, effective, and widely used in labor, they involve tradeoffs: The mother gets pain relief, but she or the fetus may experience unwanted side effects—directly, from the drug itself, or indirectly, through potential problems such as restriction of the mother's activity or the need for other interventions. Long-term detrimental effects on the baby of drugs used judiciously in labor have not been established. There may be no harm, or, in some cases, there may be subtle long-term effects. This is a subject of great debate in the medical literature, and it is unlikely to be settled in the near future.

For these reasons I advocate planning to use non-drug methods of pain relief at least for part of labor (see chapter 4, "Comfort Measures for Labor") and seeking a birth place that has the amenities (bathtub, shower, squatting bar, birthing bed, places to walk, rocking chair) that enhance a laboring woman's comfort. You may bring your own music, hot or cold packs, and birth ball (see page 145) if the hospital or birth center doesn't have them. If you're planning a home birth, you probably have furniture to lean on and hold on to for squatting and pillows to support you in various positions in bed.

By using non-drug pain-relief methods for at least part of the labor, the mother can comfortably postpone her use of pain medications. In this way, she will reduce the total amount of medications she receives and lessen the likelihood of undesirable effects and the need for additional interventions.

Many women find these non-drug methods sufficient to keep their pain at a level at which they can cope throughout the labor. Afterward, the absence of drug side effects and the ability to get up and move freely immediately after the birth contribute to a feeling that the rewards are worth the pain.

Preparing to deal with labor pain using non-drug methods is time-consuming, however, and going through labor without drugs can be a challenge. And if labor is exhausting or complicated, the benefits of pain medications will outweigh the potential risks. Many women do not have the time or inclination to master the non-drug approaches, and so plan to rely on the epidural to take away most pain in labor, or wait to see whether they need it. About 70 percent of laboring American women use an epidural today.

As you both learn more about pain medication, you will be able to help the mother make informed choices. To begin our discussion of pain medications, here are several definitions.

- *Analgesia.* Reduction of pain. Analgesics are drugs that relieve pain.

- *Anesthesia.* Loss of sensation, including pain sensation. Anesthetics are drugs that take away feeling.

- *Systemic.* Taken up by the bloodstream, affecting the entire body, and reaching the baby in concentrations similar to those reaching the mother.

- *Neuraxial.* Affecting areas of the body that are supplied by specific nerves coming from the spinal cord. (The neuraxis is the brain and spinal cord.)

- *Neuraxial analgesic.* A pain medication injected near nerve roots in the spine to block or decrease awareness of pain in the area supplied by those spinal nerves. Neuraxial analgesics are used in epidural and spinal blocks.

- *Block.* Medication that interrupts the transmission of pain impulses, creating numbness.
- *Local.* Affecting specific tissues—in childbirth, the cervix, vagina, and perineum. A local anesthetic blocks the feeling provided by nerve endings in these tissues.
- *General anesthesia.* Complete loss of consciousness caused by a systemic medication, a *general anesthetic.*

When pain medications are used, several factors influence the area where pain is relieved and the severity of side effects:

- The choice of medication—a narcotic or narcotic-like drug, a sedative, a tranquilizer, an anesthetic gas, an injected anesthetic, or an amnesiac.
- The total dose—the concentration of the drug, the volume of each dose, and the number of doses.
- The route of administration—injection into a muscle, a vein, the cervix, or the vaginal wall; inhalation into the lungs; injection into the epidural or spinal (intrathecal) space; or swallowing.
- Individual characteristics of the mother—her weight, her sensitivity to medications, her blood-clotting ability, her anatomic variations, her physical condition, the duration of her pregnancy, and her overall health.

HOW PAIN IS RELIEVED BY MEDICATIONS

Medications reduce pain by altering some part of the nervous system, the system that makes it possible to recognize, interpret, and react to pain.

Labor pain originates with pressure, stretching, or compression involving tissues in the uterus, vagina, or pelvic joints. Contractions of the uterus, dilation of the cervix, and the baby's movement through the pelvis create the pain. Nerve endings in these tissues are stimulated to send pain impulses over nerve fibers to the spinal cord and brain.

The transmission of the pain signals can be modified anywhere along this pathway—in the nerve endings, in the nerve roots (which are situated where the nerves leave the spine), in the spinal cord, or in the brain.

This is how various pain medications work:

- Local anesthetics block nerve endings in the injected areas from sending the pain impulses over the nerve fibers to the spine and brain.

- Epidural and spinal (neuraxial) medications are either injected or absorbed into the spinal fluid. They block the transmission of pain signals from the nerve fibers where they enter the spinal cord.

- Systemic medications (such as narcotics) act in the brain to reduce recognition of pain or reactions to it.

The rest of this chapter presents specific information about the various medications used during labor. You and the mother may use these pages as background for your discussions with her caregiver, for seeking further information, and for making decisions. The drugs are grouped in the text according to general characteristics (subtle differences among the drugs in each group are not described here). For more details, consult the table "Pain Medications and Their Effects" (see pages 296 to 303), which lists all the medications and techniques and important information on each. The chart "When Are Pain Medication Used?," page 293, indicates at which stages of labor the various pain-relief methods are most safely used and when the drugs' effects will ideally have worn off. When you have both read through the chapter, you will be ready to use the "Pain Medications Preference Scale," on pages 294 to 295, as a tool in your decision making.

SYSTEMIC DRUGS

Drugs that affect the whole body—the entire system—are called *systemic drugs*. Systemic analgesics (pain-relieving drugs) use the bloodstream to transport the medication to the brain, where the drug exerts its pain-relieving effect. Systemic drugs can be given in several forms: as pills, as gases to inhale, as injections into the skin or muscle, or as part of a solution fed directly into a vein.

Systemic drugs give short-term relief (one-half to two hours, depending on the specific drug and the dose). Another dose might be given after this period, or the mother might go on to have an epidural. While under the effect of a systemic drug, the mother feels groggy and dozes between contractions.

Systemic drugs circulate not only to the mother's brain but also throughout her body; they also cross the placenta to the baby. Because their effects on the baby after birth may be profound, these drugs must be given early enough in the labor to allow time for them to wear off before birth. If a systemic drug has not worn off sufficiently by the time of birth, another drug, such as a narcotic antagonist, is given to counteract the unwanted effects of the original drug.

Even when the timing is appropriate, some of a drug (or its metabolic by-products) almost certainly remains in the baby's bloodstream after birth and may subtly alter her behavior and reflexes for a few days following. How severely medication affects the baby depends on her health and maturity, the choice of drug, the size and number of doses given, and the times they are given during labor. The healthier the baby, the smaller the amount of medication used, and the greater the time between its administration and the birth, the less pronounced the effects will be on the baby.

There are three categories of systemic pain medications that may be given during prelabor or during the dilation (first) stage: tranquilizers, sedatives, and narcotics (see the table on page 296). Other systemic medications, called general anesthetics, are occasionally used during the dilation or birthing (second) stage. General anesthetics are discussed as a separate category on page 289.

The partner's role when the mother has taken a narcotic. Tranquilizers, sedatives, and morphine are used in prelabor to reduce anxiety or help the mother sleep, so when one of these drugs is given, the partner's role is to try to keep the mother from being disturbed. Narcotics, however, are given during labor to help the mother cope with pain. They require the partner's or the doula's help to work well. A narcotic may help the woman relax between contractions, and give her a slightly longer break before the next one. The peaks, however, are as painful with as without the narcotic. A common problem is that the mother dozes during the early seconds of the contraction, so the peak hits her suddenly, and she can't cope. Many women who have taken a narcotic report that it was "useless," even though they got a little more rest after taking it.

Try to remain awake after the mother takes a narcotic, so you can tell from her behavior that the contraction is coming. Although she will probably be dozing, she will wince or groan before she is fully aware of the contraction. As soon as it begins, get her attention: "Okay, here it is. Open your eyes and breathe with me. That's good." This allows her to get into a rhythm before the peak. Help her over the peak by talking and moving your hand rhythmically until she drifts off again. In this way, you can maximize the benefit of the narcotic.

NEURAXIAL ANALGESIA AND ANESTHESIA (EPIDURAL AND SPINAL)

Of all the pain-relieving medications, these provide the most effective pain relief, use the smallest amount of drug, and have the fewest effects on the mother's mental state and on the baby's well-being. Depending on the dosage, these drugs, which were formerly referred to as "regional" anesthetics and analgesics, cause partial to complete numbness, muscle weakness, decreased control over the legs, an inability to urinate, and other effects (see page 279).

As I will explain in the following pages, there are numerous varieties of neuraxial analgesia. You and the mother may want to talk with her doctor or midwife about the particular techniques used in your hospital.

Neuraxial blocks can be used for either vaginal or cesarean delivery. They usually combine a low dose of a narcotic with a low dose of an anesthetic drug. Neuraxial blocks do not alter the mother's consciousness as much as systemic drugs do, because the narcotic in a neuraxial block is a much lower dose and isn't given directly into a blood vessel. The narcotic enhances the effects of the anesthetic, and this allows for lower doses of both drugs than would be effective if they were used separately. Neuraxial blocks provide the best pain relief of all the medications for labor.

Administering a neuraxial block requires a high degree of skill, and is therefore done only by specialists—anesthesiologists or specially trained nurse-anesthetists. Neuraxial blocks are the most costly of all obstetric pain-relieving techniques, but they are also the most popular. They are great sources of revenue for hospitals, many of which actively promote the use of epidurals.

The spinal can be given as a single injection of a narcotic or an anesthetic or as a combination of the two. The effects last a few hours.

The epidural block is usually used for more prolonged analgesia. A catheter (a thin tube) is inserted into the epidural space in the woman's low back (see the illustration on page 281) and left in place. The medication is dripped into the catheter continuously, and sometimes the mother can push a button to give herself small additional doses of the medicine whenever the pain escalates. This is called "patient-controlled epidural analgesia."

Both the spinal and the epidural blocks are given in the *lumbar spine*, in the low back. The spinal injection goes in a few millimeters deeper—through the *dura* and into the *dural space*. The dura is the membrane that surrounds the spinal cord and the spinal nerves and contains the spinal fluid; the dural space is the space within the dura. The epidural injection stops just short of the dura, in the *epidural space*. The medicine is absorbed across the dura and has effects similar to a spinal, though usually with less effect on the mother's ability to move her legs.

General characteristics of neuraxial analgesia. The anesthetics used for neuraxial blocks are sometimes referred to as "caine" drugs; common examples are Carbocaine, Marcaine, Xylocaine, Nesacaine, and Ropivacaine. These drugs are quite similar in their effects on the mother, on the labor, and on the baby. Subtle differences in their biochemical makeup, however, affect the way they act in the body and the duration of their effects. The mother's caregiver and her anesthesiologist usually select the specific drug to be used. The mother should be sure to inform the anesthesiologist if she knows she has a sensitivity or allergy to any drug.

The narcotics that are used for neuraxial analgesia include morphine, fentanyl, and sufentanil. They can be given alone in early labor or after a cesarean, or in combination with the "caine" anesthetics for vaginal or cesarean birth.

Narcotics take effect more quickly than the caine drugs and interfere less with a woman's use of her legs. If narcotics are given alone in early labor, they are usually given as a spinal. The mother may be able to stand and walk a bit with help, but she may not be very steady on her feet, and she could fall. For this reason, most hospitals discourage laboring women from walking with spinal narcotics. If the mother does walk, her partner or the nurse must stay right with her whenever she is upright.

Because the spinal narcotics administered in early labor usually are inadequate by the time a woman is in active labor, a caine drug may be added in the epidural space. This gives good relief when the pain becomes more intense. The two-step approach is called a "combined spinal-epidural." It allows a woman to feel virtually no pain from early labor until pushing, when she may have perineal pain.

Narcotics administered neuraxially can cause side effects in the mother, and may affect the baby, too. In many women these drugs cause some grogginess (though less than when given systemically), itching, and nausea. Fentanyl and sufentanil, because of their biochemical properties, cross more easily to the baby than do the caine drugs, and small quantities are still present in the baby's blood at two days of age. The effects of these drugs on the newborn have not been studied.

Epidural or spinal morphine (Duramorph) is often used for pain relief after a cesarean. A dose given before the mother leaves the operating room provides very good pain relief for about 24 hours, after which she is offered other pain medications.

In general, the desired effect of the drugs is loss of pain sensation in the affected area. Reducing the mother's pain during labor relaxes her and, especially in a prolonged, exhausting labor, allows her to sleep and may result in more rapid dilation of the cervix.

Possible undesirable effects depend on the area injected, the total dosage, and the choice of drugs. The effects are listed under "Neuraxial Analgesia" in the table "Pain Medications and Their Effects" (see pages 298 to 301). The table also lists precautions used to maximize the safety of each technique.

General technique for giving a neuraxial (epidural or spinal) block. There are many similarities among the techniques for administering the various neuraxial blocks. The general procedure is described here. Please refer to the table "Pain Medications and Their Effects," page 298, for specific information about each type of block.

Neuraxial blocks numb or reduce sensation in a large portion of the mother's body—between the top of her uterus and her feet. The area affected can be controlled to a great extent by the amount and concentration of the drug given and by the placement of the injection. For example, the mother may be able to move her legs while remaining numb in her trunk. This is the procedure:

1. Before receiving the anesthetic, the mother is given intravenous fluids to reduce the chance that her blood pressure will drop.

2. The mother lies on her side or sits up and curls her body forward. An anesthesiologist scrubs the area where the injection will be given, numbs the skin with a local anesthetic, and then injects a small amount of anesthetic between the vertebrae of her low back (lumbar spine), into the epidural or dural space (see the illustrations). The anesthesiologist checks to make sure that the needle is placed correctly. Sometimes more than one attempt is needed to get the needle placed perfectly.

3. For a spinal, a full dose is given in a single injection that lasts about two hours; for an epidural, a thin tube is run through the epidural needle to allow for a continuous drip of the medicine. Within minutes the mother begins to feel the effects. She is soon numb in the desired area.

4. Sometimes pain relief is uneven or spotty, and it takes some adjustment (changing the mother's position, injecting more doses) before the pain relief is adequate.

5. A thin plastic tube (a catheter) can be left in place and taped to her back so that the medicine may drip in steadily or the mother may add some, by pushing a button, if she desires.

6. The mother's blood pressure and pulse are checked frequently.

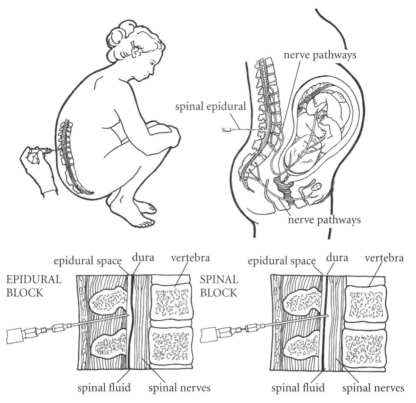

Neuraxial anesthesia. Above left: As the mother lies on her side or sits up, the anesthesiologist injects the anesthetic. Above right: The sites of injection for neuraxial analgesia. Below: These detailed drawings illustrate the placement of the needle for an epidural block (left) and a spinal block (right).

The partner's role when the woman has an epidural. Women who have epidurals are often shortchanged emotionally by their partners and the staff. It is easy to believe that when the mother no longer has pain she no longer needs support. Partners often distance themselves from the mother, by taking a break, getting a meal, going to sleep, or turning on the TV. Studies of women's thoughts and feelings before and after epidurals indicate that they want and benefit from continuous support even when their pain is relieved. An epidural not only usually relieves labor pain very effectively, but it also allows the woman to relax and rest, and, if she is exhausted, frightened, or tense, it often allows her a good sleep and adequate Pitocin to cause better labor progress. An epidural does not, however, relieve all of a woman's distress.

Following are some emotional challenges for women with epidurals, and ways the partner can help.

The decision to ask for an epidural. Women who have desired a natural childbirth may feel disappointed that they cannot handle the pain. Those who have planned in advance to use an epidural may be upset if they are asked to wait until their labor has progressed more.

The wait. The time from when a woman decides she wants the epidural until she actually gets it and has adequate pain relief is particularly difficult. Thirty to 60 minutes usually pass before the mother is prepared, the anesthesiologist arrives, the drug is administered, and the medication takes effect. The wait can be even longer if the anesthesiologist is busy with another patient or if the woman must undergo various procedures, such as admissions paperwork or administration of intravenous fluids, before she can get the epidural. In the meantime, the mother must continue coping, even though she does not want to.

If you find yourself in this situation, you may feel helpless standing by while the woman you love is in pain. You may feel ineffective and frustrated because she no longer finds the comfort techniques and your suggestions helpful, and yet you must try to persuade her to continue coping until the anesthesiologist arrives. Discuss this possible scenario together before labor, and make an agreement to continue with the coping techniques in chapter 4, especially rhythmic movements, moaning, stroking, and the Take-Charge Routine. These techniques can keep the mother from becoming panicked or overwhelmed.

Sometimes, a mother is progressing so fast in labor that she no longer needs the extra pain relief by the time it takes effect. She may be pushing her baby out by then!

Getting the epidural. Administering the epidural takes anywhere from 15 to 45 minutes, depending on the anesthesiologist's skill and experience, the mother's spinal anatomy, and her ability to cooperate by lying or sitting still while curling her back—an uncomfortable position, especially during contractions. The mother will need you to help her remain still and calm, to acknowledge the difficulty of what she is being asked to do, and to tell her how well she is doing.

Relief of pain. Within minutes after the epidural is placed, the pain of the contractions will begin to subside, and it will probably be gone within 15 to 30 minutes. The mother's mood should improve markedly; she may become chatty, optimistic, and very grateful to the anesthesiologist. If pain relief is incomplete, of course, she will be disappointed and impatient for adjustments to correct the problem.

When the mother is comfortable, you will also be relieved and grateful, and you can rest and have a snack.

"Where is everyone?" Once the mother is comfortable she will no longer need intense support and close physical contact, but she will feel suddenly alone and unimportant if you turn on the TV, leave to get a meal, or take a nap. Unless you have a doula or other family member to remain with her, don't leave the room. Continue to show support by bringing the mother things to make her comfortable— warm blankets, ice chips, her comb and toothbrush—and asking questions and making conversation with the nurse. Watch the monitor from time to time, and point out contractions when they occur. You may both find it hard to believe that the mother is really having contractions, after what she has been through.

If the mother goes to sleep, she will probably sleep lightly and fitfully. When she wakes up, she may feel quite alone if you are out of the room or sound asleep. If you are exhausted, of course, you may not be able to stay awake. Before you drift off, tell her to be sure to wake you if she needs anything or if the doctor comes in.

Almost forgetting she is in labor. It's easy for the mother to be distracted from her labor when she can no longer feel it. But she may still be able to do things to prevent the labor from slowing or to change the baby's position. Have her try the six positions of the Rollover (see page 284), changing every 20 to 30 minutes when she is awake. If the nurse finds problems with any of the positions, skip it and go to the next.

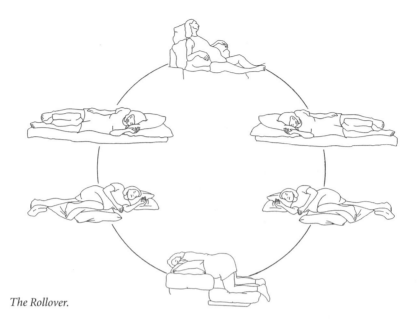

The Rollover.

When side effects occur. During this otherwise calm period, problems may occur that require action by the staff—for example, slowing of labor progress, a drop in the mother's blood pressure or the baby's heart rate, or a fever in the mother. The doctor or midwife may come to start a Pitocin drip or rupture the mother's membranes. The nurse may check her blood pressure frequently, have her change her position, or wear an oxygen mask for a while to raise the baby's heart rate. The doctor or midwife may call for antibiotics if the mother develops a fever, because it is not possible to know if the fever is a side-effect of the epidural, or due to infection.

Resting and waiting. After the epidural takes effect, the mother will hardly know that she is in labor until it is time to push. She may feel strange to be laboring without any direct experience of it, unless she presses on her belly with her hands. The nurse will check the mother's blood pressure, the fetal monitor, and, occasionally, the mother's cervix, and write in the chart while the woman waits for something to happen. If she is not sleepy, the mother may feel bored or quite helpless. She may begin to worry that the labor is taking too long or that the baby isn't tolerating the labor well. The mother needs distraction, conversation, and reassurance that a sense of detachment is expected with an epidural. This is a good time for her to prepare for the bearing-down efforts of the second stage, by gently rehearsing the bearing-down technique (breathing in, holding her breath, and gently straining) and discussing with the nurse what to expect when it is time to push.

Focusing on other discomforts. Even when the mother's pain is under good control, other discomforts may bother her, especially if she is unprepared for them. These include direct and indirect effects of the epidural: the heavy, numb feeling in her legs; heartburn or reflux; feeling too warm or too cold; trembling; pain in her upper back or shoulder; a "window" of pain in the area covered by the epidural; dry mouth; itching; nausea; or discomfort in her position. The nurse, following hospital policy or the doctor's orders, will decide whether to relieve such discomforts, and how to do it. You or the doula may be allowed to provide ice chips, sips of water or juice, changes of position, warm blankets, cool cloths, and massage. Medications for itching, nausea, heartburn, or breakthrough pain will require an order from the caregiver or anesthesiologist. Some women find it annoying to have to get permission before rolling over or taking a sip of water or chewing an antacid. You might help by addressing the nurse or doctor: "She always takes Tums for her heartburn, and it really helps. Do you think it's okay for her to take one?"

Breakthrough pain. As labor advances, some pain may return. This can be scary for the mother if she has been free of pain for hours. Let the staff know, so they can call the anesthesiologist or adjust the epidural dosage to maintain good pain relief.

Complete dilation. Even though the mother does not feel her cervix dilating, you both may feel a sense of accomplishment and optimism when the nurse tells you that the mother has reached complete dilation: a hurdle has been reached. Several options exist now: (1) to turn down the epidural to give the mother sensations to guide her bearing-down efforts; (2) to have her begin pushing by holding her breath and straining with every contraction; or (3) to delay pushing until the baby is visible at the vaginal outlet or the mother feels the urge to push.

The first option may appeal to a woman who wanted an unmedicated birth; she may see it as an opportunity to resume an active role in her labor. But because of decreases in endorphin production that occur when an epidural is in effect, the pain is greater if the epidural medication is reduced than it would be if she had never had the epidural at all. Many women who have their epidural turned down find the pain of the second stage intolerable. Endorphins are the body's own painkillers. Without them, a mother may need to turn the epidural up again, and she should not feel bad about this.

Option 2, maximal breath holding and straining, is still expected in some hospitals, but does not work very well and actually increases the need for forceps or vacuum extraction (see pages 234 to 237). Women with epidurals typically feel unable to push effectively and find it difficult to follow directions, because they can't feel what they are doing.

With option 3, the mother rests for up to an hour or more, while the staff monitors the baby, until the mother begins to feel an urge to push or the baby's head appears at her vaginal opening. Then she pushes with her contractions. Although this option may lengthen the birthing stage, it is the easiest on mother and baby, and it results in fewer instrumental deliveries. You and the mother should consider requesting option 3 in her Birth Plan and discussing it with her caregiver at a prenatal appointment. If you are lucky, you will find that her caregiver favors this option, too.

Help with pushing. When it is time for her to push, you or the doula can help the mother to push well by watching the monitor for contractions, telling her when to start pushing, and cheering her on. Tell her to push when the intensity numbers go up by 20 points or so (the nurse can tell you where to look for those numbers). As the mother holds her breath and pushes, she makes the numbers go up fast and high. You call out the increasing intensity readings from the contraction monitor to show her how effective she is: "21, 30, 40, now press that baby down . . . 60, 73, 80, 96, 100, yes! That's the way! Now breathe for the baby . . . and bear down again. You're at 73, 80, 91, 100, 120, 127! Yes! Wow! You're at the max! And breathe for the baby. Great! And now breathe your way out of the contraction. Good! Do you realize that you doubled the strength of the contraction with your pushing? That was great!" Responding this way shows the woman how well she is doing, and gives her a sense of accomplishment that she might otherwise not have. Try to have the mother hold her breath for 5 to 6 seconds, which is what women do spontaneously when they do not have an epidural. One of my clients found this so helpful that she asked me to continue calling out numbers even after the monitor was removed! (The monitor is usually removed a few contractions before the birth, because the baby is so low that the heartbeat cannot be picked up.)

"Ouch! I can feel it!" As the baby's head presses on the rectum, reaches the perineum, and distends the vaginal opening, the mother may feel much the same burning, stretching sensation that women without epidurals feel. This may come as an unwelcome shock after she has felt only numbness. To turn her fear to excitement, assure her that the baby is almost born. If the caregiver asks the mother to stop pushing as the head emerges, try to help her pant through the contractions.

Vacuum or forceps delivery. If the doctor thinks the mother may need an instrumental delivery (which is more likely with an epidural than without), she may welcome it if she is exhausted. You should implore her to "give it everything you have" to make the delivery successful. If she does, she may be able to speed the delivery and avoid the vacuum extractor or forceps.

If the doctor decides to try an instrumental delivery, the mother may be frightened that the instruments will harm the baby. The doctor should tell her that he or she will not continue with the instruments if the baby does not move with a couple of contractions. The doctor may also tell her that a cesarean will be necessary if the instruments are not successful. This prospect is added incentive for the woman to push hard.

The birth! The predominant emotions for her may be relief at not having to push any longer and fascination with the baby. You may have exactly the same emotions, along with admiration for her and powerful love for the baby.

With the sensitive support I have described here, you will contribute to a safe, satisfying birth experience that will launch you both into parenthood with a sense of competence and self-confidence.

LOCAL ANESTHESIA

The local blocks are given via injection. There are three major local blocks: the paracervical, the pudendal, and the perineal block. The paracervical block, which numbs the cervix, is rarely used in North America. The pudendal block numbs the vaginal canal, and the perineal block numbs the perineum. The perineal block is the one usually called a "local." All of the local blocks use the "caine" drugs, the same anesthetics that are used in neuraxial blocks.

Technique for giving local anesthesia. Local blocks numb smaller portions of the mother's body than do neuraxial blocks. Because local blocks are easier to administer, they do not require the skills of an anesthesiologist. The caregiver draws the anesthetic into a syringe and injects it into the appropriate sites within or near the vagina. For details about each type of block, see the table "Pain Medications and Their Effects," pages 296 to 303.

Local blocks require larger doses of medication and provide less pain relief than do neuraxial blocks. Also, with a local block more medication enters the mother's circulation; the drug may thus affect the fetus and the newborn more profoundly than it would if administered in a neuraxial block. This is why the paracervical block has almost disappeared from use in many areas of North America, and the pudendal block now tends to be reserved for late second-stage forceps deliveries. The perineal block, or "local," is given either shortly before delivery for an episiotomy, or immediately after delivery for stitching. If the anesthetic is administered close to delivery, the fetus may receive less of the drug and be less affected. With an epidural, usually, no local block is used.

GENERAL ANALGESIA AND ANESTHESIA

This form of pain relief medication comes either as a gas to be inhaled through a mask or as a liquid that is injected intravenously. It reduces pain quickly by reducing or eliminating consciousness for as little as a minute to several hours.

Inhalation analgesia: nitrous oxide. Inhaled gases are not widely used for labor pain relief in the United States, but one, nitrous oxide mixed with oxygen ("laughing gas" or "gas and air"), is widely used in Canada and many other nations for labor pain.

Nitrous oxide is self-administered by the mother. She inhales the gas via a hand-held mask or mouthpiece at the very beginning of a contraction (or a little before, if she or her partner can judge when it is about to begin). Within about 15 seconds, she feels drowsy, light-headed, or giddy. Her pain isn't eliminated, but it is reduced (as one woman said, "The pain was there, but I was not bothered by it"). The mother breathes the gas through the contraction, and then removes the mask until the next contraction. The effect disappears quickly, and she is herself between contractions.

Nitrous oxide is considered to be most effective for pain in the late dilation stage, especially transition. The gas is also useful in situations when quick pain relief is needed, such as manual removal of the placenta or some other painful procedure.

Nitrous oxide is considered safe for mothers and babies when used intermittently over a rather short time. Many women enjoy the mental effects, although others dislike them. In any case, these effects wear off quickly. Other side effects are uncommon; they include nausea or vomiting in 1 to 10 percent of women.

The greatest drawback of nitrous oxide is also its greatest advantage: Its effects are immediate and very transient, lasting one minute or so. For women who want complete pain relief over many hours, nitrous oxide is not a good choice. But for those who want a quick assist for a few contractions or a brief painful procedure, nitrous oxide might be a good choice. I wish it were more available in the United States.

General anesthetics. These are systemic drugs, affecting the whole body. Given in the form of a gas to be inhaled or as an intravenous medicine, they rapidly enter the bloodstream. They circulate to the brain, where they quickly abolish awareness of pain and cause loss of consciousness.

Though easy and quick to administer, general anesthetics carry the potential risk that the unconscious woman could vomit and inhale her vomitus, which would cause pneumonia. Although anesthesiologists place a tube in the mother's airway to prevent such a complication, neuraxial anesthesia is safer and therefore generally preferred. But general anesthesia is used today in the following circumstances:

♦ When complications that are life-threatening to the mother (such as hemorrhage) or baby (such as a prolapsed cord) require a cesarean or other surgery to be performed within minutes.

♦ When a neuraxial block cannot be performed because of specific medical conditions or anatomical anomalies in the woman.

♦ When an unexpected cesarean must be performed in a rural hospital that does not have an anesthesiologist on duty around the clock. Under such circumstances, the general anesthetic is given by the doctor doing the surgery.

♦ When the mother has expressed a strong desire to be unconscious for the birth.

See the table "Pain Medications and Their Effects" (page 302) for an explanation of the effects of different concentrations of inhaled gases.

The Mother's Decisions Regarding Pain Medications During Labor

It is important for you to know the mother's desires regarding her use of pain medications in labor, and to explore with her how you yourself feel about her using them. Many birth partners have strong personal feelings on the subject. Some believe deeply that natural, unmedicated birth is preferable; others believe that natural birth is unnecessary suffering and encourage the use of medications. The most important thing is for both of you to share your feelings in advance and then prepare together as described here. Use the "Pain Medications Preference Scale," pages 294 to 295, to thoroughly explore the way you both feel.

When you both have learned about the demands and joys of childbirth, and about the medical and nonmedical methods to manage pain, it is time to come up with a plan regarding the use of pain medication that meets the laboring woman's wishes. Both of you should examine your personal feelings about birth, pain, and the support the mother needs. How much help can she realistically expect from you? How do you honestly feel about taking on the role of the birth partner? Go through the list of questions headed "How Will I Feel?" (see page 5) to assess your reactions to some of the realities of labor. Consider having a doula to help both of you.

The "Pain Medications Preference Scale" (PMPS) offers the mother a systematic and realistic way to think about her preferred approach to pain relief and the kind of help she will need from you and others. Using the PMPS, the mother won't make a yes-no choice about the use of pain medications, but she will measure the strength of her feelings in either direction. You too should go through the PMPS, to see whether you are comfortable with the mother's feelings about pain medications.

Of course, no one knows in advance how long or painful a woman's labor will be or whether there will be complications. A flexible approach is the only sensible one. The PMPS takes this into account by including a variety of possibilities.

After thoughtful consideration of these unknowns, the mother's PMPS rating will be a good predictor of whether and under what circumstances she will or will not use pain medications. The PMPS will also be a most helpful guide to all who will be helping her.

DIRECTIONS FOR USING THE PMPS

Take plenty of time to go over the PMPS. Ask the mother to use it to help figure out the approach to pain relief that best suits her, and to discover the kind of help she will need from you, a doula, or both to make it work. In the left column, the numbers from +10 down to +3 indicate degrees of desire to use pain medication, with +10 being the highest possible (and unrealistic) desire to use them for maximum relief of pain or any other sensations. Zero indicates no opinion. The numbers from −3 to −10 indicate degrees of desire to avoid pain medication, with −10 being an impossible extreme, just as +10 is. I put the impossible extremes on the scale to give more meaning and clarity to the points in between.

After the mother picks the number that reflects her preferences, you should both look in the right-hand column for the kind of support and preparation she will need. Can you provide this kind of support? If you have doubts, she can either rethink her preferences to be more in line with the kind of support you can provide, or you can get extra help from a doula or loved one. Is she preparing adequately? Make sure she understands that avoiding pain medication requires more preparation than using it.

THE MOTHER'S CODE WORD

Many partners worry that the mother who has a strong desire (−5 to −9) to avoid pain medications may change her mind. How can the partner know when to stop encouraging her to continue without medications? The answer is to have a "code word."

You and the mother should agree on a word she can use during labor if she changes her mind about wanting an unmedicated birth. The word should be one she is unlikely to use in conversation (for example, "uncle," "pumpernickel," or "cosmic"). As long as she does not say this word, you know that you should continue helping her without suggesting pain medications, even if she says she wants them. If she says the code word, you know she really wants to change her plan, and you must respect her wishes.

This agreement allows a woman to express her discouragement ("I can't do this"; "I'm done"; "This hurts too much"; "I want drugs") without the partner's feeling a need to rescue her. With a client of mine whose preference score was −7 and who seemed very distressed in labor, I was worried. I did not want to encourage her to give up her plans for a natural birth, but I was afraid she may have forgotten about her code word. So I finally said, "You have a code word, you know." She never used it, so I continued to support her. Later she said she hadn't forgotten it and was glad she could complain as much as she needed to. Complaining—always in rhythm!—was her way of coping.

WHEN ARE PAIN MEDICATIONS USED?

MEDICATION	DILATION STAGE			BIRTHING STAGE	THIRD STAGE
	Prelabor to 3 cm	*4 to 7 cm*	*8 to 10 cm*	*(pushing, birth)*	*(placenta)*
Morphine (**S**)	▽————				
Sedatives (**S**)	▽————				
Tranquilizers (**S**)	▽————	▽————			
Narcotic-like analgesics (**S**)	▽————	▽————	▽————		
Narcotic antagonists (**S**)		▽————	▽————		▽(to baby)▽
Paracervical block (**L**)		▽————	▽————		
Self-administered inhalation analgesia (**S**)			▽————	▽————	
Epidural or spinal narcotic analgesia (**N**)	▽————	▽————	▽————	▽————	
Standard epidural anesthesia—with or without narcotics (**N**)		▽-------------			
Segmental ("light and late") epidural anesthesia (**N**)		▽-------------			
Combined spinal-epidural (**N**)	▽————	▽————			
Pudendal block (**L**)				▽————	
Perineal block (**L**)				▽————	▽
Spinal, for cesarean only (**N**)*	▽————		▽————	▽————	
General anesthesia, for cesarean only (**S**)*	▽-------------		▽————	▽————	

*These can be given whenever a cesarean is decided upon.

Key

———— Time when drug may safely remain in effect.

----------- Time when dosing may be continuous.

▽ Time when drug may be given (some must be discontinued early to allow side effects to diminish before birth).

S systemic medication   **N** neuraxial anesthesia   **L** local anesthesia

When are pain medications used?

PAIN MEDICATIONS PREFERENCE SCALE

RATING	WHAT IT MEANS FOR THE MOTHER	HOW PARTNER AND DOULA HELP
+10	• Desire that she feel nothing; desire for anesthesia before labor begins.	• This is an impossible extreme; if the mother says she is +10, help her accept that it is not wise or possible to feel nothing in labor; the risks are too high. She will have some pain and should focus on dealing with it. • Review the discussion of pain medications with her. • Help her get pain medications as soon as possible.
+9	• Fear of pain; believes she cannot cope; dependence on staff for total pain relief.	• Same as for +10 • Suggest she discuss her fears with her caregiver.
+7	• Definite desire for anesthesia as soon as the doctor will allow it, or before labor becomes painful.	• Make sure the doctor is aware of her desire. Learn whether early anesthesia is possible in her hospital. • Inform the staff of her desire when you arrive.
+5	• Desire for epidural anesthesia in active labor (at 4 to 5 cms dilation). • Willingness to cope until then, perhaps with narcotic medications.	• Encourage her in 3Rs (see pages 115–121). • Know the comfort measures (see chapter 4) and how to help. • Suggest medications as she approaches active labor.
+3	• Preference for using medication, but as little as possible, with some sensation. Desire to use self-help comfort measures. • Natural childbirth is not a goal.	• Plan to be active as a birth partner to help her keep medication use low. Use comfort measures (see chapter 4). • Help her get medications when she wants them. • Suggest low doses of narcotics or a "light" epidural (to allow some feeling).
0	• No opinion or preference. • This attitude is rare among pregnant women, though not among birth partners or doulas.	• Make sure she is informed. • Discuss medications. • Help her decide what she prefers. • If she has no preference, let the staff manage her pain.
−3	• Would like to avoid pain medications unless coping becomes difficult. Would not feel disappointed or guilty if she used medications.	• Do not suggest medications. • Emphasize coping techniques, but do not try to talk her out of pain medications if she asks.

PAIN MEDICATIONS PREFERENCE SCALE

RATING	WHAT IT MEANS FOR THE MOTHER	HOW PARTNER AND DOULA HELP
−5	• Strong preference to avoid pain medications, to avoid side effects on the baby or the labor. • Will accept medications for a long or difficult labor.	• Plan to be very active. • If possible, hire a doula to help the two of you. • When calling the hospital before going in, ask for a nurse who supports natural childbirth. • Learn and practice all the comfort measures in chapter 4 together. Know the 3Rs (see page 115). • Choose a "code word" that she can say if she really wants you to help her get pain medications. • During labor, do not suggest medications. • If she asks for medications, wait for the code word; have her checked for progress; ask her to try three more contractions before deciding; use the Take-Charge Routine (see page 166).
−7	• Very strong desire for natural childbirth, for a sense of personal gratification as well as to benefit the baby and the progress of labor. • Will be disappointed if she needs to use medication.	• Same as listed for −5, but with even greater commitment. • Interpret requests for pain medication as a need for more help. • If she doesn't use the code word, keep encouraging her. • Remind her that she will be disappointed later if she uses medications.
−9	• Desire that you and the staff deny the mother pain medication, even if she requests it.	• Same as listed for −7. • Ignoring her requests for medication is correct unless she uses her code word. If worried, remind her she has a code word. • Promise to help all you can, but remind the mother that the final decision is hers.
−10	• Desire that the mother forego all medications, even for cesarean delivery.	• Impossible choice. • Same as for −9: Help her develop a realistic understanding of the risks and benefits of pain medications.

PAIN MEDICATIONS AND THEIR EFFECTS

DRUG NAMES, AND HOW AND WHERE GIVEN	DESIRED EFFECTS	OTHER POSSIBLE EFFECTS	PRECAUTIONS AND PROCEDURES FOR SAFE USE
SYSTEMIC MEDICATIONS			
Morphine • Given by injection into muscle or vein. • Given in pre- or early labor.	• Therapeutic rest. • Temporary stop to nonproductive contractions. • Feeling of well-being.	*Mother:* Drop in blood pressure, dizziness, restlessness or excessive sedation, confusion, nausea and vomiting, urinary retention, respiratory depression. *Fetus:* Hypoxia, drop in fetal heart rate, decreased movement. *Baby:* If ill-timed, heart rate changes, respiratory depression, need for resuscitation, depression of sucking and other reflexes.	Restriction to bed, continuous fetal monitoring, oxygen for the mother or baby, administration of nalaxone (a drug to reverse side effects), timing of dosage to avoid the greatest risks to the baby. Some hospitals send mothers on morphine home (with a driver) when it is clear that they have no adverse reaction to it and are still in prelabor.
Sedatives/Barbiturates pentobarbital (Nembutal), secobarbital (Seconal) • Given by injection or pill. • Used during the first stage before 4 cm dilation to allow effects on the baby to diminish before birth.	• Sleepiness, relaxation. • Possible slowing of unproductive contractions. • Reduction in anxiety and tension.	*Mother:* Increased perception of pain, dizziness, confusion, restlessness, excitement, disorientation, nausea, nightmares after use, respiratory depression. *Fetus:* Heart-rate changes. *Baby:* Poor suckling, breathing problems, decreased alertness, decreased attention span for 2 to 4 days.	Oxygen for the mother or baby; resuscitation equipment for the baby; avoidance of concurrent use of narcotics.

Medication	Benefits	Side effects	Comments
Tranquilizers promethazine (Phenergan), promazine (Sparine), hydroxyzine (Vistaril), midazolam (Versed), diazepam (Valium) • Given by injection or pill. • Some (not Versed or Valium) are used during the first stage before 7 cm dilation. • Versed and Valium may be used for cesarean delivery for profound tranquilizing effects.	• Drowsiness, relaxation. • Reduction in tension, anxiety, nausea, and vomiting. • Reduction of side effects of some narcotics. • Possible acceleration of labor in a tense, exhausted woman.	*Mother:* Dizziness, confusion, dry mouth, blood-pressure and heart-rate changes. Versed causes amnesia of the birth and the first hours with the baby. *Fetus:* Heart-rate changes. *Baby:* Problems with breathing, temperature, and nursing; jaundice; lack of muscle tone and alertness.	Versed and Valium are considered too risky to the fetus and newborn to be used during labor. They are reserved for cesarean deliveries, and then used in small doses.
Narcotic and Narcotic-like Analgesics meperidine (Demerol), nalbuphine (Nubain), fentanyl (Sublimaze), butorphanol (Stadol), pentazocine (Talwin) • Given by injection or IV and also by patient-controlled IV device, especially after a cesarean. • Used during first stage until 7 cm dilation, or after a cesarean.	• Partial relief of pain, relaxation. • Halting, slowing, or speeding of contractions, depending on the amount, timing, and drug used.	*Mother:* Nausea, dizziness, "high" or groggy feeling, hallucinations, low heart rate and blood pressure, confusion, itching, respiratory depression, temporary slowing of labor. *Fetus:* Heart-rate changes, decreased movement. *Baby:* Heart-rate changes; depressed respiration at birth, which may require resuscitation; poor suckling; depression of other reflexes.	Oxygen for the mother or baby; naloxone (a narcotic antagonist) for the mother or baby to counter depressive effects; effort to predict the time of birth to avoid giving the drug when the risks to the baby are greatest.
Narcotic Antagonist naloxone (Narcan) • Given by injection into the muscle or vein. • May be given to the mother or baby after birth, if needed, to reverse the side effects of a narcotic.	• Reversal of some effects of narcotics on mother or baby, such as itching, hallucinations, respiratory depression, low blood pressure and heart rate, diminished newborn reflexes and poor suckling.	*Mother:* Nausea, vomiting, sweating, shivering, restlessness, increased heart rate, return of pain, high blood pressure, heart arrythmias, pulmonary edema (rarely), tremors. *Fetus:* Increased activity, improved heart rate. *Baby:* No effects observed when the drug is used to reverse respiratory depression in the newborn.	Possible supplemental doses after 30 to 45 minutes, or the effects of the narcotic may return.

continued on next page

PAIN MEDICATIONS AND THEIR EFFECTS (*continued*)

DRUG NAMES, AND HOW AND WHERE GIVEN	DESIRED EFFECTS	OTHER POSSIBLE EFFECTS	PRECAUTIONS AND PROCEDURES FOR SAFE USE
SYSTEMIC MEDICATIONS (*cont.*)			
Inhalation Analgesia nitrous oxide gas and oxygen • Self-administered by mother. • Given late in the dilation stage, in the birthing stage, and occasionally in the placental stage.	• Loss of pain awareness and consciousness for about a minute, followed by quick recovery.	*Mother:* Temporary grogginess and difficulty in bearing down during birthing contractions. *Fetus:* Transient effect. *Baby:* Little effect on newborn; long-term effects unknown.	The mother tries to begin inhaling nitrous oxide a little before the onset of a contraction, to ease pain and reduce consciousness through the peak. If she waits until the contraction begins before inhaling the gas, relief comes only after the contraction has peaked.
NEURAXIAL ANALGESIA			
Standard Lumbar Epidural mepivacaine (Carbocaine), chloroprocaine (Nesacaine), bupivacaine (Marcaine), Lidocaine (Xylocaine), Ropivacaine (Naropin) • Injected into a catheter placed in the epidural space outside the spinal canal; given as a continuous drip. • Given before 8 cm dilation, or later if labor is slow or arrested.	• Loss of pain sensation from abdomen to toes, adequate for cesarean. • Relaxation as pain is relieved. • Sleep for an exhausted mother.	*Mother:* Inability to move the lower half of her body; toxic reaction (rare); after four hours, fever that increases with the duration of the epidural; decrease in blood pressure; slowing of labor; reduced urge and ability to push; spinal headache if the drug is inadvertently injected into the dural space; prolonged birthing stage; increased chance of malpositioned baby. *Fetus:* Heart-rate changes and lack of oxygen, caused by low maternal blood pressure and fever. *Baby:* Subtle changes in reflexes, including suckling and breathing; fussiness.	*Mother:* Restriction to bed, frequent checks of blood pressure and blood oxygenation, withholding of food, limits on drinking, intravenous fluids, bladder catheter, oxygen mask, possible antibiotics for fever, continuous electronic fetal monitoring, Pitocin to augment contractions, forceps or vacuum extractor, episiotomy, possible increased chance of cesarean. *Baby:* Blood or urine cultures to detect infection, antibiotics, and 48 hours in a special-care nursery for observation if the mother has had a fever in labor (to rule out infection).

Segmental "Light" Epidural, with or without PCEA (Patient-Controlled Epidural Analgesia)

mepivacaine (Carbocaine), chloroprocaine (Nesacaine), bupivacaine (Marcaine), lidocaine (Xylocaine), ropivacaine (Naropin), mixed with low doses of narcotics (fentanyl or sufentanil)

- A lower concentration of anesthetic than for a standard epidural is injected into the epidural space outside the spinal canal.
- Given as a continuous drip into a catheter, and may have patient-controlled apparatus, which allows mother to give herself small additional doses as needed; generally reduces the total amount of medication used and its side effects.
- Given in the first stage, once labor is established.

- Loss of pain sensation in the trunk, without total loss of movement and sensation in the perineum and legs.
- Relaxation as pain is relieved.
- Sleep for an exhausted mother.

Mother (some of these are less likely with a "light" than with a standard lumbar epidural): Itching; nausea; after four hours, fever that increases with the duration of the epidural; drop in blood pressure; slowing of labor; reduced urge and ability to push; spinal headache if the needle is inadvertently injected into the dural space; increased chance of forceps, vacuum extractor delivery.
Fetus: Heart-rate changes and lack of oxygen, caused by low maternal blood pressure and fever.
Baby: Subtle changes in reflexes, including suckling and breathing; fussiness.

Mother: Restriction to bed, frequent checks of blood pressure and blood oxygenation, withholding of food and drink, intravenous fluids, bladder catheter, oxygen mask, continuous electronic fetal monitoring, Pitocin to augment contractions, forceps or vacuum extractor, episiotomy. Narcotic antagonist to control side effects; Benadryl for itching. "Lockout" mechanism controls timing of medicine (e.g., once every 10 minutes) to prevent overdose of PCEA.
Baby: Blood or urine cultures to detect infection, antibiotics, and 48 hours in a special-care nursery for observation if the mother has had a fever in labor (to rule out infection).

Epidural Narcotics and Spinal (Intrathecal) Narcotics

meperidine (Demerol), morphine (Duramorph), fentanyl (Sublimaze), sufentanil (Sufenta)

- Epidural: Given by injection or continuous drip into the epidural space outside the spinal canal.
- Spinal: Given as an injection into the dural space in the spinal canal.
- Used during the first stage or after a cesarean delivery.

- 90 minutes to 24 hours of pain relief depending on medication used, with little change in mental state.
- Retention of enough muscle function in the legs that the woman may be able to stand and walk with help, and move freely in bed.

Mother: Nausea, vomiting, urine retention, itching, spinal headache (caused by leaking of spinal fluid), "breakthrough" pain at 6 to 8 cm dilation if only narcotics are used.
Fetus: Heart-rate changes (these occur less frequently with epidural than with IV narcotics).
Baby: Narcotics are absorbed by the baby in small amounts, but the effects are unknown.

Intravenous fluids and oxytocin, narcotic antagonist to control side effects; Benadryl for itching, bladder catheter, blood patch (some of the mother's blood is injected into the dura to form a clot to stop leaking of spinal fluid and relieve a spinal headache), continuous fetal monitoring, increased chance of forceps or vacuum extractor delivery and episiotomy.

continued on next page

PAIN MEDICATIONS AND THEIR EFFECTS *(continued)*

DRUG NAMES, AND HOW AND WHERE GIVEN	DESIRED EFFECTS	OTHER POSSIBLE EFFECTS	PRECAUTIONS AND PROCEDURES FOR SAFE USE
NEURAXIAL ANALGESIA *(cont.)*			
Spinal Block mepivacaine (Carbocaine), chloroprocaine (Nesacaine), bupivacaine (Marcaine), lidocaine (Xylocaine) • Usually given as a single injection into the dural space in the spine. • Given any time before or during labor for a planned or unplanned cesarean. • Not used for vaginal births today.	• Two- to three-hour absence of sensation below chest. • Easier and quicker to administer than an epidural block. • More rapid onset of pain relief than with an epidural. • Loss of pain, other sensations, and movement from chest to toes for two to three hours after injection, with no mental effects. • Relaxation and rest as pain is relieved.	*Mother:* Toxic reaction (rare); decrease in blood pressure; spinal headache (caused by leaking of spinal fluid); impaired sensation of breathing, or actual inability to breathe, requiring artificial ventilation if the level of anesthesia rises high enough to affect the muscles in the chest. *Fetus:* Heart-rate changes, caused by low maternal blood pressure. *Baby:* Subtle changes in reflexes, including suckling; fussiness.	Frequent checks of blood pressure and blood oxygenation, electrocardiogram, intravenous fluids, bladder catheter, oxygen mask, artificial ventilation, continuous fetal monitoring until cesarean begins, blood patch (see "Epidural Narcotics and Spinal [Intrathecal] Narcotics," page 299).

Combined Spinal/Epidural (CSE) fentanyl (Sublimaze) or sufentanil (Sufenta) plus bupivacaine (Marcaine) or ropivacaine (Naropin)

- Two separate pain-relief techniques are used at one time.
- The "needle-through-needle technique": First, an epidural needle is placed in the epidural space; then, in early labor, a very thin spinal needle is run through the epidural needle into the spinal space, and narcotics are given in the spinal space. The spinal needle is removed and a catheter is run through the epidural needle into the epidural space, where, later, an anesthetic can be dripped. The epidural needle is then removed. Only a catheter remains, taped to the mother's back.
- Given as early as 2 cm dilation with narcotics and 4 to 6 cm with anesthetic.

- Very fast pain relief, lasting throughout labor, with the ability to move (and perhaps walk a bit in early labor), and without mental effects.
- Rest for an exhausted mother.

Mother: From the narcotic, itching, nausea and vomiting, retained urine, some weakness in the legs. From the anesthetic, fever, impaired movement in the legs, slowing of labor and the baby's descent, drop in blood pressure, impaired urge and ability to push.

Fetus: From the anesthetic, heart-rate changes, caused by the mother's fever and low blood pressure.

Baby: From the anesthetic, fever. Narcotics are absorbed by the baby, but their effects are unknown.

Mother: Restriction of food and drink, intravenous fluids, check of muscle strength in legs before the mother tries to walk, additional medications to control itching and nausea (these may make the mother sleepy or interfere with pain relief), bladder catheter, Pitocin to speed labor.

Baby: Blood or urine cultures to detect infection, antibiotics, and 48 hours in a special-care nursery for observation if the mother has had a fever in labor.

continued on next page

PAIN MEDICATIONS AND THEIR EFFECTS *(continued)*

DRUG NAMES, AND HOW AND WHERE GIVEN	DESIRED EFFECTS	OTHER POSSIBLE EFFECTS	PRECAUTIONS AND PROCEDURES FOR SAFE USE
GENERAL ANESTHESIA *Inhalation gas: nitrous oxide; isoflurane (Furan); injected medication: thiopental (Pentothal), ketamine* • Gases are administered by an anesthesiologist to induce total unconsciousness and total muscle inactivity in the mother. (Stronger concentrations of nitrous oxide are used for total anesthesia than for self-administration during labor.) • Injected medications are transported into a vein to rapidly induce unconsciousness and total muscle inactivity in the mother. • With either method, the anesthesiologist provides oxygen and mechanically assists with respiration. • Used before labor when an elective cesarean is planned, or during labor when an emergency cesarean becomes necessary.	• Rapid, total pain relief and loss of consciousness, for an immediate emergency cesarean.	*Mother:* Hallucinations, postoperative excitement, amnesia, vomiting and aspiration of stomach contents, respiratory depression, drops in blood pressure and heart rate. *Fetus:* Unconsciousness, slowing of movements and heart rate. *Baby:* Depression of the central nervous system and respiration, poor muscle tone, low Apgar scores, need for resuscitation.	*Mother:* Antacid given right before surgery to neutralize stomach contents; intubation (a tube is placed in the windpipe to protect against aspiration of stomach contents); intravenous muscle relaxants; taping of closed eyelids to protect the eyes from damage; electrocardiogram; monitoring of the pulse, blood gas levels, and blood pressure; assistance with breathing; electronic fetal monitoring. *Baby:* Resuscitation procedures and equipment to assist breathing and alertness.

LOCAL ANESTHESIA

Paracervical Block

mepivacaine (Carbocaine), lidocaine (Xylocaine), chloroprocaine (Nesacaine)

- Given as an injection into each side of the dilating cervix.
** Given after 5 cm and before 9 cm dilation.

- Short-term localized pain relief with no change in consciousness or ability to move freely.
- Quick administration that can be done by the mother's doctor; no anesthesiologist is needed.

Mother: Toxic reaction (rare), sudden decrease in blood pressure.
Fetus: Profound and sudden fetal heart-rate abnormalities.
Baby: Reduced muscle tone, fussiness, decreased reflexes.

Frequent blood-pressure and blood-oxygenation checks, intravenous fluids, oxygen mask, continuous electronic fetal monitoring, capability to perform rapid cesarean if the baby has an adverse reaction.
Rarely used in North America.

Pudendal Block

mepivacaine (Carbocaine), lidocaine (Xylocaine), chloroprocaine (Nesacaine)

- Given as an injection into pudendal nerve endings on each side of the vaginal canal.
- Used during the birthing stage before application of forceps or vacuum extractor.

- Numbing of the birth canal and rectum, relaxation of the pelvic floor, enabling a less painful forceps or vacuum extractor delivery.

Mother: Toxic reaction (rare), decrease in blood pressure, diminished pelvic floor muscle tone.
Fetus: Sudden drop in heart rate.
Baby: Temporary reduction in muscle tone, fussiness, decreased reflexes.

Pitocin, oxygen, episiotomy, availability of forceps or vacuum extractor for delivery.

Perineal Block

mepivacaine (Carbocaine), lidocaine (Xylocaine), chloroprocaine (Nesacaine)

- Given as several injections into the perineum and vaginal outlet.
- Used during the birthing stage, before an episiotomy, or after the birth to repair an episiotomy or tear.

- Numbing of the perineum.
- Less pain during an episiotomy or stitching.

Mother: Pain from injections, tearing from swelling if injections are given during the second rather than third stage.

Fetus and Baby: Risks unlikely, since the injections are given just before or after birth.

None

CHAPTER 9

Cesarean Birth, and Vaginal Birth After Cesarean

She dilated from 5 centimeters to complete in two hours, and the baby was pretty low in her birth canal, but then she pushed and pushed. We tried every position, but the contractions spaced out. She got an epidural, we tried Pitocin, but she made no progress. We waited. Then there was nothing left but a cesarean. His head was tilted at an angle, and it was huge. She worked so damn hard—she could even see his dark hair when pushing! But he couldn't come through. She's my goddess, and we're blissed out with our baby. But we just wish . . .

—PAUL, FIRST-TIME FATHER

I wish I had read the chapter on cesareans!

—KEVIN, FIRST-TIME FATHER

Sometimes a baby is delivered surgically, through an incision in the mother's abdomen, instead of vaginally. This procedure is a cesarean section, also called a cesarean delivery, a cesarean birth, a C-section, or, simply, a cesarean. The cesarean section is the most common surgery performed in the United States. The rate has risen steadily since 1996, when about 1 in 5 women had their babies by cesarean. Today the rate is about 1 in 3, or over 1.3 million cesarean births per year.

This rapid rise has taken place in all categories of cesareans: first-time cesareans, repeat cesareans, cesareans without medical indications, cesareans with medical indications, planned cesareans, and unplanned cesareans performed during labor. The causes for the increase are numerous, complex, and controversial. In general, though, the prevailing attitude toward cesareans is much more accepting and unquestioning than it has ever been before.

Over the past four decades, there has been ongoing debate in the medical literature over the appropriate use of the cesarean section. The public has joined in, with organizations formed, on the one hand, to halt unnecessary cesareans by teaching about the overuse of the procedure and, on the other hand, to argue for a woman's right to choose whether she will avoid labor by having a cesarean. The obstetric profession is divided on the issue; some obstetricians advocate even higher cesarean rates, and others try very hard to perform cesareans only when necessary for the health of mother or baby. Individual doctors' cesarean rates range from 10 to 50 percent of deliveries. Midwives and family physicians generally have lower cesarean rates than do most obstetricians, even if only the obstetricians' "low-risk" cases (healthy women with healthy pregnancies) are counted. Many obstetricians, however, also combine excellent outcomes with low cesarean rates.

I am saddened, discouraged, and frustrated by this trend, but I am certain there will be a reversal as we learn more about the risks of this major surgery and its lack of benefits for healthy mothers and babies. In the meantime, however, we must not lose sight of the fact that the cesarean operation has, over the years, saved or improved the lives of millions of mothers and babies, and continues to do so.

You need to be able to recognize when a cesarean will improve the chances of a healthy mother and baby, and when it is optional. Clear communication with a caregiver whom both you and the mother trust and a birth setting that has a relatively low cesarean rate are probably your most important assurances that the mother will not have an unnecessary or ill-advised cesarean.

REASONS DOCTORS AND MOTHERS CHOOSE CESAREANS

The most highly publicized reason to choose a cesarean is that the woman's pelvic floor will remain undamaged and that this will save her from being incontinent of urine or feces. Although it may seem logical, at first, to assume that stretching the vagina would cause permanent damage, this is a misleading assumption. The way vaginal birth is managed, rather than vaginal birth itself, *can* increase incontinence and other pelvic-floor problems. For example, difficult forceps deliveries and large episiotomies, with or without the use of forceps, increase the rate of immediate incontinence in the weeks after birth. A caregiver can usually avoid a difficult and damaging vaginal delivery by predicting, from the labor pattern and the size, position, and station of the baby, whether a vaginal birth with forceps or vacuum will cause pelvic-floor damage. Even while using forceps or a vacuum extractor during delivery, the doctor can simply remove the device if he or she recognizes that the baby is not moving. In such cases, a cesarean is the solution. Pushing with prolonged breath holding and straining for a very long time while lying on the back can also increase incontinence by stretching the ligaments that support the bladder, cervix, and rectum (thankfully, this sort of directed pushing is giving way to more physiological bearing-down techniques, as described on page 130).

Studies have found that by middle age, there is no difference in the rate of incontinence among women who have had cesareans, women who have had vaginal deliveries, and those who have never given birth at all. This suggests that factors other than birth management (such as physical fitness and congenital structural differences) contribute to incontinence in later life. When birth-related incontinence occurs, it usually resolves within several months, except in rare cases in which damage is severe.

Another reason women choose to plan cesareans is that their doctors (ones with very high cesarean rates) coerce them into it. These doctors may suggest fearful possibilities, such as a baby too large to deliver vaginally, a failed induction leading to an unplanned cesarean, a delay in getting an epidural, an overdue labor, or a uterine rupture during a VBAC attempt. If the woman then decides to have a cesarean, it will be recorded in her chart as being done on "maternal request."

A desire to avoid all possible complications that can arise with vaginal birth—such as long duration, exhaustion, fetal distress, and a need for forceps or a vacuum extractor—may lead some women to choose to bypass the vagina. They may perceive the risks and unpredictability that come with vaginal birth to be more frightening than those accompanying cesarean birth. Sometimes a woman will rethink her desire for a cesarean if she learns about ways to minimize possible difficulties with vaginal birth and about undesirable outcomes of cesarean birth, and if her caregiver promises to personalize her care in a way that takes her fears into account. But she may not change her mind.

A woman who asks for a cesarean may have an extremely deep fear of labor pain and vaginal birth ("tocophobia"). Although sensitive counseling often alleviates this fear, if there is no such counseling available, or if she cannot come to terms with the fear and is informed of the consequences of each choice, she should have the right to a cesarean.

"Social" reasons for choosing a cesarean—convenience, control over timing, apparent simplicity (you just schedule it and have your baby in an hour), and others—are often based on naiveté and a lack of information about the short- and long-term risks of the cesarean and the realities of recovery. Social reasons often disappear when women hear both sides of the issue, but the number of women opting for an elective cesarean, though small, seems to be on the increase. The following discussion explores some of the key issues in this controversy.

Risks of a cesarean, especially one done without a clear medical reason. Because a cesarean is major surgery, it carries all the same possible risks—including hemorrhage, infection, prolonged healing, and adhesions (overgrowth of scar tissue to involve neighboring structures and organs)—as other types of major surgery. Furthermore, prolonged and painful recovery from a cesarean adds challenges (though not insurmountable ones) for the new mother, whose baby needs her night and day. In the long term, a cesarean increases the mother's risk of problems with future pregnancies and deliveries, such as the uterine scar giving way, another cesarean, and placenta previa and abruption (see page 248). A cesarean poses risks to the baby, too; babies born by elective cesarean are more likely to be premature and to have breathing problems and other difficulties. See "Recommended Resources" for more information on the risks of elective cesareans.

It makes sense to avoid these risks when there is little or no benefit to be gained. Sometimes, however, the benefits of a cesarean are clear. These situations are discussed on pages 306 to 308.

Avoiding a cesarean. Many women, if they have a choice, seek caregivers and birth settings in which cesarean rates are low. They practice a lifestyle to maintain or improve their health. They eat well; address any mental health issues; exercise; practice stress management; and avoid tobacco, alcohol, and recreational drugs—all to improve the chances of an excellent outcome. If the woman and her baby are strong and healthy, some reasons for a cesarean (subnormal fetal growth, fetal distress, maternal exhaustion) are less likely to arise. The woman and her partner also learn techniques to relieve pain and enhance labor progress, and participate in decision making (see the "Key Questions for Informed Decision Making" on page 202) to improve the chances of a vaginal birth. Many arrange for a doula, too; studies have found lower rates of cesareans and fewer interventions among doula-attended births. The reasons are not well understood, but may have to do with a doula's contributions to a calmer, less stressful atmosphere and her encouragement and guidance, which instill greater confidence in the parents to choose options that include fewer unnecessary interventions and improve the chances for a normal labor. See chapter 5 for discussion of these options.

Preparing for a possible cesarean. As you both look forward to the upcoming birth, please think about the possibility of the mother's having a cesarean. Even with your best efforts to establish the most favorable conditions for a vaginal birth, a cesarean may become necessary.

To help you in your role as birth partner, you need answers to the following questions: Under what circumstances might the mother need a cesarean after you have done all you can to lessen the likelihood of this? If the need for a cesarean arises during labor, how can you help the mother adjust to the shift and get through the surgery and the recovery period? What can you do to ensure that she has as good an experience as possible, despite this unexpected turn of events? How might you feel during this mysterious, highly technological procedure involving the woman and baby you care for so deeply? This chapter will give you some answers to these questions.

Know the Medical Reasons for Cesarean Birth

Both you and the mother should understand the reasons for the cesarean before it is done and agree that it is the right thing to do. If she finds out in advance that she or the baby has a medical problem that requires a cesarean delivery or makes it highly likely, she can learn all about the surgery and adjust emotionally beforehand. If the need for the cesarean arises in labor, she will have to do much of the adjusting afterward. Either way, she should have plenty of opportunity to talk about the experience with you, your doula, the doctor, and the nurses.

See chapters 6 and 7 for information about problems that sometimes arise in labor and how they are detected and treated; a cesarean becomes the solution if other treatments are unsuccessful.

Following are the most likely reasons for a cesarean. Although cesareans are not always necessary in these circumstances, they are always considered and very often done.

1. *Emergencies.* These include the following:

   ◆ Prolapsed cord (see page 256).

   ◆ Serious hemorrhage (excessive bleeding) in the mother (see page 248). In these situations there is no time for questions. Rapid action is essential.

2. *Arrested labor.* This is the most common reason for a woman's first cesarean. A failure to progress in labor may be caused by the following:

   ◆ Abnormal position or presentation of the baby.

   ◆ Uterine inertia (inadequate contractions).

   ◆ A poor fit between the baby's head and the mother's pelvis (see page 253).

   ◆ A combination of these.

According to many experts, far too many cesareans are performed because of arrested labor, or "failure to progress" (see "Complications with Labor Progress," page 252). Many of these cesareans are actually done because of failure to *wait* rather than failure to progress.

3. *Problems with the fetus.* These include the following:

    ◆ Fetal distress. Many experts believe this is another reason for which cesareans are too often performed (see "Fetal Distress," page 259).

    ◆ Breech presentation (see "A Breech Baby," page 190).

    ◆ Prematurity, postmaturity (when the baby is overdue), or other conditions that might make vaginal birth too stressful for the baby. Through fetal movement counting, by which the mother keeps track of how much the baby moves (see page 22), nonstress testing (see page 208), and ultrasound (see page 207), the caregiver predicts whether the baby can tolerate labor.

4. *Problems with the mother.* These include the following:

    ◆ Serious illness (such as heart disease, diabetes, or preeclampsia) or injury. Sometimes, in these cases, a cesarean section is planned in advance. Otherwise, a "trial of labor" is allowed. The mother is watched carefully and, if all goes well, she gives birth vaginally. If the problem worsens, she has a cesarean.

    ◆ A genital herpes sore (see page 247).

    ◆ A previous cesarean delivery. This is one major reason for the increasing cesarean rate in the United States and Canada. Today, more than 90 percent of women who have had a cesarean before will have another, even though few truly need one. The VBAC (vaginal birth after cesarean) rate has plummeted over the past decade, even though the risks of VBAC are very low. With the right doctor and hospital, however, a VBAC is still possible. If the mother wants to try for one, you both should read "A Previous Disappointing or Traumatic Birth Experience," page 194, and "Vaginal Birth After Cesarean," page 321.

Once the decision to perform a cesarean is made, concentrate on helping the mother and greeting the baby as lovingly and gently as you can.

Know What to Expect During Cesarean Birth

You may be surprised by how quickly the staff moves once the decision is made to do a cesarean, and by the number of people involved: There is the doctor who will do the surgery; an assisting doctor or midwife; a "scrub nurse," who gives instruments to the doctor; a "floating nurse," who prepares the room and looks after the surgical team; an anesthesiologist; a pediatric nurse or two to look after the baby; and possibly a pediatrician or neonatologist, if problems with the baby are anticipated. They all work together as an efficient, businesslike team.

You may feel frightened and worried for the mother or baby. You may feel relieved to know that the end is in sight, especially after a long, difficult labor. You may be impressed and reassured by the teamwork and competence of the staff. You may feel left out or even shocked by their apparently casual attitude. They may talk and even joke among themselves, paying little attention to you and the mother, as if you are not there. You may feel overwhelmed by the sounds, smells, and sights of the operating room. You may be confused over your role. Should you ask questions and try to make sure that the mother's wishes are being followed, or should you stay out of the way and let them proceed in their customary manner? Just a few minutes before, your role was essential to the mother's ability to handle her contractions; now you feel much less important. Be assured that you are still most important to the mother, but in a different way. The following descriptions of the surgery and of your role will help you to help the mother.

PREPARATIONS FOR SURGERY

Preparations for cesarean delivery include the following steps:

- The mother signs a consent form.

- A nurse starts intravenous fluids in the mother's arm, which is placed on a board that extends out to the side of the operating table. The nurse checks the mother's blood pressure frequently.

- The mother may be given a sedative. She can refuse it if she wants to remain aware during the surgery and immediately after birth.

- An anesthesiologist, nurse-anesthetist, or, rarely, the obstetrician gives the anesthetic (spinal, epidural, or general; see chapter 8). The choice of anesthesia depends on the mother's situation, the training and qualifications of the staff, and the facilities. General anesthesia, being fastest, is chosen if the cesarean must be done immediately, but neuraxial anesthesia is much safer to use if time allows. Regulating bodies require that hospitals be able to provide general anesthesia, but not necessarily neuraxial anesthesia, around the clock.

- The mother will probably receive oxygen, administered with a face mask or nasal prongs (tubes that blow oxygen into the nose).

- A pulse oximeter, a small device that measures the oxygen content in the mother's blood, will be clipped to her finger or toe.

- Electrocardiogram (EKG or ECG) leads are placed on her chest. These keep track of the mother's heart rate throughout the surgery.

- The mother's body is draped so that only her abdomen can be seen. The end of the drape is raised to form a screen between her head and her abdomen. Even if she is conscious, she cannot see the surgery.

- Most hospitals now welcome the mother's birth partner (and a doula or other person) in the operating room for a cesarean. You sit on a stool at her head. The anesthesiologist remains at her head also.

- Some birth partners want to watch and even photograph the surgery. Discuss this option with the mother and her caregiver, if it interests you. If you remain sitting on the stool, you will see nothing. You will have to stand up and look over the drape or hold your camera high in order to see or photograph the surgery.

- The mother's abdomen is scrubbed and shaved. Some pubic hair is usually removed.

- A catheter is placed in her bladder to keep it empty.

Know what to expect during cesarean birth

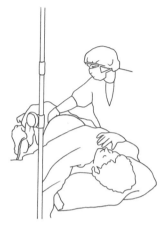

The mother's abdomen is scrubbed in preparation for the surgery.

SURGERY BEGINS

This is how a cesarean delivery starts:

- ◆ Once the anesthetic takes effect, the doctor makes the incisions with a scalpel.

- ◆ The skin incision is usually low and horizontal, or *transverse* (this is called a "bikini incision"), but occasionally it is vertical and in the midabdomen.

- ◆ The muscles of the abdomen are not cut; they are separated from each other and spread apart. The muscles therefore heal very well.

- ◆ The uterine incision is usually horizontal, or *transverse*, in the lower segment of the uterus, but it can be made higher if speed is essential or if the higher opening is needed to get the baby out (for example, in the case of twins, a premature baby, or an unusual presentation).

- ◆ The amniotic fluid is suctioned from the uterus with a plastic tube. You will hear the sucking sound.

- ◆ To prevent excessive bleeding, the cut blood vessels are cauterized. You may hear the high-pitched tone of the cautery device or notice a slight odor as it burns the ends of the blood vessels to close them. The mother cannot feel this.

◆ If at any time during the procedure the mother indicates that she is feeling pain, make sure the doctor knows it and stops working until more anesthetic can be given. This does not happen often, but sometimes the anesthesia is spotty and the mother is not numb where she needs to be.

THE BABY IS BORN!

The baby is usually delivered within 15 minutes after the surgery has begun. This is how:

◆ The doctor either places one hand in the uterus to grasp the baby's head or buttocks, or attaches a vacuum extractor to the baby's head if it is accessible (vacuum extraction allows for a smaller incision in the mother's abdomen). The assisting doctor pushes on the mother's abdomen to move the baby to the incision. The first doctor removes the baby. The mother may feel pressure and tugging, but she should not feel pain. Help her to use relaxation and slow rhythmic breathing (see page 127). Make sure the doctor and anesthesiologist know if she complains of pain, so she can have more anesthetic.

◆ The doctor or nurse suctions the baby's airways, and clamps and cuts the cord. You may want to ask the doctor to lower the drape so the mother can see the baby, or the baby may be briefly held up for you both to admire. Then he is taken to an infant-care area in the corner of the delivery room, or in an adjacent room, for evaluation and any necessary treatment. By this time he is probably crying lustily. You may wish to go over and take a look at the baby, especially if your doula can remain with the mother.

◆ The oxygen apparatus is removed from the mother's face.

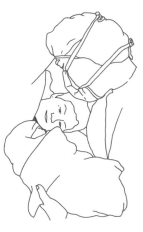

While the mother's incision is being repaired, you may hold the baby so she can see and talk to him.

Know what to expect during cesarean birth

THE PLACENTA IS REMOVED

While you are greeting the baby, the doctor reaches into the uterus, separates the placenta from the wall of the uterus, and removes it.

Some doctors then lift the uterus out of the abdomen to check it thoroughly before doing the repair. The mother may feel this as uncomfortable pressure. She may feel nauseated and vomit, turning her head to the side and using the basin that you, the doula, or the anesthesiologist holds for her. Because the benefit of removing the uterus is questionable, and because it causes the mother discomfort, many physicians have stopped doing it. You might discuss this with the doctor ahead of time, and the mother might state in her Birth Plan that she would prefer not to have her uterus lifted out for inspection.

THE REPAIR BEGINS

The repair phase takes 30 to 45 minutes. These procedures are involved:

- The uterus and other internal layers are sutured with absorbable suture thread. You might ask ahead of time whether the caregiver does a single-layer or double-layer repair of the uterine incision. Doctors began using the single-layer repair in the mid-1990s because it is quicker, but studies have found that it leaves the uterine scar weaker and more likely to separate in a future pregnancy. Consider asking for a double-layer repair in the mother's Birth Plan.

- The skin is closed with stitches or stainless-steel clips. You may hear the clicking of the stapler as the clips are placed.

- A bandage is applied over the incision.

- The mother may develop a pain up in her shoulder. This is "referred pain"—pain that is felt nowhere near where the problem lies. Shoulder pain is usually caused by air entering the mother's internal pelvic area. The anesthesiologist may be able to help by raising the head of the operating table slightly, which sometimes moves the air bubble. There is little else that can be done—rubbing the shoulder is unlikely to help much—but the pain will fade away as the air disperses.

◆ Since the mother may be very shaky, trembling all over, or nause-ated—normal reactions after major surgery—she might be given a relaxing, sleep-inducing medication via her intravenous line, with-out either of you knowing about it. If it is important to her to be awake after the birth so she can experience the first hours with her baby, you should ask ahead of time, and again just after the birth, that these medications not be given without first checking with her. The nausea and trembling usually subside within a half hour.

If the nausea and trembling are extreme, she can always change her mind and ask for some medication. It takes effect within 2 minutes.

There is one medication, Versed, that she should be warned about. Along with being an effective sedative, it is also a potent am-nesiac. It wipes out all memory of the birth and events for hours af-terward. The mother will not remember having the baby, nor will she remember her first impressions or the first feeding. The ab-sence of memory of the momentous event might haunt her and cause much regret.

Zofran is a very good anti-nausea medication that does not make a woman groggy. Ask about it.

◆ The mother is cleaned up and taken to the recovery area.

THE RECOVERY PERIOD

This is what you can expect during the recovery period:

◆ The mother remains in the recovery room or back in her labor room for a few hours with a nurse close by, until it is clear that she is recovering well and that the anesthetic is wearing off as expected.

◆ The nurse frequently checks the mother's pulse, temperature, blood pressure, uterine tone, and state of anesthesia.

◆ The baby may remain with the mother or go to the nursery for ob-servation or treatment, depending on the baby's condition and hospital custom.

◆ A pain medication regimen will be established. See pages 297 and 299 for explanations of narcotics used after a cesarean.

◆ The mother can breastfeed the baby now or as soon as he returns from the nursery. She will need her doula or the nurses to help her position the baby and get started. It is a good idea for her to begin breastfeeding before the anesthesia wears off, since it will be a little easier for her to get started when she is not in pain.

◆ If she is asleep or groggy from the medication for nausea and trembling, it will be hard for her to nurse. This is why some women refuse medication for nausea and trembling, preferring to put up with it for a half hour to an hour: They do not want to miss the first few hours with the baby.

◆ If the mother is unable to nurse or hold the baby, you take him. Hold the baby close and talk to him.

◆ The nurse checks the baby's breathing, skin color, temperature, and heart rate frequently.

◆ Once the anesthesia wears off and the mother's condition is stable, she is taken to her postpartum room, where she will stay until she goes home. See chapter 10 for information about the first few days after birth.

Your Role During and After a Cesarean Birth

For the woman who plans a vaginal birth, a cesarean is unexpected and disappointing, even if she knows the surgery has made it possible to have a healthy baby. Some women get over these feelings quickly; others do not. A woman often needs time afterward to adjust emotionally, to talk about and even grieve over the experience, especially if she had a strong desire to give birth vaginally. It is sometimes surprising to loved ones, nurses, and caregivers how deeply disappointed some mothers are. The mother may need much patience and understanding from you to help her come to terms with her baby's cesarean birth.

The mother is less likely to grieve for a long time if she has been able to participate thoroughly in her labor and in the decision to have a cesarean. Prolonged anger, depression, or guilt may result if the

Know what to expect during cesarean birth

mother is caught by surprise and can do nothing to help herself or questions the need for it. How you respond to the mother, both during and after the cesarean, can make a big difference in how well she adjusts. Here are guidelines:

◆ Your perceptions of what has happened will be very important to the mother as she puts the pieces together. You will be able to help her come to terms with the experience later if you stay with her during the surgery, ask questions, hold her hand, and tell her what is happening. She may want you to take some pictures; check with the staff before doing so. Many women, especially if they were unaware during the surgery, treasure photographs of it later, because the photos help to fill them in on the parts they missed. Even if the mother has no interest in photos of the surgery, early pictures of her baby will probably mean a great deal to her.

◆ The mother, if aware, will probably feel some discomfort during the surgery. If she feels pain, not just pressure or tugging, ask that she be given more anesthetic. You should help her continue her relaxation and slow rhythmic breathing to handle the sensations of pressure and tugging.

◆ After the birth, you will probably be allowed to get close to the baby, to see her, talk to her, and possibly stroke her or hold her hand. The thought of talking or singing to the baby in the operating room may seem strange, but, if you are the baby's father or the mother's lover, the baby knows your voice and will respond when she hears it. You may be able to soothe the baby as no one else can besides her mother. Think of this birth from the baby's point of view—an abrupt tug out of her mother's warm and familiar womb to a bright, cold, noisy place. She is handled competently but perfunctorily and hears only strangers' voices. Then you come close and say, "Hi, Baby! I'm so glad to see you. Everything is all right, and I'm here to take care of you." Or you sing a song, perhaps one you sang aloud often during the pregnancy. You stroke her arm and put your finger into the palm of her hand. She stares into your eyes and clings to your finger. At last, a familiar voice and loving touch for the baby! You will always cherish this moment.

◆ Bring the baby to the mother as soon as possible, so she can see, touch, and kiss her. I will never forget one of the most beautiful welcomes I ever witnessed for a cesarean-born baby. When the couple had learned early in the pregnancy that their baby was a boy, they sang the song, "Here Comes the Sun!" to him every day. When their baby emerged, the father was so overcome that he began singing loudly, in a choked-up voice, "Here Comes the Son!" The mother joined in weakly, despite her nausea and trembling. The baby stopped crying and looked right at his dad. Everyone in the operating room was very moved, and I was in tears. What a lucky child!

◆ Help the mother breastfeed in the recovery room. She may need your help in holding the baby up to the breast.

If the baby has to go to the nursery for special care, you may want to go along so that you can see for yourself what is being done and fill in these gaps for the mother later. Or you can stay with the mother, to comfort her and ease your worries about her. This is a difficult choice. If a family member or doula can stay with one, then you can be with the other, and have some peace of mind.

◆ Physical recovery from a cesarean takes a matter of weeks or months. Pain, weakness, and fatigue are great at first, and she may require narcotics or other pain medication (injections, pills, or IV) for days or more. It may take weeks or months for the last step—from functioning fairly well to returning to how she was before she became pregnant. Encourage her to rest and focus on feeding the baby while you take over the housework or get help from others.

◆ It may take the mother longer to recover emotionally than it takes her to recover physically. Be patient. Give her time, and fill in any gaps in her memory or understanding of what happened and why.

Women vary in how long it takes them to integrate and accept the cesarean birth experience. For some, a cesarean is a positive experience; for others it is not. If the mother is disappointed, accept her feelings as valid and normal. Too often a woman's loved ones try to distract her from thinking about the birth by pointing out that "all that matters" is that she has a healthy baby. But that is not all that matters. How she gave birth matters. Her feelings also matter, and her loved ones' patience, acceptance, and concern for these feelings will help her work through them.

- If the mother's birth experience was particularly negative, she may benefit from professional counseling or therapy. Call her caregiver or childbirth educator or doula for referrals. See "Unhappiness After Childbirth," page 355.
- See chapter 7 for more suggestions about the birth partner's role when problems arise during labor.

Despite her possible disappointment with the birth experience, the mother will rejoice in her baby. A cesarean birth is, after all, a birth, and all the emotions that come with birth also come with cesarean birth. The mother's ability to love, feed, enjoy, and care for her baby are not altered by the fact that the baby was born by cesarean. You will enjoy this child together.

Vaginal Birth After Cesarean (VBAC)

Attitudes toward VBACs have changed more since the year 2000 than attitudes toward any other aspect of maternity care. The VBAC rate in the United States has dropped to a third of what it was in the mid-1990s; at this writing the rate is less than 9 percent. Hundreds of hospitals have stopped doing VBACs altogether. Many readers of this book will not have an option for a VBAC unless they are willing to travel long distances or risk having one at home with or without a midwife or doctor in attendance. While a woman's right to have a cesarean without medical justification is often unquestioned, her right to a vaginal birth is seriously jeopardized. This "VBAC-lash" is a very appropriate area for consumer activism, and I would recommend contacting the International Cesarean Awareness Network (ICAN) and checking the Web site at www.VBAC.com for information, support, and an opportunity to make a difference on this issue.

The reasons for the sudden downturn in the VBAC rate are not clear. No new evidence has revealed that VBACs are more dangerous than they were in the mid-1990s, when VBACS were promoted by insurance companies, government agencies, and many organizations of medical professionals. Researchers *have* found that uterine scars are more likely to separate with two recent practices: the use of a single-layer rather than a stronger double-layer closure after a cesarean delivery (see page 316) and the use of prostaglandins to induce a VBAC labor. Provided that women have had double-layer suturing with their cesareans and that prostaglandins are avoided in their subsequent labors, VBACs are as safe as they were when they were very common.

Even though VBACs are becoming very rare, if the mother wants one you may be able to find a supportive caregiver. With modern surgical techniques and a supportive birth environment and caregiver, between 60 and 70 percent of women who attempt a VBAC will have one.

Major benefits of VBAC. After a vaginal birth, recovery is easier and faster than after a cesarean; this is a blessing especially when a couple have a toddler as well as a newborn to look after.

If her cesarean was a great disappointment for her, a woman may find a VBAC emotionally healing.

Improving Her Chances for a Vaginal Birth

Obstetricians vary widely in their support of VBACs, and their attitudes are reflected in their rates of repeat cesareans. An unsupportive doctor or midwife is likely to warn the woman against getting her hopes up, or to emphasize potential complications, instead of encouraging her. Such a negative attitude may undermine her confidence and lead her, in the words of one woman, "down the garden path to another cesarean."

It is wise for the mother to learn which hospitals maintain relatively low cesarean rates, and to interview some doctors and midwives who work there. She should check her health plan to find out which caregivers are covered by her insurance. She might also ask a childbirth educator (preferably one who is self-employed, or one who is employed by the hospital she is considering) for advice on which caregivers to interview.

Try to attend these interviews with her, to give her moral support and to help her ask such questions as these: Do you support VBACs?

What percentage of your clients who have had cesareans plan to have VBACs? What percentage succeed? What are the most likely reasons for a VBAC attempt to end in a cesarean? Can you recommend ways I can improve my chances for a VBAC? Do your associates share your opinions about VBACs?

After comparing the attitudes of the various caregivers, she can choose one who seems most supportive.

It helps if the mother is surrounded by people who respect her desire for a VBAC and assume that she can and will do it. Her family and friends, her professional caregiver, and you most of all should have confidence in her. A doula can supply a lot of emotional support and concrete practical advice. A doula with experience supporting VBACs will inspire confidence in both of you.

Knowledge of ways to deal with some of the challenges inherent to VBAC labors will arm both of you with self-confidence and helpful coping strategies. Childbirth classes are valuable preparation. A good refresher class should cover the unique challenges that come with VBACs. There are also valuable books, Web sites, and Internet news groups centering on VBAC (see "Recommended Resources"). Lastly, if the woman suffered emotional or physical trauma in her previous birth experience, counseling with a perinatal social worker, a trauma therapist, a seasoned doula or childbirth educator, or a sensitive midwife or doctor may help her develop strategies to prevent troubling thoughts and feelings from undermining her self-confidence (see page 194).

FEARS ABOUT VBAC

Although most VBAC labors proceed normally, they carry a small extra risk due to the fact that the uterus bears a scar from the cesarean. The greatest fear about a VBAC is the risk of scar separation, sometimes referred to as uterine rupture. The risk of scar separation is about 0.5 percent, or 1 in 200 VBAC labors, and may be somewhat higher in women who have had more than one cesarean. With careful monitoring of the fetal heart rate and observation of the mother, however, a scar separation can usually be detected in time for a cesarean to be performed and the separation mended. Though worrisome when they occur, most scar separations end well, with a healthy mother and baby, because of immediate and appropriate action. On very rare occasions, the scar separates enough to cause a fetal crisis (or death) and/or serious bleeding in the mother.

A uterine scar sometimes thins during labor without separating, but in this case the uterus heals itself as it returns to its nonpregnant state.

EMOTIONAL CONCERNS SURROUNDING VBAC

Once a woman becomes pregnant after having had a cesarean, she may feel less confident about giving birth than she did the first time. She may feel that she was naive before, and is now realistic enough to recognize that she might have another cesarean this time. Her preparation for a vaginal birth should include exploring emotions involving the cesarean and the upcoming birth, and also seeking out resources that will give her the best chance of a safe and satisfying experience.

Once the mother has prepared as well as she can to optimize her chances for a VBAC, she will know that she will give birth vaginally unless a cesarean is truly appropriate.

You can help the mother prepare for a VBAC in the following ways:

- ◆ Explore any strong emotions associated with the first cesarean. Was it necessary? Was it traumatic? Was she well cared for?

- ◆ Explore any fears about the next labor—a fear of pain or exhaustion, or a fear that something could go wrong (the scar could separate, she could have another cesarean, or she could encounter a lack of support from her caregiver, the nurses, or even from you).

- ◆ Explore her feelings about her caregiver and the hospital where she gave birth to her first child. Does she want to go back to them? Were they a part of the problem? Can she find a caregiver whom she trusts?

- ◆ Explore how much she wants a VBAC. Is she willing to prepare herself not only with these steps, but also by learning self-help measures for comfort and aiding labor progress? Is she willing to use medications and other interventions very judiciously? Will she surround herself with truly supportive friends and relatives?

◆ For a woman who has had a long, exhausting labor that ended in a cesarean, the thought of attempting a VBAC may raise all kinds of fear. "I can't put myself through all that again," she may say. "I'd rather just plan a cesarean." After a traumatic or disappointing first labor, she may be very reluctant to try again, even though she may dread the thought of having to recover from major surgery while taking care of an infant and an older child.

In such a situation, you might suggest that she think about conditions under which she would be willing to labor—for example, if she doesn't have to push again for three hours, or if she doesn't have to keep going after her labor stalls for more than two hours. If she concludes that she would prefer to try for a VBAC as long as she does not have to go through an ordeal like the first birth, then she might discuss the idea of setting limits with her caregiver, and prepare a Birth Plan for a VBAC that reflects these limits. Knowing that this labor will not be allowed to happen as the first one did, she then can put her mind at rest and focus on a positive birth experience over which she has some control. If the labor does exceed the limits she and her caregiver have set, she will have the option of going with a cesarean. After a traumatic birth, setting limits for an upcoming labor frees a woman to go ahead with a positive attitude, unafraid that the same trauma will be repeated. Even if the woman ends up needing another cesarean, her position of control, not helplessness, will save her from emotional trauma.

As the birth partner, you may have mixed feelings about the mother's trying for a vaginal birth, especially if her first labor was distressing for you. It will help to prepare yourself so that you can fully support the mother's efforts, by reading this chapter, getting answers to your questions from the mother's caregiver, attending a VBAC support group or class, and sharing your concerns with a doula.

THE SPECIAL CHALLENGE OF A VBAC

Beyond the usual emotional challenges that come with most labors (see chapter 3), a woman having a VBAC may have to deal with other challenges. See chapter 5, page 194, for a description of these challenges and how to deal with them.

If, during labor, you become worried or are reminded of some of the unhappy events of the previous labor that ended in cesarean, it is best that you talk to someone else about this. Do not increase the mother's anxiety with your own. If you have a doula, you might talk with her; if not, you might talk to the nurse, out of earshot of the laboring woman. If the doula or nurse knows you are troubled, she can reassure you in nonverbal ways.

We are in an era in which the cesarean rate is rising rapidly, and not because cesareans have proven to be safer than vaginal birth, except with a few conditions. If you and the mother want the best chance of a vaginal birth without giving up the option of a cesarean when it is truly indicated, you may have to actively seek out the right caregiver and setting and prepare well for the experience. With the right caregiver, setting, and preparation, your odds for a vaginal birth are very good.

PART FOUR
After the Birth

Once the baby and the placenta are born, the pace seems to slow down. Everyone relaxes. The caregiver and the staff seem preoccupied with finishing the medical tasks and with cleaning up. You, the mother, and the baby are almost in your own world, engrossed with the appearance, the touch, and the smell of one another. The doula is busy getting the all-important photos, helping with breastfeeding, bringing beverages and snacks, and making mother and baby comfortable.

The baby's every gurgle, every grimace, every squirming stretch brings fascinated exclamations and surprised looks from both of you. Some babies are quiet, calm, and alert, drinking in all the new sights and sounds, the most captivating being your faces and your voices. Other babies fuss and cry a lot at first as they discover themselves in strange new surroundings. They seem to need soothing and reassurance right away.

Phone calls go out to those near and dear, answering the same questions over and over: the gender (if it wasn't known before the birth), the name, the weight and height, whom the baby looks like (it depends on whom you are talking to!), how the labor went, how the mother is feeling, and, oh, yes, how you are feeling. The same message over and over—it never gets old.

If you are the father of the baby or the mother's life partner, this is the beginning of a honeymoon for the three of you. What happens is much like a honeymoon for lovers: withdrawal from the everyday events of the world, intense preoccupation and fascination with one another, profound feelings of love, lack of sleep, and deep contentment.

CHAPTER 10

The First Few Days Postpartum

*Through the labor, I was struck by the thought that I would
be meeting my child later that day. I had done a lot of
thinking about the birth ahead of time and about being a
parent, but I was surprised at how instantly we moved from
one to the other. I realized afterward that it was as if I had
expected someone to hit the pause button, let us relax, check
in with each other, get some sleep, and then start parenting.
This was obviously not the case.*

—MATT, FIRST-TIME FATHER

During the first few days after the birth, there is much going on physically, medically, and emotionally with both the mother and the baby. This chapter explains what to expect at this time—what the caregiver does, what happens with the mother and baby, and your role in all this. Your primary duty, of course, is to stay with the mother and give her as much emotional support and practical help as possible.

The First Few Hours

Immediately after the birth, the baby is quickly checked and, assuming all is well, dried and placed naked against the mother's skin. Both are covered with warm blankets. This skin-to-skin contact is really the best way to keep the baby warm—better than wrapping the baby or placing her under warming lights. The baby may be crying or accustoming herself quietly to her new surroundings. You and the mother will probably be focused completely on the baby, except when reality reenters in the form of the caregiver or nurse's necessary intrusions. Their agenda is a little different from yours: Their main concern is the physical well-being of the mother and the baby. So, while the two of you are engrossed in the baby, they are dealing with the following immediate clinical concerns.

THE MOTHER'S PERINEUM

After a vaginal birth, the caregiver carefully inspects the mother's vagina and perineum to determine whether stitches are necessary. This examination is often somewhat painful if the mother has had no anesthesia. An episiotomy (see page 231) or a sizeable tear will require stitches. The caregiver gives the mother a local anesthetic if she needs stitches and is not already anesthetized. The stitches will be gradually absorbed as the incision heals; they do not have to be removed.

AFTER A CESAREAN

Following a cesarean birth (described in chapter 9), the mother leaves the operating room and spends a few hours in a recovery room or in her labor room while the anesthetic wears off. She may be very sleepy, depending on the drugs she has been given. There will be a nurse close by all the time. You can remain with the mother, and unless the baby has a problem that requires care in the nursery, he will be with you, too.

THE MOTHER'S UTERUS

The mother's uterus is checked frequently by the nurse to make sure it is contracting tightly. If it is soft and relaxed, it will bleed too much. There are three ways to make it contract:

- *Nipple stimulation.* When the baby suckles at the breast, the hormone oxytocin is released, which makes the uterus contract. If the baby is not ready for a feeding, you or the mother can stroke or roll the mother's nipples, which has a similar effect.

- *Fundal massage.* The nurse or the midwife does this, but the mother can learn to do it, too. This massage involves firmly kneading the low abdomen until the uterus contracts to the size and consistency of a large grapefruit. This is painful for the mother, which is one reason she should learn to do it herself: She can do it less vigorously and get the same results.

◆ *Injection or intravenous administration of Pitocin or Methergine.*
This is the most reliable way to contract the uterus; it may be used along with the methods described above, although it is not needed in most cases.

THE MOTHER'S AND BABY'S VITAL SIGNS

The caregiver frequently checks the vital signs (pulse, respiration, temperature, and blood pressure) of the mother and the baby, and performs other routine assessments. If the mother or the baby had medical problems during the pregnancy or labor, the nurse or caregiver watches even more closely. The nurse or midwife will also check the mother's lochia (see page 250).

CORD BLOOD REMOVAL AND STORAGE

Umbilical cord blood contains stem cells that can be used for the same conditions that bone marrow is used for: leukemia, various anemias, and genetic and metabolic disorders. Some public blood banks accept donated umbilical cord blood for research and for treatment of people with these conditions. You may instead arrange to have your baby's cord blood stored privately for possible later use by the child or other family members. For more information, see "Recommended Resources."

COMMON PROCEDURES IN NEWBORN CARE

In the first few minutes or hours after birth, the baby is examined and a number of procedures are done. Many of these are routine; others are optional. Some are required by law to detect or prevent certain serious conditions. Because the mother may be exhausted or preoccupied with the things that are still happening to her, it will be up to you to keep track of what is being done to the baby, remind the staff of the mother's preferences regarding newborn care, and help the mother make decisions, if necessary.

Suctioning the baby's nose and mouth. The baby's airway may contain mucus, amniotic fluid with or without meconium, or blood. There are two ways to suck away this fluid. In the most common method, the tip of a rubber bulb syringe is inserted into the baby's nostrils and mouth, as soon as the head is out or when the baby is born. Most caregivers do this to all newborns, because it is quick and simple and may take less time than determining whether the baby has excessive airway excretions and needs help coughing them out. Some caregivers, including most home-birth and birth-center midwives, wait to see whether the baby needs suctioning.

Sometimes, if the amniotic fluid was stained with meconium, deeper suctioning is done, with a long tube that is passed through a nostril and down the baby's trachea (windpipe).

Purposes of suctioning. Suctioning is done to clear the airway of secretions, especially if the baby is unable to cough or sneeze to remove them, or to assist the baby who is not breathing.

Deeper suctioning may be done if the baby has had a meconium bowel movement while still in the uterus. When this happens, the meconium mixes with the amniotic fluid. Because the meconium may be in the baby's airway, the caregiver tries to suction it out before the baby's first breath, to keep the baby from breathing the meconium into her lungs, and again as soon as possible after the birth. A recent large scientific trial of early deep suctioning, when the baby's head is out, compared with no suctioning, found no difference in the number of babies who inhaled meconium. This finding comes as a relief to caregivers, because sometimes the baby comes out too quickly to accomplish the first suctioning.

Disadvantages of suctioning. These are (1) brief discomfort and stress for the baby, who may flinch or struggle, and (2) possible abrasions of mucous membranes in the baby's nose and throat if the tip scrapes them. Usually suctioning is unnecessary, because most healthy babies are fully capable of coughing or sneezing the fluids out.

Alternatives to consider. You and the mother can ask the caregiver to withhold suctioning of the mouth and nose unless the baby is unable to rid his airway of secretions. If suctioning is necessary, the caregiver can use the syringe gently. If there is meconium in the amniotic fluid, however, most caregivers will want to do deep suctioning as soon as the baby is out.

Cutting the umbilical cord. Once the baby is out, the cord is clamped in two places and cut with scissors. You might like to cut the cord. The nurse will give you the scissors and show you exactly where to cut.

The cord is often cut immediately, but a recent scientific analysis has found benefit to waiting for at least two minutes or until it stops pulsating—in five minutes or so. Less likelihood of anemia for as much as six months exists in babies whose cords are cut late. Until the cord is clamped or stops pulsating, blood passes back and forth between the baby and the placenta. It goes from placenta to baby whenever the uterus contracts, squeezing blood from the placenta through the umbilical cord to the baby. Betweeen these contractions, with each beat of the baby's heart, blood is pumped from the baby through the umbilical cord and back to the placenta. This transfer stops when the cord is clamped or stops pulsating, which occurs when the blood vessels close down. The best way to make sure that the baby has the right amount may be to place the baby on the mother's belly and wait for the cord to stop pulsating. Exceptions to this are when the baby needs immediate medical attention (because of meconium in the amniotic fluid or a low Apgar score; see page 210), when the cord is tightly wrapped around the baby's neck, preventing delivery, and when you have decided on cord blood removal and storage (see page 104).

Eye medication. An antibiotic (usually erythromycin ointment) is placed in the baby's eyes within the first hour after birth.

Purposes of eye medication. The antibiotic prevents serious eye infection or even blindness due to bacteria that cause gonorrhea or chlamydia, two common sexually transmitted diseases. These bacteria are sometimes present in the vagina and can be transmitted to the baby during birth.

Eye medication is medically indicated if the mother tests positive for chlamydia or gonorrhea or if either parent may have been exposed to the diseases (by having sex with someone else). Because the lab tests are not 100 percent reliable, and the organisms can appear after the lab tests were done, the eye medication is required by all states and provinces unless the parent refuses it and the nurse or midwife (or other person required to give it) agrees to withhold it from the baby.

Disadvantages of eye medication. The medicine blurs the baby's vision for a short time, until the warmth of the baby's eyes melts the ointment.

Alternatives to eye medication. Getting the doctor or nurse to accept your refusal may be difficult, because the most worrisome organisms, chlamydia and gonococcus, although tested for during early pregnancy, sometimes are present at birth. Because these do not always cause symptoms in adults, they sometimes go untreated. Unfortunately, the newborn can be seriously infected by these organisms. But if you and your partner have both been tested and found negative for them, and you both have been monogamous, the odds of having these organisms are extremely low. Still, your nurse or caregiver may feel very uncomfortable if you refuse the eye treatment, since most states and provinces may hold the caregiver, not the parents, responsible if the treatment is not given and the baby develops one of these infections.

A very popular alternative is to ask the nurse or midwife to postpone putting the ointment in the baby's eyes until an hour after birth, so the baby will be able to see your faces clearly in the meantime.

Vitamin K. Required in most U.S. states and Canadian provinces, vitamin K is given as an injection within an hour after birth. This vitamin is essential in the clotting of blood. Newborns are relatively slow in clotting their blood for the first week or so, although once they start consuming and digesting colostrum and milk they begin making their own vitamin K. Until then, they are at a small risk for excessive bleeding (called vitamin K deficiency bleeding, or VKDB). Giving vitamin K to tide them over reduces the risk of bleeding problems.

Vitamin K is given by injection. Until recently it was sometimes given by mouth, but it was found that oral vitamin K does not prevent later onset of VKDB, so the American Academy of Pediatrics now recommends only injectable vitamin K. The injection is given once, in the thigh within an hour after birth.

Purposes of giving vitamin K. The injection is quick, easy, and inexpensive to give, and it is very effective in preventing VKDB. Giving vitamin K is especially important when a baby is at greater risk of bleeding, because of a difficult or forceps-assisted birth, prematurity, plans for circumcision, or before the baby is a week old.

Disadvantages of giving vitamin K. The injection is briefly painful. Concerns that vitamin K may be linked to childhood cancer and jaundice have been allayed by research confirming the safety of the low dose given to newborns.

Alternatives to giving vitamin K. Refusing vitamin K altogether is a somewhat risky option, because it is not possible to predict which babies will or will not develop VKDB. The disease is rare, however.

Blood tests.   Blood samples are obtained in two ways:

1. A few drops of the baby's blood are drawn from the heel or a vein to check for:

   ◆ The level of bilirubin, a yellowish blood pigment that at high levels causes jaundice (see page 265).

   ◆ Blood sugar (glucose) levels.

   ◆ Infection, if the mother had a fever in labor or if the baby has one now.

   ◆ Numerous genetic or congenital disorders (see "Newborn Screening Tests," page 340).

2. Blood from the baby's umbilical cord may also be collected at birth for:

   ◆ Blood typing.

   ◆ Rh determination.

   ◆ Storage or donation to a blood bank (see page 104 and "Recommended Resources").

Purposes of blood tests. The general purpose of testing the newborn's blood is to detect potentially serious problems early enough to treat them and prevent dangerous effects on the baby.

Disadvantages of blood tests. The heel stick is painful to the baby, and some of the tests (such as those for bilirubin and blood glucose) may have to be repeated many times.

Also, results of blood tests are sometimes confusing and can lead to overtreatment. Caregivers sometimes disagree on when bilirubin and blood glucose levels require treatment. Ask the Key Questions (see page 202) to learn enough to make a good decision about any recommended tests.

Alternatives to consider. You and the mother can ask the caregiver about less painful ways to gain the information provided by blood tests. For example, you can observe the baby's skin and the whites of his eyes, and have a blood test for jaundice done only if they appear yellow. Or, if your baby is at low risk of hypoglycemia (if he was born at full term and the mother is not diabetic), ask whether the nurse can look for early symptoms of hypoglycemia (such as jitteriness and low body temperature) before doing the blood test, and have the mother nurse the baby as soon as possible. If the caregiver prefers the blood test to these other approaches, he or she should explain why. Weigh the benefits of the recommended test and treatment against the risks of the test and the problem it is designed to detect. Then make informed choices.

Warming unit. A warming unit is a special bed with a heater above it. A baby who is placed in a warming unit has a small thermostat taped to her abdomen; the thermostat automatically turns up the heat if the baby gets chilled. Small or premature babies get chilled more easily than average-sized or full-term babies.

Purposes of the warming unit. The unit is used to prevent a temperature drop and its harmful aftereffects (sluggishness, abnormal blood sugar levels, lung problems, and others), or to warm a baby who has become chilled.

Disadvantages of the warming unit. The baby is separated from her parents. Also, warming units are not risk-free; they may cause the baby to lose fluids through evaporation of moisture from the skin and lungs (breathing out moist air). This is a greater potential problem for premature babies, but fluid loss and signs of dehydration must be monitored carefully. Nursing often, feeding water or formula, or giving IV fluids to the baby, and adjusting the heat in the warming unit, are the most common solutions, but being held skin-to-skin with the mother is the best solution (see below).

Alternatives to consider. Prevent chills in the baby by drying her with towels right after the birth and protecting her from the air. She should be kept warm by placing her skin-to-skin with her mother, putting a hat on her, and covering mother and baby with a warm blanket. Her temperature should be checked frequently with a quick-action thermometer. If it is not possible to do these things because the baby needs medical attention, the warming unit becomes a necessity. If the mother is not ready to hold the baby, you might hold the baby skin-to-skin with a blanket around the two of you.

Cleanup. The mother's bed linen is changed; the caregiver or the nurse helps the mother wash up and put on a clean gown. The gown should open in the front for convenient breastfeeding. The mother wears a sanitary pad to catch the bloody vaginal discharge (see page 344), which will be present for several days or weeks. The baby is wiped clean and dry, diapered, and dressed. The baby should wear a hat (which you or the hospital supplies). A hat helps keep the baby warm all over; when his head is uncovered, a lot of heat is lost, and he can get a chill.

During all this cleanup activity, the mother should hold the baby close to her breast so that he can nurse as soon as he is ready. The nurse, doula, or midwife can be a great help in getting the baby to "latch on" to the breast correctly. Ask for help if the baby is having difficulty or if the mother is unsure of what to do. See chapter 11 for more on breastfeeding.

When the immediate postpartum care is over, you, the mother, and the baby may be left in privacy for a while. Dim the lights to encourage the baby to open his eyes; enjoy these quiet moments together. You and the mother both will soon be ready for a meal.

If the mother had a cesarean delivery she may be allowed small amounts of solid food when she wants it, or she may have to wait for several hours before she is offered anything more than clear liquids; caregivers' orders vary. She may continue receiving intravenous fluids for up to a day after the cesarean.

The First Few Days for the Baby

Once both mother and baby are settled, the three of you can relax together, cooing, cuddling, exploring, and nursing—or simply sleeping. There is usually no reason for mothers and babies to be separated after birth, although for a long time it was (and still is in some places) a hospital custom to separate them. If the mother or baby is not well, the baby may go to the nursery or may stay in the room but the mother may be unable to hold her.

You are the perfect person to hold the baby if the mother cannot (and even if she can), or to remain with the baby in the nursery, as long as both you and the mother wish for you to do so. If you cuddle with the baby sometime during the first day or so after birth, you will have even stronger feelings for your child. There is something magical about holding your baby close—especially skin-to-skin—gazing at him while he gazes back, and talking or singing to him. I overheard one father saying to his baby as he held him close, "And when you're six, we'll take you horseback riding in Montana!" The baby seemed to approve. They were planning their lives together.

PHYSICAL EXAM AND ASSESSMENT

A doctor or a midwife will give the baby a thorough physical exam, checking her entire body and all her systems. It is interesting to watch the exam, which can teach you a great deal about the baby. Over the next few days you, the mother, or the staff will make certain observations of the baby: the number and quality of bowel movements, frequency of urination, frequency and length of time in feeding, respiration, temperature, pulse, and so forth. The staff will teach you more about these observations, because they will be your responsibility for the first few days at home with the baby.

Bowel Movements

The baby will have a bowel movement within a few hours after birth. This and the next several bowel movements are called meconium, and they are different from later bowel movements. Meconium is thick, black, sticky, and hard to clean. If you think of it, soon after birth, rub some vegetable oil or massage oil all over the baby's buttocks and genitals. This will make cleaning off the meconium easier, and you will thank me.

Over the next few days, as the mother's milk shifts from colostrum (see page 340) to mature milk, the baby's bowel movements will change from black to brown to green to yellow and will become very runny and almost odorless or slightly sweet-smelling. After the first few days, the baby may have a bowel movement almost every time she eats, and she should have at least four per day. This is a good sign that she is getting enough to eat.

Bathing the Baby

The baby will have a bath within the first couple of days. Unless you or the mother is accustomed to bathing newborns, the nurse or midwife will probably give the bath, teaching you both at the same time. The usual advice is to start at the top and work down, always holding the baby securely with your arm around the baby and your hand holding the baby's upper arm.

Caring for the Cord

The cord stump needs to be kept clean and dry. Arrange the baby's diaper so that it does not touch the cord. Clean the cord with tap or bottled water. The nurse or midwife will show you how to do this. The cord clamp is removed by the nurse or midwife, usually on the second day, leaving a black, dry stump that remains for a week or two and then drops off. The cord usually has a faintly foul smell, but call the baby's doctor if pus or red blood oozes from it.

FEEDING THE BABY

For the first six months, breastfed babies need no food but colostrum (the first "milk" to come from the breasts) and breast milk. They do not need formula or water, and they do not need glucose water unless they have low blood sugar that is not corrected by breastfeeding. It is a good idea to begin breastfeeding as soon after birth as the baby is interested, usually within 20 to 60 minutes.

Babies who are to be formula-fed should begin receiving formula when they seem ready to suck and when their condition is stable.

For more information about your role in feeding the baby, see chapter 11, "Getting Started with Breastfeeding."

NEWBORN SCREENING TESTS

Every state and province has a newborn screening programs. Through the "heel-stick test," these programs can detect numerous rare endocrinological, metabolic, and hematologic disorders, most of which, if detected early, can be treated to prevent mental or developmental retardation and other serious disabilities or early death. As of this writing, the March of Dimes recommends that a minimum of nine disorders be tested for, but the number that various states actually screen for varies from 4 to 31. One heel stick can usually provide enough blood for the tiny samples needed for all these tests. The nine disorders that the March of Dimes recommends testing for are PKU (phenylketonuria), congenital hypothyroidism, congenital adrenal hyperplasia (CAH), biotinidase deficiency, maple-syrup urine disease, galactosemia, homocystinuria, sickle-cell anemia, and medium-chain acyl-CoA dehydrogenase deficiency (MCAD). You might check with your state or provincial public-health department to see whether it screens for all of these.

Hearing screening test. Within the first few days, your baby will probably be given a hearing test. This test will identify any hearing problem much earlier than you and the mother would notice it (the average age at which hearing problems are identified without the screening test is 14 months, by which time the child already has fallen behind in speech development). Identifying hearing problems early allows for early therapy.

Most hospitals do the hearing test routinely, but if you give birth outside the hospital you may want to arrange a test yourself. Ask your midwife how and where to do this, and check whether your insurance company will cover the cost.

The test is done while the baby is asleep. The baby wears head-phones, and several electrodes are placed around his head. They record brain-wave activity and middle-ear activity in response to sounds that are transmitted into the baby's ears and via the bones of his head.

If the test indicates a problem or the results are unclear, there will be more testing. If repeat tests indicate that the baby has impaired hearing, you will be referred to a hearing specialist and speech ther-apist so you can begin a program to maximize your child's hearing and communication skills.

CIRCUMCISION

Nonreligious circumcision of the newborn is an extremely controver-sial subject, and the decision whether to circumcise a baby is a highly personal one. I will try to present a fair discussion of this topic. Most major medical groups, including the American Academy of Pedi-atrics and the Canadian Paediatric Society, are officially neutral on the subject of circumcision. They advise that parents should learn about the pros and cons and decide as they see fit.

If the baby is going to be circumcised, the procedure will be done in the hospital on the first or second day after birth, or, in the Jewish tradition, in the home or synagogue on the eighth day. When circum-cision is done in the hospital, the penis is usually numbed with local anesthetic. The foreskin is separated from the underlying glans (the end of the penis) and removed from the glans with a scalpel.

The incidence of circumcision in the United States is now esti-mated at about 65 percent, with much regional variation. Rates range from 37 percent in the western United States to 81 percent in the Midwest. In Canada the rate is considerably lower, about 20 percent.

Purposes of circumcision. The surgery is done:

◆ To change the appearance of the penis according to the parents' preferences.

◆ To observe Jewish or other religious custom.

◆ To reduce the child's chances of acquiring some sexually transmitted diseases (STDs) after he becomes sexually active. Studies in Africa and New Zealand indicate that circumcised men have a lower incidence of STDs of all kinds. There is much controversy over the applicability of these studies to North America.

◆ To reduce the risk of cancer of the penis, although this cancer is very rare, affecting only 1 to 2 men in 100,000. Penile cancer is more common in elderly uncircumcised men with long-term poor hygiene, and it is almost unheard of in elderly circumcised men with poor hygiene. The American Cancer Society does not recommend newborn circumcision as way to prevent cancer of the penis.

Other health-related reasons for circumcision have been less well studied, and their validity hasn't been established. For more information about these, see "Recommended Resources."

Disadvantages of circumcision. Circumcision carries the same risks as all surgery: infection, hemorrhage, adhesions, pain, and injury due to human error.

◆ The procedure is very painful unless anesthesia is used. A local anesthetic is usually injected in several places at the base of the penis to reduce the pain. Although the injections are painful, they prevent pain during the circumcision itself. Sometimes, instead of being injected, anesthetic is applied as a cream to the penis. But a wait of 20 minutes is needed for the cream to take effect, so it is not widely used.

◆ Infection or hemorrhage occurs in about 1 in every 200 circumcisions. These conditions can usually be well controlled with medications and extra time in the hospital.

- There is a small possibility, especially with an inexperienced, unsupervised doctor, that the surgery will be done poorly—too much or too little foreskin may be removed.
- The circumcised penis usually takes seven to 10 days to heal. Parents must take special care of the penis during this time, avoid wet diapers and other irritations, and observe the penis for signs of poor healing.
- If the newborn child is ill or if his penis is abnormal in structure, circumcision may be very harmful.

Alternatives to consider. You and the mother can:

- Leave the baby uncircumcised. If you do, learn proper care of the uncircumcised penis (see "Recommended Resources"). Do not try to pull your son's foreskin back to clean it or for any other reason. When most baby boys are born, their foreskin adheres to the glans. Over a period of months or years, it gradually loosens and becomes easily retractable. A lot of the problems attributed to being uncircumcised are really caused by parents and others who do not know to leave the foreskin alone. As your child grows up, teach the child proper hygiene; washing the penis is about as complicated as washing the ears.
- Decide to have the baby circumcised, but request anesthesia for the procedure and an experienced doctor. If possible, remain with the baby to comfort him. Learn proper care for the newly circumcised penis to promote healing.
- Leave the decision for the child to make himself when he reaches adulthood.

Whether you choose to circumcise your son or not, you will later want to teach him responsible sexual practices to protect himself and his partners from sexually transmitted infections.

BABY CARE

The nurse or midwife can teach you baby skills not covered in this book, such as changing diapers, bathing, and soothing the baby when she is fussy. Books, videos, and classes are also available. See "Recommended Resources."

The First Few Days for the Mother

For the mother, the early postpartum period is marked by fatigue, emotional highs and lows, preoccupation with the baby, some pain, and an array of physical changes that affect most parts of her body.

She may be tired and excited at the same time, finding it difficult to sleep, but unable to exert herself very much without feeling worn out. A shower or a short walk is enough to send her straight back to bed.

The mother may be surprised by the variety of physical changes she experiences; these physical changes will require more attention than she ever expected.

HER UTERUS

The nurse or midwife and the mother herself should check the uterus frequently in the first few days to make sure it remains contracted (see page 330). Remind the mother to continue checking until it feels contracted at every check over two or three days.

AFTERPAINS

These are uterine contractions that come and go. Especially if she has had a child before, the mother's afterpains may be quite intense when she suckles the baby. Afterpains are a good sign that the mother's uterus is returning to its prepregnant size. Remind her to use her relaxation and breathing techniques. If the pains are severe, she can request pain medications. Afterpains go away in a few days.

VAGINAL DISCHARGE

The mother will have a vaginal discharge, called *lochia*, which is similar to a menstrual period. It starts out as a heavy red flow containing some clots, and gradually diminishes; it lasts from two to six weeks.

In the first few days after birth, the mother may notice that she bleeds very little while lying down, but when she stands up after a few hours in bed she may suddenly lose a lot of blood. This can be alarming, but it is probably due to the fact that blood has been collecting in the vagina until gravity causes it to flow out. If heavy bleeding continues longer than a few minutes, however, or if the mother feels faint, call her caregiver or the hospital's maternity floor.

After the lochia has clearly subsided, if it suddenly increases, or if the mother passes large, golf ball–sized clots, call her caregiver, because she may be bleeding from a blood vessel at the former site of the placenta. Sometimes heavy physical exertion causes a woman to bleed heavily after her lochia had decreased. Rest usually puts an end to the heavy bleeding, but you should call the mother's caregiver if you are concerned.

THE PERINEUM

After a vaginal birth, the mother's perineum will be sore, especially if she has had stitches. In any case, she may have swelling and bruising. You can suggest the following comfort measures:

- Applying an ice pack helps, especially during the first 24 hours.

- Sitting in a bath of warm water for 20 minutes, two or three times a day, is soothing. She should not wash in this water; it should be kept clean.

- Carefully patting her perineum dry (starting at the front, and moving toward the anus) or squirting it with warm water from a bottle after urinating or having a bowel movement is less irritating than wiping with toilet paper.

- Applying witch hazel–soaked pads to stitches and hemorrhoids is soothing.

- Doing the pelvic-floor contraction exercise ("super-Kegel") promotes healing, reduces swelling, and restores strength. The mother tightens the muscles around her vagina and urethra as she would if she were trying to hold back urine (see page 19). She should try to do 10 super-Kegels per day, and she should always do one as she sits down. She may find she cannot hold the super-Kegel for a full 20 seconds at first. She should hold it as long as she can; her ability will steadily improve.

Emptying Bowels and Bladder

You may be surprised at how preoccupied the mother becomes with bowel movements and urination! These functions are more difficult than usual because her perineum is sore, her abdominal muscles are temporarily weak (making straining to move her bowels difficult), and the interruption in her food and fluid intake during labor may have caused constipation.

If she is unable to urinate, try all the tricks—run a faucet, have her urinate in the bath (and get out when she is done) or shower, and have her press in on her low abdomen just above her pubic bone (as long as she didn't have a cesarean). These almost always work, but in the unlikely event that she does not urinate within a half day or so, you should call her caregiver. The mother may have to have a catheter placed in her bladder to empty it. This is unpleasant, but it is better than letting her bladder become distended.

On a positive note, one very welcome change is that her bladder, no longer crowded by the baby, has much greater capacity than during pregnancy, so she will have to urinate much less frequently.

To help the mother avoid or reduce difficulties with the first bowel movement after giving birth, remind her to eat and drink high-fiber foods: prune juice, other juices, raw fruits and vegetables, bran breads or cereals, and so forth. Bulk-producing stool softeners or laxatives may also help. In addition, she might support her sore perineum by pressing toilet paper against it as she has a bowel movement. These measures also help if a woman has painful hemorrhoids.

It may take a week or two for the mother to resume her usual bowel patterns. If she feels uncomfortable or constipated despite the measures described in the preceding paragraph, she probably ought to contact her caregiver.

Pain Following Cesarean Delivery

Post-cesarean pain results from the incision, from the stitches or clamps closing it, and from gas that commonly builds up in the mother's abdomen after this surgery. Activities such as turning over, getting out of bed, walking, and nursing the baby are usually very painful for a few days, but they hasten recovery. Help as much as you can to make these activities easier for the mother, by reminding her of how to roll from back to side, giving her a hand as she gets out of bed, offering a supportive arm as she walks, providing a pillow for her lap as she nurses the baby. The mother will gradually begin feeling better each day.

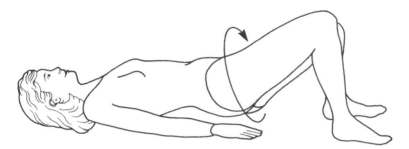

To reduce pain when rolling from her back to her side, the mother who has had a cesarean should raise her hips and rotate her hips and legs to the side before turning her shoulders.

Clamps are removed on the second or third day after the delivery. The procedure is not very painful, and the pain from the incision will then decrease.

To help her reduce abdominal pain, encourage the mother to do the following:

◆ When rolling from her back to her side, she should first bend her knees so that her feet are flat on the bed. Then she should raise her hips (so that only her head, shoulders and feet are on the bed), twist them to one side, and roll her shoulders to the side. See the illustration. This is much easier and far less painful than rolling over the usual way. To sit up from the side-lying position, she should push herself up with her hands. These techniques avoid strain on her incision.

◆ She should avoid gas-producing foods (lentils and beans, foods in the cabbage family, and cold or carbonated beverages).

◆ To avoid feeling faint when she gets out of bed the first few times, she should first circle her ankles, raise her arms above her head several times, and then sit up and raise her arms several more times. As she stands, you should stand next to her so she can hold on to you.

◆ When holding the baby on her lap, she should place a pillow over the incision to protect it.

◆ She should ask the nurse to show her other ways to hold the baby to avoid pressure on her incision.

Homecoming

Check the mother's insurance plan ahead of time to learn what to expect and what options she has after the birth. The usual hospital stay after a normal vaginal birth is 24 to 48 hours; after a cesarean, it is 72 hours. If the birth takes place in a birth center, the mother will probably go home three to six hours afterward. After a home birth, the midwife usually stays for three to four hours.

The mother's caregiver should make sure you both have clear instructions about observations to make of the mother and baby, special care needs of each of them, and numbers to call in case you have any concerns. Make sure you know the name and phone number of the baby's doctor. Ask for these if you do not have them.

A follow-up appointment should be scheduled within the first week (preferably three or four days) after birth to check on breast-feeding and on the mother's and baby's health and well-being. Unfortunately, with all the cutbacks in services that hospitals and insurance companies are making to save money, a follow-up appointment may not be offered. In this case, it is especially important to make sure you know whom to call if the mother has any problems before her first scheduled postpartum checkup.

If the baby was born at home, the midwife will make two or more home visits within the first several days.

Before the mother and the baby come home from the hospital, take a moment to think about what they are coming home to. Is the house a mess? Is the sink full of dishes? Is the bed unmade? Is the baby's place (basket, bassinet, cradle or crib, and changing area) ready? There is nothing more disheartening for the mother than returning home to chaos. You want her to feel glad to get home, so try to provide a pleasant homecoming.

Consider going home alone for a few hours to prepare the home. Better yet, get friends and family to help. These are things they might do:

◆ Make the bed with fresh linens.

◆ Tidy up the house, and wash any dirty dishes.

◆ Make sure good food is available.

◆ Have a stack of fresh diapers ready (call a diaper service or buy some).

◆ Have a few welcoming touches around the house—fresh flowers, a "Welcome Home" poster.

Prepare for the ride home:

◆ Install the infant car seat (see page 15) if this hasn't been done already.

◆ Tidy up the inside of the car.

◆ Have enough gas so that you don't have to stop on the way home.

◆ Make sure the mother and the baby have clothes to wear home and that the baby has a blanket or two.

When the mother and baby arrive home, you and she may feel like celebrating. And with good reason! You're introducing the baby to his own new world. The mother may feel she has been away a long time (even though it probably has been only a few days!) and may be relieved to be in familiar surroundings once again. Fatigue is likely to set in very soon. Perhaps the best thing for her to do is get right into bed, snuggle with her loved ones, and bask in the warm feelings. Ask visitors not to come until at least the next day.

After a Home Birth

If the baby has been born at home, there may be a cleanup operation ahead—dishes, laundry, trash, a bed to make with fresh linens. The midwives, doula, and others who have attended the birth should leave things reasonably clean, but after they leave to give you and your family some quiet time together, you may still have a lot to do. Plan in advance, so you can avoid this situation:

◆ Ask the caregiver about cleanup ahead of time: (1) How much does she or he do? (2) What will need to be done? (3) What happens to the placenta? Sometimes the caregiver takes it and disposes of it. Some families bury it and plant a tree or a bush over it. You might store it in the freezer (mark it well, so no one will open the package, expecting food!), until you have time to do this.

◆ Have large trash bags available during labor—one for trash, one for laundry. As items are used, they can go right into the appropriate bags.

◆ If extra people are available, assign ongoing and after-birth cleanup tasks: picking up and washing dishes, putting food away, doing laundry, taking out trash, and straightening up the house.

Getting Help and Advice

The two of you will have your hands full, maintaining the household, feeding yourselves, and getting to know and care for the new family member, especially since all these tasks must be carried out in the midst of disrupted sleep schedules and the mother's postpartum adjustments. The brightest spot in all this is the deep and overwhelming love you feel toward your baby. The baby certainly makes it all worthwhile, but is there anything that could also make it a bit easier? The answer is yes: help!

Accept any and all offers of help from family and friends. Errand running, meal preparation, phone calls, housework—all these can be done by someone else. The best kind of help, however, is availability whenever you need it—day or night. Getting such help may not be possible unless you are fortunate enough to have a relative or close friend who can fit comfortably into the chaos. If you are very lucky, grandparents or other helpful relatives or friends will come every day to help as needed. Or maybe the baby's grandmother or aunt can come to stay for a week or two. She can keep the household running smoothly, feed you both, and answer your questions about baby care.

You will want to make sure this person can foster the mother's self-confidence in meeting her baby's needs. This is no time for mother-daughter strife to rear its ugly head.

One way to ensure harmony is to invite the person most preferred by the mother, and to plan the visit for when the mother would prefer it—perhaps immediately after the birth, perhaps one or two weeks later. It also makes sense to spell out what you think you need from this person: "We are going to need help with running the household and cooking, because Jane gets really upset when the place gets messy. Knowing her, she'll run herself ragged trying to do everything even though the most important things are for her to spend lots of time with the baby, to get a good start with breastfeeding, and to get plenty of rest. Will you come and help us, so that she can devote herself to being a mother?"

Postpartum doulas are a great solution to the problem of new family adjustment. These trained women can be hired for blocks of several hours every day or every other day for a period of a week or many weeks. See page 36 for more on postpartum doulas, and check "Recommended Resources" to locate one.

The Mother's Postpartum Emotions

During the early postpartum period, the mother's emotions are changeable and unpredictable. One moment she may be rapturous and full of energy; the next, tired, frustrated, and in tears. The sudden changes in hormone production and body functions—as she goes from supporting the growth of a fetus during pregnancy to expelling the baby and to breastfeeding while returning to a nonpregnant state—take an emotional toll. Add to that her inevitable fatigue from loss of sleep during labor and for weeks after the birth, as well as the stress of a profound role change, and it is not surprising that she is volatile.

If you are the mother's life partner as well as her birth partner, you have your own share of emotional adjustments—the role change to parenthood, your own fatigue, and a complete disruption in lifestyle. Even if you are a relative or a friend helping out temporarily, you are probably tired from the birth experience and from the strain of caring for the mother and the new baby.

As two tired people with a great many needs, you will be sustained through this stressful time by your underlying feelings for each other and by the joy and commitment you share in having your new baby. It helps to know that this situation *will* get better. Following are suggestions for getting through the emotional ups and downs of the first few days after the baby is born.

POSTPARTUM BLUES

You may be caught off guard if the mother seems sad or cries a lot. You may feel helpless or guilty, believing that you are to blame or that it is up to you to make things right. You may worry about her; you may feel angry with her; or you may wonder whether this situation is going to be permanent.

What can you do about postpartum blues? Here are some suggestions:

- First of all, ask what you can do to help. She may or may not have an answer. She may not know why she is crying. She may simply need to cry without you and other people feeling you must help her get over it. Accept her need to cry with patience, tenderness, and empathy. She might appreciate it if you hold her quietly while she lets the tears flow.

- Do not blame yourself if you did nothing to make her cry.

- Know that almost every woman sheds tears and goes on an emotional roller coaster for a few days after childbirth. Emotions are close to the surface at this time, probably because of the abrupt changes in hormone production that take place with birth.

- Realize that this will probably pass after a few days. Give her time. Encourage her to nap and to rest (see "Recipe for Getting Enough Sleep," page 356).

- Ask her friends and relatives, especially those who have given birth, to visit.

- Call the mother's caregiver, childbirth educator, or lactation consultant if you are worried.

- Enlist the assistance of a postpartum doula or someone else who understands and can both help the mother and give you perspective.
- Look into mothers' groups or postpartum classes. They are becoming very popular as settings where feelings can be shared and discussed.

Sometimes blue feelings continue without letup for more than a week. If this is happening, or if you feel under undue pressure, the mother may have postpartum depression or another mood disorder. Discuss your concerns with the mother, and call the resource people already mentioned. Ask the mother to go over "Unhappiness After Childbirth: A Self-Assessment" (see page 355) with you, as a way to clarify her feelings. A referral from the mother's caregiver to a social worker, psychologist, or psychiatrist for counseling or therapy may be appropriate and very helpful. A complete physical exam, with blood tests to check levels of various hormones, including thyroid tests, might reveal a physical condition that could be contributing to depression. Or a support group alone might help the mother recover from her depressed feelings. Consider these options if the mother is unhappy most of the time.

What about Your Feelings?

Becoming a parent has its thrills and joys, but if you are the mother's life partner you are also making huge emotional adjustments and lifestyle changes in a state of fatigue and constant demands. How are you doing? Are you overwhelmed? Are your needs being met? Many partners do very well during this rather chaotic and unpredictable time, but others feel depressed or angry at times. Even though your needs seem to be low in the hierarchy, you deserve time for yourself—to sleep, see your friends, and get a break. Why don't you and the mother plan for you to take a few hours' break when someone else is with her? Make a date with yourself, and do something that you like to do. You'll be refreshed and glad to reconnect with your family!

Practical Matters at Home

Much of the turmoil of the postpartum period can be avoided if you're prepared for it in advance and if you can simplify your lives for a while. The following suggestions will help all of you get through these first days until the household becomes more settled.

FATIGUE AND SLEEP DEPRIVATION

The mother is tired. You are probably tired, too. If after being her birth partner you are now her "at home" support person, you are probably running out of energy. Sleep deprivation is a serious problem among new parents that is often ignored. In the mother, it may cause inadequate milk supply; severe mood swings (including postpartum mood disorders); and inability to deal with the baby's crying, other minor annoyances, and even simple decision making (about what to have for dinner, for instance). Fatigue makes *everything* worse, and adequate rest makes *everything* better—the mother's appetite, her feelings toward the baby and toward you, her mood, her milk supply, her patience, and so on.

And yet people simply resign themselves to the belief that all new parents, especially mothers, cannot possibly get enough sleep. This is not true. It is possible for most new parents to get enough sleep. To do so, however, you must give sleep a very high priority (right next to making sure the baby is fed and cared for), and restructure your lives to ensure you both get enough. It does not work for the mother to simply "sleep when the baby sleeps," as most women are advised to do. If the baby is often wide awake when the mother needs to sleep, you might help out by looking after the baby.

Until things have settled into a comfortable routine, give a high priority to getting enough sleep. Unplug the phone, and keep a "Do Not Disturb" sign on the front door until one of you is ready to get up. For the first several weeks after birth, try very hard not to schedule any appointments before noon. Any earlier would be too early!

Of course, if she already has a child or children, it may be impossible to avoid morning activities. Then you will have to adapt in other ways, such as urging the mother to go to bed 11 or 12 hours before she needs to get up in the morning.

Unhappiness After Childbirth: A Self-Assessment

Circle the answer that comes closest to how you have felt in the past seven days, not just how you feel today.

1. I have been able to laugh and see the funny side of things . . .
   a. As much as I always could.   b. Not quite as much as I used to.
   c. Definitely not as much as I used to.   d. Not at all.

2. I have looked forward with enjoyment to things . . .
   a. As much as I always did.   b. Not quite as much as I used to.
   c. Definitely not as much as I used to.   d. Not at all.

3. I have blamed myself unnecessarily when things went wrong . . .
   a. Not at all.   b. Very little.   c. Some of the time.   d. Most of the time.

4. I have been anxious or worried for no good reason . . .
   a. Not at all.   b. Very little.   c. Some of the time.   d. Most of the time.

5. I have felt scared or panicked for no good reason . . .
   a. Not at all.   b. Very little.   c. Some of the time.   d. Most of the time.

6. I have been feeling overwhelmed . . .
   a. Not at all; I've been coping very well.
   b. Very little; I've been coping pretty well.
   c. Some of the time; I haven't been coping as well as usual.
   d. Quite a lot; I haven't been able to cope at all.

7. I have been so unhappy that I've had difficulty sleeping, even when the baby is asleep and the house is quiet . . .
   a. Not at all.   b. Very little.   c. Some of the time.   d. Most of the time.

8. I have felt sad or miserable . . .
   a. Not at all.   b. Very little.   c. Some of the time.   d. Most of the time.

9. I have been so unhappy that I've been crying . . .
   a. Not at all.   b. Very little.   c. Some of the time.   d. Most of the time.

10. The thought of harming myself or my baby has occurred to me . . .
   a. Not at all.   b. Very little.   c. Some of the time.   d. Most of the time.

If you have a feeling after completing this form that something isn't right, or if you have any questions about your emotional well-being, please contact your caregiver, childbirth educator or doula, or a mental-health therapist.

Adapted from Cox, J. L. and J. M. Holden, "Detection of Postnatal Depression: Development of the 10-Item Edinburgh Postnatal Depression Scale," *British Journal of Psychiatry* 150 (1987): 782–86.

RECIPE FOR GETTING ENOUGH SLEEP

This applies to both parents until the breadwinner returns to employment. Then he or she will have to get more sleep at night and less during the day. Start right off with this technique the first night you are at home.

Each of you should think about how many hours of sleep you need every 24 hours in order to function well. Six hours? Eight hours? Nine? That is the amount of sleep you now owe yourself every day.

Since you cannot get this amount of sleep in one stretch, because of interruptions for feedings and baby care, you will require more hours in bed to get your allotted amount of sleep. Plan to stay in bed or keep going back to bed until you have slept your allotted number of hours. This means that except for meals and trips to the bathroom, you do not get up in the early morning. Keep a mental note of approximately how much time you have slept at each stretch, and stay in your nightclothes until you have slept the required number of hours. You may have to stay in bed from ten at night until noon the next day to get eight hours of sleep! If that's what it takes, do it. Then brush your teeth, take a shower, get dressed, and greet the day! You might even want to stay in bed all day for the first few days after birth.

Many parents find it easier to follow this advice if the baby sleeps with them or nearby.

As your baby grows and begins to sleep for longer stretches, it will take you less time to get enough sleep.

The "Recipe for Getting Enough Sleep" will help if the baby is the only child in your family. You can combine it with "platoon sleeping," if you wish. If you have an older child, one of you may have to look after her while the other sleeps. In this case, "platoon sleeping" may be the best way to increase sleep for both of you.

Platoon sleeping. It works this way: Right after the baby is fed in the early evening, one parent is in charge of the baby (awake or asleep) and any older children while the other parent sleeps in the evening, and the parent who sleeps in the evening gets up early so the other can sleep in the morning. When it is your turn to stay up, rock and talk and bounce and walk and soothe the baby as long as she is awake. If the baby is asleep, you can doze, watch TV, or get something done. Try to give the mother two to three hours of sleep, but when the baby really wants to eat, then take the baby to the mother. Then you both sleep, or try to, with intermittent feedings and diaper changes. You carry on in this way until the mother has had the amount of sleep she is supposed to get. She then gets up with the baby, allowing you a few extra hours of sleep.

With platoon sleeping—theoretically, at least—you each get a stretch of unbroken sleep, plus several hours of intermittent sleep.

FUSSY, CRYING BABY

Entire books have been written about fussy babies (see "Recommended Resources"). In the first few days, a fussy baby can usually be soothed by:

- Feeding or burping.
- Changing her diaper.
- Letting the baby suck on your (clean) little finger: Place your finger in her mouth with the nail down on her tongue and the soft pad touching the roof of her mouth. She might take your finger more eagerly at first if you wet it. (Offer your finger only if she has been fed within the past hour. At any other time, she may be crying because she needs to be fed.)
- Swaddling the baby snugly in a blanket.
- Picking her up, rocking, or walking her. "Wear" the baby by carrying her close to your body in a baby carrier or sling.
- Holding the baby against your shoulder while bouncing on a birth ball (see the illustration on page 147). This works wonders.
- Reclining on your back, holding the baby with her belly against your chest, and singing to her.
- Creating "white noise"—the sounds of a dishwasher or a washing machine, "shushing" (that is, saying "shhhh, shhhh," for a few minutes very close to her ear), peaceful recorded music, or crooning lullabies in the baby's ear.

To learn a successful step-by-step approach to soothing a crying baby, see "Recommended Resources."

Don't leave a tiny baby crying. The first few days after birth are a time of major adjustment for the baby, as they are for the mother and for you. A newborn needs the comfort and security of feeling your bodies and hearing your voices nearby. Do not worry about spoiling the baby: You cannot spoil her by meeting her basic needs.

SCHEDULING THE BABY'S SLEEPING AND FEEDING

Don't even try to get the baby on a schedule in the first few weeks. Instead, discover the baby's own schedule, and pattern your life around that. Focus on meeting the baby's needs; try to figure out how he tells you he is hungry, curious, interested, bored, uncomfortable, or over-stimulated. Let the baby call the shots. It is much easier for the household to adjust to the baby at first than to make the baby adjust to the household. Make it your goal to meet the baby's needs, as he expresses them—you will all be happier if you do. Read *Your Amazing Newborn* (see "Recommended Resources") to help you understand the baby.

MEALS

Time for meal preparation hardly exists during the busy first days at home, yet good food, quickly available, is a must. Try the following:

- *Prepare meals in advance.* Before the birth, prepare a few dishes—such as soups, casseroles, and stews—that will either keep for several days or will freeze.

- *Purchase quick, nutritious, tasty foods.* Foods that need little or no preparation—that you can grab and eat—are good choices for the first few weeks. Such foods include yogurt, fruit, granola and nuts, cottage cheese, hard cheese, raw vegetables, cold cuts, and whole-grain breads and crackers. Try to have these on hand before the birth so you won't have to go shopping right away. This is the time, too, to search the deli counter and frozen food section at the grocery store for nourishing, delicious prepared food.

◆ *Fix dishes that last for a while.* For example, you can roast a turkey and pick from it for a week; or wash, cut, and chill raw vegetables to keep in the refrigerator for munching.

◆ *Accept food from friends and relatives.* If people ask how they can help, tell them you'd love a main dish. Sometimes a group of friends establishes a "meal train," in which each signs up to provide one or more meals over the course of a week or two. One hint: Ask your friends to bring food only every other day. People usually bring more than one meal's worth, so you can find your refrigerator overflowing after a few days of daily contributions. Besides, if you ask for meals only every other day, your friends may keep the meal train going for a longer period.

◆ *Remember the mother's dietary needs.* Her postpartum diet should be as good as her pregnancy diet was. If she is breastfeeding, she will need 200 to 300 calories more than normal each day. She will also need at least two quarts of liquids each day.

HOUSEHOLD CHORES

The first few days at home are busy and full of adjustments. Do the mother and yourself a big favor: If you have no help, plan to do the minimum in the way of household chores—just enough to maintain sanity. It may be easier if you have "super-cleaned" before the baby was born; if you haven't, just close your eyes and let things accumulate for a while. Simplify your lives so you are free to care for and enjoy the baby and to get enough rest.

If you do have help, do not be shy about asking for what you and the mother really want done. One advantage of a postpartum doula is that she is there to do what you need done, not to enjoy the new baby and your company, and you don't need to worry about offending her. She won't even mind wearing the baby in a sling while she does some chores or prepares a meal, allowing the two of you a chance for a nap!

In conclusion, the first days and weeks postpartum are a time of adjustment: for the mother, as her body returns to a nonpregnant state and begins lactating, and for you both, as you learn your parenting roles, take on a new lifestyle, and explore your relationship with each other. You will never be the same, nor will you want to be.

CHAPTER 11

Getting Started with Breastfeeding

Before Elliot's arrival, we could never understand why
anyone wouldn't breastfeed her baby. One session with
a bad latch, and Heather's nipple hurt terribly. Dread
and fear of feeding led to brief moments of resentment.
We stayed with it, though, and feel wonderful about the
quality and quantity of his intake. It is a great relief to us
to know he is getting the best thing for him.

—MATT, FIRST-TIME FATHER

Your role when the mother breastfeeds may seem unclear, because it is not as simple as taking over the feeding for her when she is tired. It is more a matter of supporting her decision to breastfeed and helping simplify her life while she does it. It really helps if you have some knowledge and conviction about the advantages of breastfeeding.

Advantages of Breastfeeding

The advantages of breastfeeding are many, for everyone involved. For the family:

- It costs much less to breastfeed than to formula-feed.
- Formula preparation and bottle washing are avoided.

  For the mother:

- Breastfeeding hastens the return of her uterus to normal, by causing it to contract with every feeding.

◆ Hormones associated with breastfeeding cause relaxation and feelings of contentment.

◆ Once the initial learning period has passed, most women find breastfeeding very satisfying.

◆ Breastfeeding is quick and convenient; the mother simply lifts her shirt and offers her breast. She doesn't have to frantically prepare a bottle while her baby cries impatiently.

For the baby:

◆ Breast milk is perfectly suited to the baby's nutritional requirements.

◆ Breast milk contains substances (immunoglobulins and antibodies from the mother) that provide important protection against illness.

◆ Breast milk changes in composition as the baby grows and his nutritional requirements change.

◆ Problems with allergies, indigestion, and overfeeding are fewer with breast milk than with formula.

◆ The milk is always at the right temperature and instantly available.

◆ Breastfeeding provides protection against adult obesity.

◆ Breastfeeding has other long-term health benefits, such as superior jaw development, reduced likelihood of asthma, and better ability to handle dietary fats.

Because of all these advantages, most mothers today decide to breastfeed. There are challenges to overcome, however, before breastfeeding becomes easy, quick, and convenient. A lack of experience may lead parents to doubt whether the baby is getting enough milk, and to worry that the baby nurses too often or not enough. They may not feel they can trust the process.

There is much to know to get off to a good start with breastfeeding. Before the baby is born, identify helpful resources:

◆ A good breastfeeding book can be a godsend in the middle of the night! (See "Recommended Resources.")

◆ Most hospitals have lactation consultants, but they may not be available for ongoing support. The baby's doctor or your childbirth educator can probably refer you to a lactation consultant who can provide later or longer-term help.

◆ Mother-infant groups, La Leche League chapters, and other support groups meet regularly in most communities. La Leche League leaders are listed in the white pages (in the business section, if there is one) and sometimes in the yellow pages of phone books. You can also locate them through the League's Web site; see "Recommended Resources."

◆ The baby's doctor will help the mother know whether her baby is thriving on breast milk and can suggest helpful resources, if needed.

◆ Friends who have breastfed can advise on helpful products and resources, and can empathize and assist with problems.

◆ Internet sites provide products and information, and news groups offer advice and support (see "Recommended Resources").

◆ Videotapes are available that teach and illustrate basic principles (see "Recommended Resources").

Make a list of names, phone numbers, and addresses of all these helpful resources. Post it on the refrigerator for the mother's reference.

If possible, you should both take a breastfeeding class to learn the basics before the birth. Most organizations and hospitals offering childbirth classes also offer breastfeeding classes.

As a supportive partner, you are the nursing mother's best resource, even if you do not know very much about breastfeeding. She needs your belief that she can breastfeed and your help in making it easier, by providing an extra pair of hands to help position the baby for feeding; keeping the mother fed and her thirst quenched; helping her stay as rested as she can; changing diapers; bathing, soothing, rocking, or bouncing the baby; taking the baby for short walks or rides outside; and being patient and loving through the early adjustments. Above all, she needs you to recognize that she is giving your baby the best possible food for the best possible start. Show the mother how much you appreciate that she is breastfeeding by helping as much as you can and encouraging her to continue if she encounters problems. Help her find professional help, if needed.

Getting Off to a Good Start

A good start with breastfeeding depends on:

◆ Frequent feeding of the baby on cue (whenever the baby gives indications that she wants the breast), beginning as soon after birth as the baby will suck. Babies need to nurse at least eight times per day.

◆ Recognition of the baby's feeding cues: bringing a hand to her mouth, opening her mouth and turning her head toward anything that brushes her cheek ("rooting"), making sucking sounds and motions with her mouth and tongue, fussing, or sucking avidly on a finger placed in her mouth. A baby usually indicates her desire for the breast long before she cries from hunger.

◆ A good "latch" between the baby's mouth and the breast.

◆ Availability of advice from a lactation consultant or other knowledgeable person.

◆ *Your* help and positive support.

◆ Freedom from excessive difficulty.

I mention the last item because, on rare occasions, a woman who wants very much to breastfeed has one problem after another, even when working closely with a breastfeeding counselor. If breastfeeding is the way most of her friends and family choose to feed their babies, a woman may feel a great deal of pressure to do the same. If she finally gives up in exasperation and disappointment, she may feel depressed, uncertain, and ashamed over her decision. But only she can balance the advantages and disadvantages of her situation. She should get the best support and advice available, and if feeding problems are still insurmountable she is correct to formula-feed. And she should be forgiving of herself.

Your understanding and support of her decision will help her immensely. Most important, try to deal with overzealous advocates of breastfeeding who may not understand that the mother has made her best effort to breastfeed. Such people sometimes become judgmental, and increase a woman's guilt and disappointment.

Early Concerns

Breastfeeding does not come easily at first to most women. It takes two to four weeks to reach the point where all the mother has to do is put the baby near her breast to get him to latch on and suck. In the meantime, problems such as temporary nipple soreness, lack of sleep, and concern about the milk supply may have to be overcome. Both you and the mother need information and guidelines on what is normal and how to solve these problems. The resources you have lined up (see pages 362 to 363) will help with these concerns.

MILK SUPPLY

How can you know whether the mother is making enough milk? If the baby needs to nurse frequently, does it mean the mother is not making enough milk to satisfy the baby's hunger? It sometimes is difficult to trust such an imprecise process as breastfeeding. Knowing these facts may help:

- The mother makes a very small quantity of colostrum for the first two to four days after birth. It is enough to satisfy all the baby's nutritional requirements for the first few days.

- The colostrum is replaced by milk on the third or fourth day after birth. The frequency and total amount of time spent suckling help determine when the milk "comes in" and how much milk the mother makes.

- Young babies normally nurse often—8 to 18 times a day. This may come as a surprise to the mother, who will spend many hours every day breastfeeding. Generally, the more she suckles the baby, the more milk the mother will make.

- Babies do not nurse at regular intervals; they "bunch up" several feedings in a row, and then go without feeding for a relatively long stretch. It is normal for a baby to nurse four times in six hours, then sleep for three to four hours before the next feeding.

- An ample milk supply is indicated by these signs: how the breasts feel (more heavy and full before a feeding than afterward); whether milk can be expressed or drips from the breasts; whether the baby is wetting her diapers and having bowel movements (after the milk comes in, six to eight wet diapers and four or more bowel movements a day are good signs for the first four weeks); and whether the baby noticeably swallows after every few sucks. Weight gain is a clear sign that the baby is getting enough milk, although the baby may not begin to gain until he is a few days old.

If the baby appears not to be getting enough milk, try the 24-Hour Cure (see page 369).

FATIGUE AND LACK OF SLEEP

Because young babies nurse frequently and sometimes fuss during the night, long stretches of sleep are no longer possible for the mother, or for you if you're trying to help at night. Sleep tends to come in the form of two- to three-hour naps between feedings. This normal change in sleep patterns is not a major problem if you and the mother can catch up during the day with a nap or two. If not, fatigue sets in, and it interferes with all aspects of parenting and daily living. Follow the instructions for "Recipe for Getting Enough Sleep" on page 356.

The mother may get more sleep, and the baby may fuss less, if she nurses him in bed at night and naps or sleeps with or near him. This way she can doze as she feeds the baby and does not have to get up as much. (A good discussion of this subject appears in *Sleeping with Your Baby* by James McKenna.) But if the mother is uncomfortable having the baby in bed with her, this solution will not work. If fatigue (or other problems, such as inadequate milk supply or a baby who will not take the mother's nipple) becomes a major concern for the mother, try the 24-Hour Cure (see page 369).

BREAST AND NIPPLE PAIN

Breast pain in the first few days may be caused by:

Engorgement. Replacing colostrum after two to four days, breast milk usually "comes in" over a period of 8 to 12 hours. Some women's breasts become extremely full and painful, or engorged, making it difficult for the baby to latch on.

Frequent breastfeeding, even before the milk comes in, helps to prevent severe engorgement, but the baby's appetite and ability at the breast may not match the milk supply at first. If the breasts are too firm to allow the baby to get a good latch, the mother should soften her nipples by expressing a small amount of milk before she feeds the baby, either by hand or with a mechanical pump. She can apply warm compresses or let the shower run over her breasts to start the flow of milk. She should express just enough milk to soften her nipples so the baby can take them into her mouth.

After the feeding, the mother may want to apply a cold pack to her breasts to reduce the pain and the engorgement. A pain reliever such as ibuprofen may also help (it is a good idea to check this with her caregiver).

After a few days, the engorgement will subside, and a balance will eventually be reached between the amount of milk needed by the baby and the amount produced by the mother.

Engorgement occurs even in women who do not breastfeed, but a lack of suckling and a pressure binder (an elastic bandage wrapped around the chest to flatten the breasts) will stop milk production.

Nipple pain may be caused by the following:

Prolonged, vigorous suckling with a poor latch. Some babies suck harder and longer than others. Early nipple soreness may be greater with such babies, but it passes after the milk comes in or within a week or so if the latch (the connection between mouth and breast) is good. Soreness is considered within normal limits if it occurs in the first minute of the feeding but then subsides for the rest of the feeding. If soreness persists throughout a feeding, it may be caused by a poor latch (see "A Poor Latch," page 368).

Trying to limit suckling time to 3 or 5 minutes per breast does not reduce soreness. If the baby sucks steadily at one breast for 15 minutes, however, the mother can switch breasts, since the first breast is likely to be empty.

It is important not to fall into the trap of giving a bottle to "rest" the breasts, unless the soreness is extreme. In cases of extreme soreness or cracked, bleeding nipples, the mother should seek help from a professional lactation consultant, one of the recommended books on breastfeeding (see "Recommended Resources"), or a woman experienced with breastfeeding.

A poor latch. Improper suckling is the number-one cause of nipple soreness. If the baby nibbles or "clicks" (breaks the suction with each suck), the mother's nipples will hurt more than is normally expected, and she may not produce enough milk. Her nurse or midwife, a lactation consultant, her childbirth educator, or a good book on breastfeeding (see "Recommended Resources") can help with the latch.

A good latch means the baby takes a large amount of the *areola* (the dark circle around the nipple) into her mouth. When held in the mother's arms, the baby should lie on her side ("tummy to tummy") rather than on her back. Other good positions are lying side by side and the "football" or "clutch" hold, in which the mother sits up, holding the baby beside and facing her. The baby's feet are behind the mother, and the baby's head is held by the mother at her breast. In all positions, ordinary pillows, or the now popular horseshoe-shaped nursing pillows, are useful for comfortably propping the baby and the mother's arms. In all positions, too, the baby's face is held very close to the breast, so that she doesn't pull hard on the nipple with every suck. Her mouth should open wide as she latches on.

Thrush. A yeast infection in the baby's mouth can spread to the mother's nipples, causing deep, severe pain during nursing. If the mother has this kind of pain, check the baby's mouth for patches of white film on his gums, his tongue, or the roof of his mouth. Check the mother's nipples, as well, for irritated or whitish patches. A thrush infection is most likely to occur if the mother or the baby has recently taken antibiotics or if the mother is prone to yeast infections. Call the baby's doctor if you suspect thrush. There are good treatments for this problem.

Treating sore nipples. The mother can treat her sore nipples in the following ways:

◆ Rub a little colostrum or milk into the nipples and allow them to air-dry.

◆ Dry the nipples after each feeding with a hair dryer (on its lowest setting) held at arm's length. This feels wonderful, and thoroughly dries the nipples.

◆ Apply ice (in a plastic bag) to the nipples just before a feeding to reduce sensation.

◆ Rub unscented purified lanolin (or another ointment recommended by a knowledgeable caregiver) into the nipples.

◆ Avoid washing the nipples with soap, even if they are protected by a coating of lanolin. Soap makes soreness worse. Rinsing with water is sufficient for cleanliness.

◆ Expose the breasts to the air by lowering the flaps of her bra, or by wearing no bra.

◆ Begin each nursing on the less sore side.

◆ Reduce suckling time to 15 minutes per side until the soreness begins to subside.

◆ If the soreness is extreme and the nipples are bleeding, stop breastfeeding, and pump milk for a day or so to get healing started. During this time, give the baby pumped breast milk from a bottle.

◆ Try breast shields, thin silicone nipple covers with holes that allow the milk to flow out. They may protect the nipples from further damage during nursings. It is best to consult a breastfeeding expert or at least a good breastfeeding book if you are considering using these shields (see "Recommended Resources").

◆ Check with her caregiver about pain medications, if the mother needs them.

If these measures fail, consult a lactation consultant, childbirth educator, the baby's physician, or a good book on breastfeeding (see "Recommended Resources").

THE 24-HOUR "CURE"

During the first few weeks after birth, the mother and baby are mastering the art of breastfeeding. The 24-Hour Cure can solve some of the problems that arise, such as the following:

◆ Doubts about whether the mother is making enough milk.

- Fatigue, lack of sleep, or anxiety in the mother.

- Lack of appetite, poor nourishment, or low fluid intake in the mother.

- Slow weight gain in the baby.

- "Nipple confusion"—that is, the baby seems to prefer a rubber nipple or nipple shield to the mother's breast.

The "cure" promotes frequent, efficient suckling and an abundant milk supply by nurturing both the mother and the baby. The mother gets complete rest, plenty of good food and drink, and freedom from all responsibility other than feeding and cuddling her baby. The baby gets prolonged skin-to-skin contact with the mother and constant access to her breast and nurturance.

Before starting the cure, make sure that the baby is gaining weight—slowly, at least—by comparing weights recorded over a few days. If he isn't gaining weight, consult the baby's doctor or a lactation consultant before beginning the cure. Make sure, too, that the mother does not have sore, blistered, or cracked nipples. The causes of any soreness should be addressed before the cure begins (see "Treating Sore Nipples," page 368).

Here is how to do the cure:

- Set aside a full 24 hours when the mother can have help. Use your day off, or get a friend or relative to take your place for part of the 24 hours. Around-the-clock help is essential.

- The mother goes to bed with the baby. They both wear as little clothing as practical under the bedcovers so the baby can get lots of warm skin-to-skin contact, which will stimulate his suckling reflex and interest in feeding.

- The mother may read, watch TV, chat with you (no visitors, please), or, most important, doze. The extra sleep will make a big difference for her, although it will come in short snatches. Even if it takes the mother a long time to fall asleep, she should stay in bed; some sleep-deprived women take a long time to relax and give in to sleep. She should get out of bed *only to go to the bathroom*—not to eat, answer the phone, do housework, or anything else.

- Supply her with liquids; place water or juice within her reach. She should drink about two to three quarts of liquid during the 24 hours.

- Fix tasty, nutritious meals for her. Tempt her appetite with foods she is unlikely to prepare for herself. If she has been relying on take-out fast foods or cold ready-to-eat foods, she will love a hot, home-cooked meal or two.

- The baby should stay in bed with her, except when a diaper change is necessary, or when the baby is fussy (but not willing to nurse) and needs to be briefly walked or rocked. Then you should take care of the baby.

- Whenever the baby awakens or seems at all interested in suckling, the mother should offer her breast. Do not give the baby a bottle of either formula or breast milk, unless the baby's doctor or a lactation consultant has advised doing so because the baby is underweight.

The combination of rest and nourishment for the mother and skin-to-skin contact and unlimited suckling for the baby almost always results in a marked increase in milk production, improved sucking by the baby, and a much happier mother.

If the mother is unable to closely follow the 24-Hour Cure, or if it fails to solve the problem, consult the baby's doctor, a lactation consultant, or La Leche League.

When to Give the Baby a Bottle

Most parents want their babies to be able to get milk from a bottle sooner or later, especially if the mother will be away from home regularly. You may have heard stories about babies who won't take a bottle, and about how distraught the parents become when they need the baby to do so. For a smooth introduction to bottle feeding, timing is crucial. Too-early bottle feeding may interfere with the baby's learning to breastfeed. But if the bottle is introduced too late, the baby may refuse it.

It is wise not to rush bottle-feeding with a breastfed baby, for two reasons. First, while the baby is getting used to the human nipple, it may be confusing for him to suck from a rubber nipple. Different sucking techniques—different mouth and jaw motions—are required for human and rubber nipples. The baby may not be able to go from one to the other. (Of course, there are circumstances when a very young infant must be bottle-fed. A lactation consultant can be very helpful in teaching a baby who has been bottle-fed to suck at the breast, when he is able to do so.)

Second, when a baby skips breastfeedings and takes milk from a bottle, he spends less time suckling at the breast. This may slow milk production, especially at the time when breastfeeding is still becoming established, because it is the suckling that stimulates the breasts to produce. A shortage of breast milk may result. Pumping during these gaps between breastfeedings will help maintain the milk supply.

If you will need to feed the baby with a bottle at some time, wait until the baby is able to latch on and suckle at the breast easily, without coaxing, and until the milk supply is clearly plentiful. Most babies are good latchers and sucklers by three to four weeks of age (although some may need several more weeks). If the bottle is introduced at this time, the baby will probably adjust easily. You must continue to offer the bottle regularly after that, however—about three to five times a week—or the baby may "forget" that he was willing to take the rubber nipple and may come to prefer the breast so strongly that you will have to struggle to get him to take a bottle.

It is usually preferable that someone other than the mother give the bottle to the baby; he may insist on the mother's breast if she is right there. Feed the baby the mother's expressed milk, preferably, or formula.

If the baby is reluctant to take the bottle after becoming accustomed to the breast, allow a couple of weeks for the baby to learn to use the bottle before the mother leaves him for a significant length of time with you or a babysitter. Don't wait until two days before she will go back to work!

Many people advise introducing a bottle when the baby is really hungry. This doesn't always work, however. If he is really hungry, he may be so upset that he just wants Mom and has difficulty adjusting to the different sucking required with a bottle. Instead, try offering the bottle when the baby is full but awake and content. Stroke the baby's lips with the bottle, and let him "play" with it. Out of curiosity, he may suck on it a bit. Do this several times. Then he may be ready to take the bottle when he is hungry.

With persistence on your part, the baby will eventually take the bottle. But if it ever happens that the mother is unavailable to nurse and the baby will not take the bottle, you can try squirting milk into a corner of his mouth with an eyedropper, or even using a tiny cup, such as a shot glass.

Once Breastfeeding Is Established

By three to six weeks of age, most babies and their mothers find breastfeeding to be a pleasant, quick, convenient method of feeding. By this time you and the mother probably function as an efficient team as you divide the work and pleasure of integrating the baby into your lives. Although there are more hurdles to come, the greatest breastfeeding challenges are behind you, and the closeness and joy you all share are most satisfying.

Parting Words

The family is launched. The baby is born and getting used to the world; the mother is no longer pregnant and is adjusting to being on constant call. Your job as birth partner is over, and your new role has begun. The excitement is over, and you may feel strangely let down.

Now what? It will take a while to absorb and integrate all that has happened. This birth has transformed you into a parent, or grandparent, or more-special-than-ever friend. You will never be the same, and you will always treasure this experience.

I wish you well.

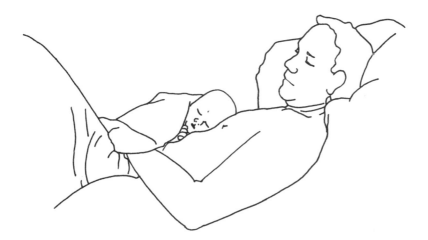

Recommended Resources

The topics are listed here in the order in which they are mentioned in the text, along with names of books, video recordings, and Web sites that provide helpful information to supplement this book. I have added publisher's names only for publications that are hard to find without this information. Everything else should be easy to track down at a bookstore or via the Internet.

To contact Penny Simkin:
> www.pennysimkin.com, info@pennysimkin.com

Locating a doula — chapter 1, page 11
> www.dona.org
> www.doulaworld.com
> www.doulanetwork.com
> Klaus, Marshall, John Kennell, and Phyllis Klaus. *The Doula Book: How a Trained Labor Companion Can Help You Have a Shorter, Easier, and Healthier Birth.* 2002.

Building strength and stamina for assisting in labor — chapter 1, page 19
> Fitness Digest Online (www.fitnessdigest.com)
> Mayo Clinic (www.mayoclinic.com/health/fitness)
> Roizen, Michael, and Tracy Hafen. *The Real Age Workout: Maximum Health, Minimum Work.* 2006.

Preparing older children for the birth of a sibling — chapter 1, page 25
> Overend, Jenni, and Julie Vivas. *Welcome with Love.* 1999.
> Simkin, Penny, Janet Whalley, and Ann Keppler. *Pregnancy, Childbirth, and the Newborn: The Complete Guide,* 3rd ed. (chapter 16). 2001.
> Van Dam Anderson, Sandra, and Georgeanne Del Giudice. *Siblings, Birth, and the Newborn.* Minneapolis: International Childbirth Education Association, 1983.

Baby care and infant development — chapter 1, page 31
Johnson & Johnson Pediatric Institute (www.jjpi.com).
The Amazing Talents of the Newborn. VHS. 2000.
Klaus, Marshall, and Phyllis H. Klaus. *Your Amazing Newborn.*
2000.
Leach, Penelope. *Your Baby and Child.* 2003.
McKenna, James. *Sleeping with Your Baby.* 2007.
Pantley, Elizabeth. *Gentle Baby Care.* 2004.
Sears, William, and Martha Sears. *The Baby Book.* 2003.
www.kidshealth.org

Aids for relaxation — chapter 4, page 115
Schardt, Dana. *Pregnancy Relaxation: A Guide to Peaceful
Beginnings.* 2000.
Simkin, Penny. *Comfort Measures for Childbirth.* DVD. Seattle:
Penny Simkin, Inc., 2007.
Simkin, Penny. *Relax for Childbirth.* CD with music and
narration. Minneapolis: International Childbirth Education
Association, 1988.

Hypnosis for birth — chapter 4, page 123
Mongan, Marie. *HypnoBirthing: The Mongan Method:
A Natural Approach to a Safe, Easier, More Comfortable
Birthing,* 3rd ed. 2005.
O'Neill, Michelle Leclaire. *Hypnobirthing: The Original Method:
Mindful Pregnancy and Easy Labor Using the Leclaire
Childbirth Method.* 2007.

Birthing tub rental and sales — chapter 4, page 142
AquaDoula (www.aquadoula.com)
Waterbirth International (www.waterbirth.org)
www.yourwaterbirth.com

TENS unit rental — chapter 4, page 150
www.babycaretens.com

Aromatherapy — chapter 4, page 160

Worwood, Valerie Ann. *The Pampered Pregnancy Bliss Box: An Aromatherapy Kit for Wellness and Comfort.* 2004.

Baby's positions in utero and ways to identify and change them — chapter 5, page 185

www.spinningbabies.com

Simkin, Penny, and Ruth Ancheta. *The Labor Progress Handbook,* 2nd ed. 2005.

Grieving a baby's stillbirth, death, or disability; recovery after a traumatic birth; pregnancy after the loss of a baby — chapter 5, page 194

Church, Lisa, and Ann Prescott. *Hope Is Like the Sun: Finding Hope and Healing After Miscarriage, Stillbirth, or Infant Death.* 2004.

Schweibert, Pat, and Paul Kirk. *When Hello Means Goodbye.* 1993.

www.HopeXchange.com (on miscarriage, stillbirth, and infant death)

Kitzinger, Sheila. *Birth Crisis.* 2006.

Madsen, Lynn. *Rebounding from Childbirth—Toward Emotional Recovery.* 1994.

Simkin, Penny, and Phyllis Klaus. *When Survivors Give Birth: Understanding and Healing the Effects of Early Sexual Abuse on Childbearing Women.* 2004.

International Cesarean Awareness Network (www.ican-online.org)

www.sheilakitzinger.com/BirthCrisis.htm (on birth trauma)

Trauma and Birth Stress (www.tabs.org.nz/)

Douglas, Ann, John Sussman, and Deborah Davis. *Trying Again: A Guide to Pregnancy After Miscarriage, Stillbirth, and Infant Loss.* 2000.

Gestational diabetes — chapter 7, page 244

Geil, Patti Bazel, Patricia Geil, and Laura Hieronymus. *101 Tips for a Healthy Pregnancy with Diabetes.* 2004.

www.diabeticmommy.com

Prematurity and Kangaroo Care — chapter 7, page 263

Bradford, Nikki, Jonathan Hellman, Sharyn Gibbins, and Sandra Lousada. *Your Premature Baby: The First Five Years.* 2003.

Ludington-Hoe, Susan M., and Susan K. Golant. *Kangaroo Care: The Best You Can Do for Your Preterm Infant.* 1993.

Sears, William, Robert Sears, James Sears, and Martha Sears. *The Premature Baby Book: Everything You Need to Know About Your Premature Baby from Birth to Age One.* 2004.

Risks of elective cesarean — chapter 9, page 308

Childbirth Connection. *What Every Woman Needs to Know About Cesarean Section.* Rev. ed. 2006.

Childbirth Connection (www.childbirthconnection.org)

Vaginal birth after cesarean — chapter 9, page 321

Korte, Diana. *The VBAC Companion.* 1997.

www.VBAC.com

Cord-blood storage — chapter 10, page 331

American Academy of Pediatrics. "Cord Blood Banking for Potential Future Transplantation." Policy Statement, 2007. http://aappolicy.aappublications.org/cgi/content/full/pediatrics;119/1/165

www.keepkidshealthy.com/pregnancy/cord_blood_banking.html

Circumcision — chapter 10, page 341

American Academy of Pediatrics Task Force on Circumcision. "Circumcision Policy Statement." 1999, reaffirmed 2005. http://aappolicy.aappublications.org/cgi/content/abstract/pediatrics;103/3/686

Proper care of the uncircumcised penis — chapter 10, page 343

Wallerstein, Edward. *When Your Baby Boy Is Not Circumcised.* Pamphlet. Minneapolis: International Childbirth Education Association, 1982.

(Also, most comprehensive infant-care books contain a section on this topic.)

Videos, books, and classes on baby care –— chapter 10, page 343
See the resources on baby care and infant development listed
for chapter 1.

Postpartum doulas — chapter 1, page 36 and chapter 10, page 351
Kelleher, Jacqueline. *Nurturing the Family: The Guide for
Postpartum Doulas.* Jasper, Ind.: DONA International, 2002.

Fussy, crying babies — chapter 10, page 357
Brazelton, T. Berry, and Joshua Sparrow. *Calming Your Fussy
Baby: The Brazelton Way.* 2003.
Karp, Harvey. *The Happiest Baby on the Block.* 2002. (Also
available on VHS and DVD.)
Pantley, Elizabeth. *The No-Cry Sleep Solution.* 2002.
Sears, William, and Martha Sears. *The Fussy Baby Book:
Parenting Your High Need Child from Birth to Age Five.* 1996.

Breastfeeding — chapter 11, pages 361, 364, and 365
Huggins, Kathleen. *The Nursing Mother's Companion.* 5th ed.
2005.
Mohrbacher, Nancy, and Kathleen Kendal-Tacket. *Breastfeeding
Made Simple: Seven Natural Laws for Nursing Mothers.* 2005.
Newman, Jack. *Dr. Jack Newman's Visual Guide to
Breastfeeding.* DVD.
Newman, Jack, and Teresa Pitman. *The Ultimate
Breastfeeding Book of Answers.* 2000.
Available from www.drjacknewman.com.
www.breastfeeding.com
The Breastfeeding Café (www.breastfeedingcafe.com)
Dr. Jack Newman's Web site (www.drjacknewman.com)
La Leche League (www.lalecheleague.org)

Index